BIGGER
LEANER
STRONGER

THE SIMPLE SCIENCE OF BUILDING
THE ULTIMATE MALE BODY

SECOND EDITION

Michael Matthews

oculus

Cover Designed by Damon Za

Edited by Kristin Wallinski

Published by Oculus Publishers, Inc.

www.oculuspublishers.com

Visit the author's website:

www.muscleforlife.com

GET MY WEEKLY NEWSLETTER AND FREE GOODIES YOU'RE GOING TO LOVE

Sign up for my weekly newsletter and every Monday I'll send you awesome, science-based health and fitness tips, delicious "guilt-free" recipes, thoughts that will keep you motivated, and more…plus you'll get a free 7-part email course that debunks the biggest health and fitness lies *and* 3 free eBooks of mine.

Sign Up Here and Get Instant Access:

www.muscleforlife.com/signup

BIGGER LEANER STRONGER SUCCESS STORIES

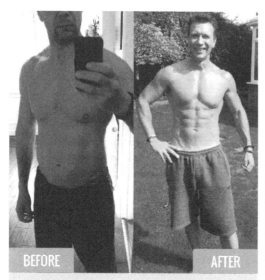

BEFORE   AFTER

"It still feels strange that my stomach is always flat; I do not miss having to suck it in."

DARREN B.

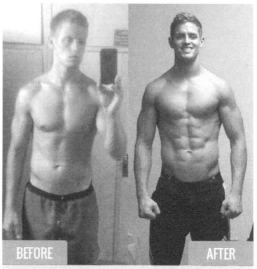

BEFORE   AFTER

"I haven't seen anything close to the results I have accomplished on Bigger Leaner Stronger!"

COREY N.

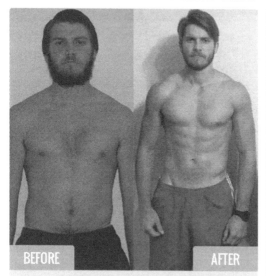

BEFORE   AFTER

"I have seen my body go from 16% to around 10!"

MARK V.

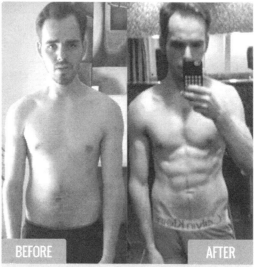

BEFORE   AFTER

"I'm living proof that your recommendations and studies are true!"

RICARDO G.

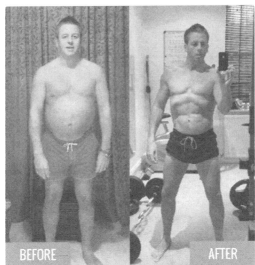

BEFORE — AFTER

"EVERYONE I see comments on how much better I am looking!"

JASON S.

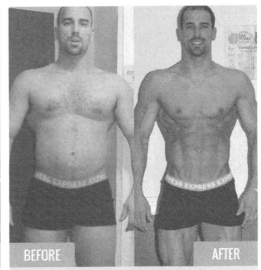

BEFORE — AFTER

"My self confidence is higher than it has ever been!"

SCOTT L.

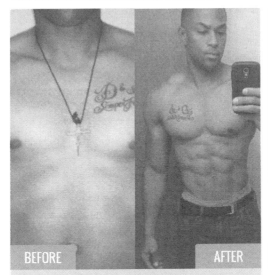

BEFORE — AFTER

I've never experienced so much change in my body with any other program!

DELANDO B.

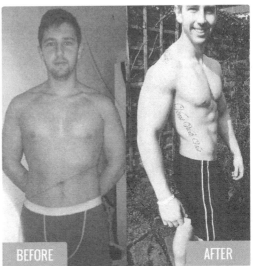

BEFORE — AFTER

"My mental focus, energy, strength, and self confidence have all gone up!"

LUKE M.

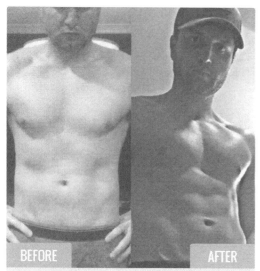

BEFORE | AFTER

*"My strength skyrocketed
as soon as I started!"*

JUSTIN E.

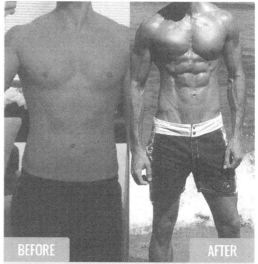

BEFORE | AFTER

*"I've gotten the results I dreamed
about my whole life, sounds
cheesy, but it's the truth!"*

ROMAN T.

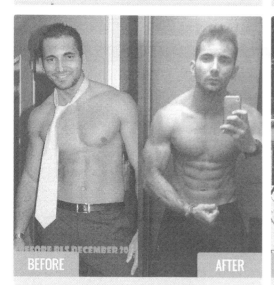

BEFORE | AFTER

*"My strength has skyrocketed and
it's encouraging to see men at the
gym lifting less weight than me."*

HECTOR C.

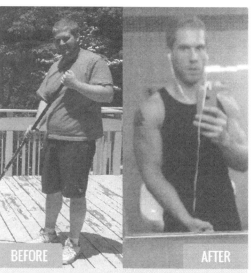

BEFORE | AFTER

*"It doesn't burn you out and it
doesn't get boring!"*

CALEB H.

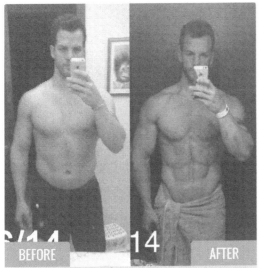

BEFORE | AFTER

"I've been able to get in the best overall shape of my life."

RYAN P.

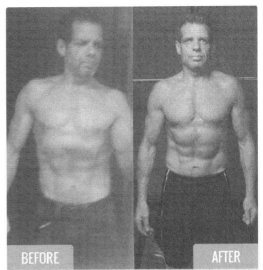

BEFORE | AFTER

"Within 5 weeks I had begun seeing my six pack for the first time!"

THOMAS T.

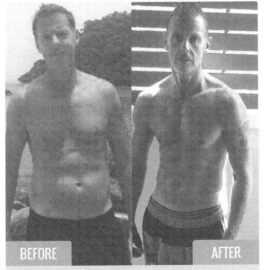

BEFORE | AFTER

"I went from 25% body fat down to 10%!"

TONY H.

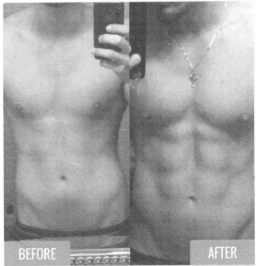

BEFORE | AFTER

"In 9 months I gained 45 pounds."

JEREMY B.

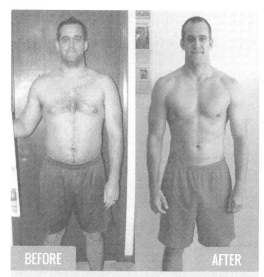

BEFORE AFTER

*"I lost 26 pounds and 11%
bodyfat in 3 months on the
BLS program!"*

SAM R.

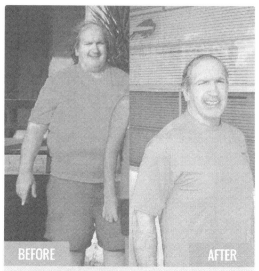

BEFORE AFTER

*"I lost 75 lbs and beat type 2
diabetes as a result of
Bigger Leaner Stronger!"*

JOHN S.

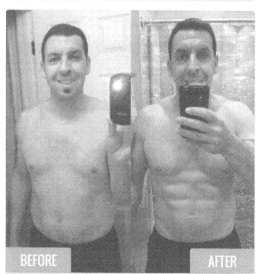

BEFORE AFTER

*"The program is just plain
easy and fun to follow,
enjoy the journey!"*

ANDREW M.

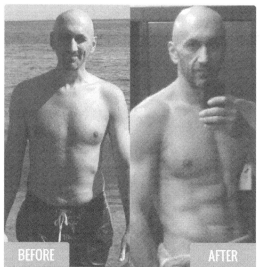

BEFORE AFTER

*"I got results much faster
compared to everything
else I tried!"*

ANDRIY Y.

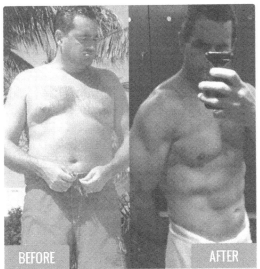

BEFORE

AFTER

"I have gained almost 25 lbs of lean muscle and significantly increased my strength across the board."

STUART M.

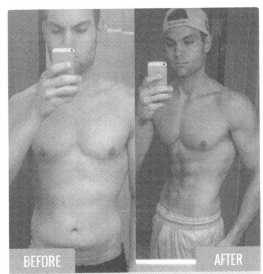

BEFORE

AFTER

" It really give me the burst of strength im not used to!"

CARTER G.

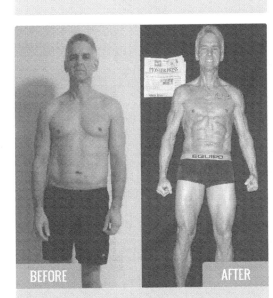

BEFORE

AFTER

"At age 54 I have lost almost 20 pounds and 9% body fat."

JAY P.

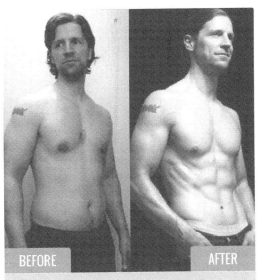

BEFORE

AFTER

"I lost 29 pounds while cutting!"

DYLAN M.

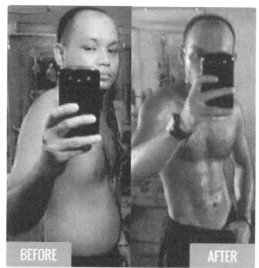

BEFORE AFTER

"The intensity to volume ratio is perfect and I never feel burned out, but that I got a great workout!"

EL G.

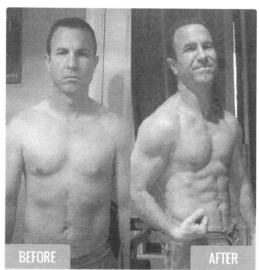

BEFORE AFTER

"I am stronger, healthier, and look better than any other time in my life!"

GARY L.

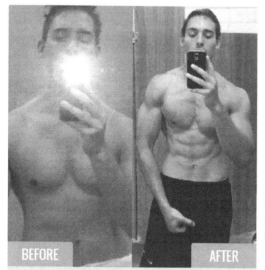

BEFORE AFTER

"Since I started the program I dropped 19 lbs!"

JP I.

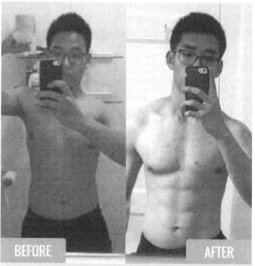

BEFORE AFTER

"I dropped 25 pounds in 6 months!"

NGUYEN H.

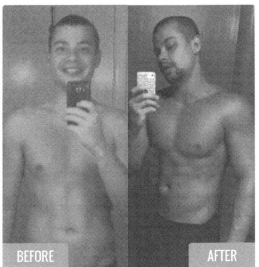

BEFORE AFTER

"This program keeps its promise. Following it quickly gave me size, strength and definition."

NICO R.

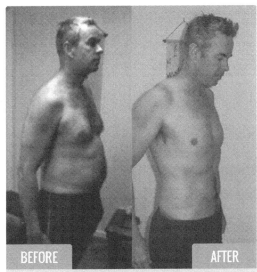

BEFORE AFTER

"I was just going through the motions for the last few years until I found BLS."

PETER V.

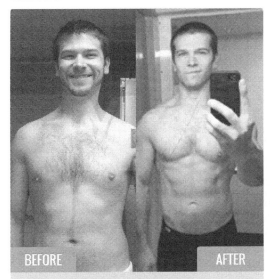

BEFORE AFTER

"Challenging yourself to improve becomes its own game with a reward every day!"

ROB N.

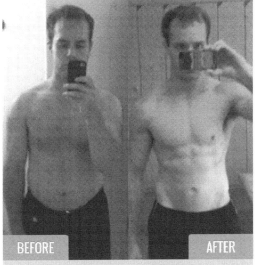

BEFORE AFTER

"This program makes dieting easy to follow and the results are quick!"

SCOTT S.

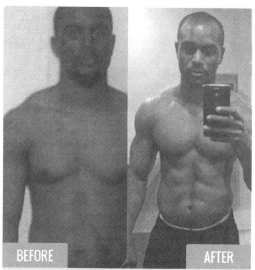

BEFORE   AFTER

*"I don't feel like
I'm wasting my time on
ineffective exercises"*

SHAWN L.

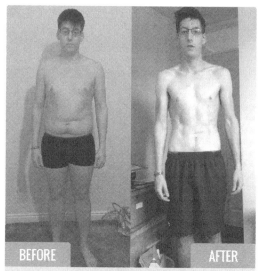

BEFORE   AFTER

*"I have seen dramatic
improvements all around both
mentally and physically!"*

STEPHEN B.

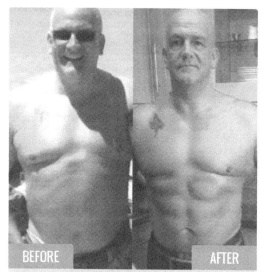

BEFORE   AFTER

*"I have been on average losing
around 1.5 lbs per week and have
lost 19 lbs so far and am continuing
to lose fat!"*

STEVE B.

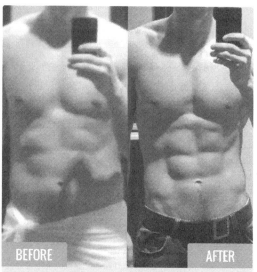

BEFORE   AFTER

"I have lost 12 kg in 3 months!"

TOMAS P.

ABOUT THE AUTHOR

Common sense will not accomplish great things. Simply become insane and desperate.
— LORD NAOSHIGE

I'M MIKE. I BELIEVE THAT EVERY person can achieve the body of his or her dreams, and I work hard to give everyone that chance by providing workable, proven advice grounded in science.

I've been training for more than a decade now and have tried just about every type of workout program, diet regimen, and supplement you can imagine. While I don't know everything, I know what works and what doesn't.

Like most guys, I had no clue what I was doing when I started out. I turned to magazines for help, which had me spending a couple of hours in the gym every day and wasting hundreds of dollars on worthless supplements each month, only to make mediocre gains.

This went on for years, and I jumped from workout program to workout program. I tried all kinds of splits and routines, exercises, rep ranges, and other schemes, and while I made some progress during this time (it's impossible not to if you just keep at it), it was slow going and eventually put me in a rut.

My weight remained stuck for over a year, and I wasn't building any strength to speak of. I had no idea what to do with my nutrition beyond "eating clean" and making sure I was getting a lot of protein. I turned to various trainers for guidance, but they had me do more of the same. I liked working out too much to quit, but I wasn't happy with my body, and I didn't know what I was doing wrong.

Here's a picture of me after almost six years of lifting regularly:

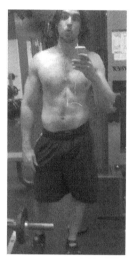

Not very impressive. Something had to change.

TIME TO GET SMART

I finally decided that it was time to get educated—to throw the magazines away, get off the forums, and learn the actual physiology of muscle growth and fat loss and figure out what it takes to build a big, lean, and strong body.

I searched out the work of top strength and bodybuilding coaches, talked to scores of natural bodybuilders, and read hundreds of scientific papers, and a clear picture emerged.

The real science of getting into incredible shape is very simple—much simpler than the health and fitness and supplement industries want us to believe. It flies in the face of almost all the crap that we hear on TV, read in magazines, and see in the gym.

As a result of what I learned, I completely changed the way I trained and ate. And my body responded in ways I couldn't believe. My strength skyrocketed. My muscles were growing again for the first time in years. My energy levels went through the roof.

That was just over five years ago, and here's how my body has changed since:

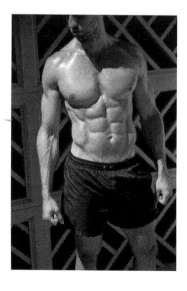

Quite a difference.

THE BIRTH OF MY CAREER

Along the way, my friends noticed the improvements in my physique and began asking for advice. I became their unofficial trainer.

I took "hardgainers" and put 30 pounds on them in a year. I took people who were absolutely baffled as to why they couldn't lose weight, stripped 30 pounds of fat off them, *and* helped them build noticeable muscle at the same time. I took people in their fifties who believed their hormones were too bottomed out to accomplish anything with exercise and helped them turn back the clock 20 years in terms of body fat percentage and muscle definition.

After doing this over and over for years, my "clients" (I never asked for money—I just had them come train with me) started urging me to write a book. I dismissed the idea at first, but it began to grow on me.

"What if I had such a book when I had started training?" I thought. I would've saved an untold amount of money, time, and frustration, and I would've achieved my ideal physique years ago. I enjoyed helping people with what I had learned, and if I wrote books and they became popular, what if I could help thousands or even hundreds of thousands of people? *That* got me excited.

I acted on the impulse and the result was the first edition of *Bigger Leaner Stronger*, which was published in January 2012. Sales were slow at first, but within a month or two, I began receiving e-mails from readers with high praise. I was floored. I immediately started on my next book and outlined several more.

I've now published seven books, including this second edition, which have sold more than 200,000 copies. More importantly, every day I get scores of e-mails and social media messages from readers who are blown away by the results they're seeing. They're just as shocked as I was years ago when I learned just how simple building lean, healthy muscle and losing fat, without ever feeling starved or miserable, is.

It's motivating to see the impact I'm having on people's lives, and I'm incredibly inspired by the dedication of my readers and followers. You guys and gals rock.

WHERE TO NOW?

My true love is researching and writing, so I'll always be working on another book, my website (www.muscleforlife.com), and whatever other types of literary adventures come my way.

My big, evil master plan has three major targets:

1. **Help a million people get fit and healthy.** "Help a million people" just has a sexy ring to it, don't you think? It's a big goal, but I think I can do it. And it goes beyond just helping people look good—I want to make a dent in alarmingly negative trends we're seeing in people's overall physical and mental health.

2. **Lead the fight against broscience and BS.** Unfortunately, this industry is full of idiots, liars, and hucksters who prey on people's fears and insecurities, and I want to do something about it. In fact, I'd like to become known as the go-to guy for practical, easy-to-understand advice grounded in *real* science and results.

3. **Help reform the sport supplement industry.** The dishonest pill and powder pushers are the people I despise the most in this space. The scams are numerous: using fancy-sounding but worthless ingredients, cutting products with junk fillers like maltodextrin

and even stuff like flour and sawdust (yes, this happens), using bogus science and ridiculous marketing claims to sell, underdosing the important ingredients and covering it up with the label "proprietary blend," sponsoring steroid-fueled athletes so they pretend supplements are the secret to their gains, and more.

I hope you enjoy this book, and I'm positive that if you apply what you're about to learn, you too can dramatically transform your physique without hating your "diet" or beating yourself to death in the gym every day.

So, are you ready? Great. Let's get to it.

CONTENTS

SECTION II:
INNER GAME

SECTION III:
NUTRITION & DIET

THE PROMISE

No matter how bad you might think your genetics are, and no matter how lost you might feel after trying and abandoning many types of workouts, you absolutely, positively can have the lean, ripped body that you dream about.

WHAT IF I COULD SHOW YOU how to dramatically transform your body faster than you ever thought possible?

What if I gave you the exact formula of exercise and eating that makes putting on 5 to 10 pounds of *quality lean mass* a breeze…and it would only take 8 to 12 weeks?

What if I showed you how to get a lean, cut physique that you love (and that women drool over) by investing no more than *5 percent* of your time each day?

What if I told you that you can achieve that "Hollywood hunk" body without having your life revolve around it—no long hours in the gym, no starving yourself, and no grueling cardio that turns your stomach? I'll even show you how to get shredded while still indulging in the "cheat" foods that you love every week like pasta, pizza, and ice cream.

And what if I promised to be at your side the entire way, helping you avoid the scams, pitfalls, and problems that most guys fall into, helping you systematically achieve your true genetic potential, and basically doing everything I can to see you achieve the best body you've ever had?

Imagine if you got up every morning, looked in the mirror, and couldn't help but smile at your reflection. Imagine the boost in confidence you'd feel if you didn't have that belly fat anymore or if you were no longer "that skinny guy" but instead had six-pack abs and were "that ripped guy."

Imagine, just 12 weeks from now, being constantly complimented on how you look and asked what the *heck* you're doing to make such startling gains. Imagine enjoying the added benefits of having higher energy levels, better spirits, and fewer aches and pains and of knowing that you're getting healthier every day.

Well, you *can* have all of these things, and it's not nearly as complicated as the fitness industry wants you to believe. It doesn't matter whether you're 21 or 61 or whether you're in shape or completely not. No matter who you are, I promise that you can change your body into whatever you desire.

So, would you like my help?

If you answered "Yes!" then you've taken a *leap*, not a step, toward your goals to become a leaner, more muscular you.

Your journey to the ultimate male body begins as soon as you turn to the next page.

INTRODUCTION:
WHY *BIGGER LEANER STRONGER* IS DIFFERENT

All truth passes through three stages. First, it is ridiculed. Second, it is violently opposed. Third, it is accepted as being self-evident.
— ARTHUR SCHOPENHAUER

I'M GOING TO TELL YOU SOMETHING that the kings of the multibillion-dollar health and fitness industry don't want you to know:

You don't need any of their crap to get ripped and to look better than you ever have before.

- You don't need to spend hundreds of dollars per month on the worthless supplements that steroid freaks shill in advertisements.

- You don't need to constantly change up your exercise routines to "confuse" your muscles. I'm pretty sure that muscles lack cognitive abilities, so this approach is a good way to just confuse yourself instead.

- You don't need to burn through buckets of protein powder every month, stuffing down enough protein each day to feed a Third World village.

- You don't need to toil away in the gym for a couple of hours per day doing tons of sets, supersets, drop sets, giant sets, etc. (As a matter of fact, this is a great way to stunt your gains and get nowhere.)

- You don't need to grind out hours and hours of boring cardio every week to shed ugly belly fat and love handles and get a shredded six-pack. (How many flabby treadmillers have you come across over the years?)

- You don't need to completely abstain from "cheat" foods while getting down to single-digit body fat percentages. To the contrary, if you cheat correctly, you can *accelerate* fat loss.

These are just a small sampling of the harmful fallacies that many people believe, and they will bury you in a rut of frustration with no real results, which will inevitably lead to quitting.

That was my motivation for creating *Bigger Leaner Stronger*. For many years now, I've had friends, family, acquaintances, and co-workers approach me for fitness advice, and they were almost always convinced of many strange, unnecessary, or unworkable ideas about diet and exercise.

By educating them in the same way as I'm about to educate you, I've helped many people melt away fat; build lean, attractive muscle; and not only look great but *feel* great too. And, while helping friends, friends of friends, and family is fulfilling, I wanted to be able to help thousands (or tens or even hundreds of thousands!). Thus, *Bigger Leaner Stronger* was born.

Now, where did the many fitness and nutrition myths come from? Well, I don't want to waste your time with the boring details, but the long story short is this:

When people are motivated to solve a problem and are willing to spend large amounts of money to do it, there will never be a scarcity of *stuff* for them to buy, and there will always be scores of brilliant marketers inventing new schemes to keep people spending.

It's pretty simple. All we have to do is look to the sources that most people turn to for their training and nutritional advice. Almost everyone gets it from one or more of these three sources: magazines, personal trainers, or friends…and most of what you'll learn from them is basically useless.

How can I make such bold claims, you wonder? Well, let's talk about bodybuilding magazines for a minute.

Last time I looked, close to a dozen of these magazines were waiting on the shelves of Barnes & Noble featuring bodybuilders ready to lure in victims like juiced-up Venus flytraps.

The bottom line is this: every time you buy one of the big bodybuilding magazines, you're paying to be lied to.

Here's a fun fact that you probably didn't know: the majority of mainstream bodybuilding magazines are little more than mouthpieces for supplement companies that either own them outright or control them financially by buying all the ad space.

In almost all cases, the primary goal of these magazines is to sell supplements, and they work damn well. The magazines push products in various ways: they have pretty advertisements all over the place, they regularly run "advertorials" (advertisements disguised as informative articles), and they balance the myriad sales pitches with some actual articles that provide workout and nutrition advice (which also, in many cases, end with product recommendations of one kind or another).

So, this is the first blow that magazines deal to you: They give you a lot of "advice" that is geared first and foremost to selling you products, not helping you achieve your goals.

"But wait," you might be thinking. "Don't supplements help me reach my goals?"

Well, we'll be talking all about supplements later, but here's all you need to know right now: most supplements are a complete waste of money and will do absolutely nothing to help you build muscle or strength and get lean.

Don't believe for a *second* that these pills and powders did anything special for the shredded bodybuilders and fitness models hawking them. If you knew the sheer amount of drugs many of these guys are on, your head would spin. These guys' bodies are basically chemistry experiments.

So, the supplement companies know that if they can just keep getting these magazines into people's hands, they will keep selling products, and all will be right in the world.

How can they ensure that you will keep buying? By coming up with a never-ending flow of new advice, of course. You know, new training methodologies, diet "tricks," supplement research (of course), and the like.

And this is the second, probably more harmful, blow dealt by the magazines: they inundate you with all kinds of false ideas about what it takes to get into great shape. If they told the simple truth every month, they would have maybe 20 articles or so that they could reprint over and over. There isn't that much to getting strong, fit, and healthy.

Instead, they get quite creative with selling you on all kinds of workout routines, diet regimens and "hacks," and, of course, supplement recommendations. And while letting magazines guide your training and diet is better than just sitting on the couch eating pork rinds, it won't get you to your ultimate goal.

So that's the story of the magazines. Let's now move on to an unfortunate truth about personal trainers:

Most of them are just a waste of money. End of story.

Their hearts can be in the right place, but the truth is that most trainers just don't have the drive or know-how to get their clients into great shape.

Their poor people are paying between $50 and 75 per hour to do the same type of silly, ineffective workout routines found in the magazines, usually with poor form to boot, and they often see no real results for their efforts.

You've probably also noticed that many trainers aren't even in good shape themselves. How can you honestly sell yourself as a fitness expert when you're a skinny-fat weakling? Who could possibly believe you?

Well, for some reason, these types of trainers get business all the time, and their clients almost always stay flabby and out of shape too.

Compounding the disservice is the fact that most trainers don't give their clients proper diet plans, which is basically the kiss of death and guarantees no results. The fact is, how you look is just as much a reflection of how you eat as how you train. Fat, skinny, ripped, whatever—your diet determines this just as much as your workouts.

Eat wrong, and you will stay fat no matter how much cardio you do. Eat wrong, and you will stay skinny and weak no matter how much you struggle with weights.

Eat right, however, and you can unlock the maximum potential gains from working out: rapid, long-term fat loss and muscle growth that will turn heads and get your friends and family talking.

Chances are, this isn't news to you. We've all heard the importance of proper dieting. Well, if you're dreading the "diet" talk, rest easy. I have good news for you: eating correctly does *not* mean dramatically restricting your food intake or cutting out everything that tastes good.

As you'll soon learn, you can actually *enjoy* "dieting." Yes, you read that right. You can eat plenty of carbs every day. You should never feel starved. Your energy levels will remain high.

Eating correctly means nothing more than following simple, flexible nutritional targets that allow you to eat foods you like while building muscle and losing fat.

But we'll dive into that later. Let's get back to trainers.

You might be wondering why these trainers know so little as certified professionals. Well, passing a PT certification test does *not* require you to be a fitness expert with proven results—

you just have to memorize and regurgitate some basic information about nutrition, anatomy, and exercise. You can even do it all online, where answers are just a Google search away.

Another problem with trainers is a simple dilemma they have to face every day: they have to keep their clients convinced that they're needed so they keep paying.

While some people are happy to pay a trainer just to force them to show up every day, most want to feel like they're getting more for their money. And the easiest way to give them this experience is to regularly change up routines and talk about "sophisticated" diet and workout principles.

The bottom line is that when all is said and done, most personal training clients waste thousands of dollars to make poor gains and quit out of disappointment.

It's not all gloom and doom, though. There absolutely *are* great trainers out there who are in awesome shape themselves, who *do* know how to quickly and effectively get results in others, and who do care about their clients.

If you're one of them and you're reading this book, I applaud you, because you're carrying the weight of the entire profession on your shoulders.

So, the title of this chapter is "Why *Bigger Leaner Stronger* Is Different." How so?

Well, I don't know about you, but I don't train to have fun or hang out with the guys—I train to look and feel better, and I want to get the most from my efforts.

If I can get better results by working out half as long as the other guy, that's what I want to do. If I were new to weightlifting and my options were to gain 10 pounds in a couple of months by doing the same exercises every week (done with correct form, intensity, and weight progression) or to squeeze out half of those gains by doing the latest fancy, overhyped muscle confusion routine, I'd choose the former.

Bigger Leaner Stronger is all about training and getting results. It gives you a precise training and eating regimen that delivers maximum gains in the least time.

The diet and training principles are nothing new or sophisticated, but you've probably never put them all together like how I'm going to teach you. There's nothing cutting-edge or complicated about how to eat and train correctly, but most people have it all wrong.

With *Bigger Leaner Stronger*, you can gain 10 to 15 pounds in your first three months of lifting weights. That's a pretty drastic change. People are going to start asking you for workout advice. Even if you're not new to lifting, you can gain somewhere between half a pound to a pound per week, every week, until you're happy with your size.

If your goal is to simply lose fat, I'm going to show you how to lose between 1 and 2 pounds of fat per week like clockwork…without starving yourself…without having to completely abstain from foods…and without gaining it all back after the suffering has ended.

So, are you ready?

Here's the first step: *Forget what you think you know about getting fit.*

I know, it might sound a little harsh, but trust me: it's for your own good. Just let it all go, approaching *Bigger Leaner Stronger* with an open mind. Along the way, you'll find that certain things you believed or did were right while others were wrong, and that's okay.

As I said earlier, I've made every mistake you can possibly make, so you're in good company.

Just follow the program exactly as I lay it out, and then let the results speak for themselves.

So, let's get started!

SECTION I:

FUNDAMENTALS

1

THE HIDDEN BARRIER TO ACHIEVING YOUR FITNESS AND HEALTH GOALS

The beginning of wisdom is the definition of terms.
— SOCRATES

YOU MAY HAVE WONDERED WHY SO many people are utterly confused about the subjects of health and fitness. Ask around one day, and you'll hear all kinds of conflicting, illogical advice and opinions.

Counting calories doesn't work. Broccoli has more protein than chicken. Any carbs you eat at night will automatically turn into body fat. If you eat dietary fat, you'll get fat. If you eat "good" dietary fat, you won't. You have to eat a lot of small meals every day to lose weight.

This is a *very* small sampling of the many, many false ideas I've heard in my travels.

So how does this happen? Why are people so susceptible to false information, lies, and weird claims?

While that question might sound like it has a deep, philosophical answer, it's pretty simple.

The next time you hear people saying that counting calories isn't necessary or doesn't work, ask them this simple question:

What *is* a calorie?

One for one, they will just stand there with a confused look on their faces. Or maybe they'll stammer out a strange definition. They don't have a clue what the word means. And that's only the beginning, of course.

What is a carbohydrate?

What is protein?

What is fat?

What is muscle?

What is a hormone?

What is a vitamin?

What is an amino acid?

Few people can answer these questions simply and definitively, so of course they'll believe nearly anything they're told. How can you gain a full and proper understanding of a subject when you don't understand the basic words used to explain it? This goes all the way back to Socrates, who said that the beginning of wisdom is the definition of terms.

That's why *words* are the biggest hidden barrier to understanding that almost everyone completely overlooks.

Simply put, if you have misunderstandings about the words being used to communicate specific concepts, a proper duplication of those concepts will not occur in your mind. You will reach your own distorted conclusions due to misinterpretation.

If I were to tell you, "The children have to leave in the gloaming," you might wonder what I am talking about.

Well, "gloaming" simply means the time of the day when the sun is just below the horizon, especially the period between sunset and dark. The sentence now makes sense, doesn't it?

In school, many of us were taught to simply guess at the meanings of words by looking at the surrounding context or by comparing them to other words in our vocabularies.

This is, of course, an unreliable method of study because the person writing the text had specific concepts to communicate and chose exact words to do so, based on, we hope, generally accepted understandings that you would find in a dictionary.

 If you want to receive the information in the same light, then you must share the same understanding of the words used to convey it, not come to subjective understandings based on what you *think* the words might mean.

With "gloaming" in the example above, context only reveals that the word might be a time of the day, which isn't enough information to guess its meaning. Then, you're left with looking at the word itself, maybe thinking, "Well, 'gloaming' looks like 'glowing,' and the sun glows, so I guess it means 'in the morning'?"

That's why the first part of *Bigger Leaner Stronger* is going to be unique: I'm going to share with you the proper definitions of the keywords of the subject matter. These are basic words that I will use throughout the book and that you *must* understand properly to have everything click in the way it should.

I know that reading the definitions of words is dry and unsexy, but trust me, it will help a lot. It's the only way you can be sure that we're on the same page and that you're understanding things the way I mean you to.

I took care in putting together these "keyword lists" to build your understanding from the simple to the more complex, and I think you'll find the learning curve mild. I'm sure you will breeze right through it and have quite a few light bulbs turn on.

By the end of the next few chapters of this book, you will know more about health, nutrition, and fitness than most. It's that bad out there.

Not only that, but you'll also protect yourself against the downright scary amount of false information floating around. Just by knowing the proper meanings of many of the words used, you can make fairly good snap judgments on the validity of many opinions or ideas presented.

So let's get started with the first list of keywords.

2

WHAT MOST PEOPLE DON'T KNOW ABOUT HEALTH, NUTRITION, AND FITNESS
PART ONE: PHYSIOLOGY 101

Being ignorant is not so much a shame, as being unwilling to learn.
— BENJAMIN FRANKLIN

ENERGY: 1. Energy is the power received from electricity, fuel, food, and other sources to do work or produce motion.

2. Energy is the physical or mental strength of a person that can be directed toward some activity.

MATTER: Matter is any material in the universe that has mass and size.

CHEMISTRY: Chemistry is the branch of science that deals with the identification of the substances that matter is composed of, the study of their characteristics, and the ways that they interact, combine, and change.

CHEMICAL: 1. Chemical means having to do with chemistry or the way that substances are made up and the reactions and changes they go through.

2. A chemical is any substance that can undergo a chemical process or change.

When people refer to chemicals, they are usually talking about man-made substances, but the definition isn't limited to just this meaning.

ORGANISM: An organism is a single living thing, such as a person, animal, or plant.

CELL: A cell is the basic unit of all living organisms.

Some living organisms exist only as a single cell. An average-sized man consists of 60 to 100 trillion cells.

Cells keep themselves alive, produce energy, exchange information with neighboring cells, multiply, and die eventually when their time has come.

TISSUE: Tissue is body material in animals and plants that consists of large numbers of cells that are similar in form and function.

MUSCLE: Muscles are masses of tissue in the body, often attached to bones, that can tighten and relax to produce movement.

SKELETAL MUSCLE: A skeletal muscle is connected to the skeleton to form part of the mechanical system that moves the limbs and other parts of the body.

FAT: 1. Fat is a natural oily or greasy substance found in animal bodies, especially when deposited as a layer under the skin or around certain organs.

2. Fat is a substance of this type made from animal or plant products that is used in cooking.

SATURATED FAT: Saturated fat is a form of fat found in animal fat products such as cream, cheese, butter, lard, and fatty meats as well as in certain vegetable products such as coconut oil, cottonseed oil, palm kernel oil, and chocolate.

Saturated fat is solid at room temperature. While it has long been believed that eating foods high in saturated fat increases the risk of cardiovascular disease, more recent research has shown this to be untrue.[1]

UNSATURATED FAT: Unsaturated fat is a form of fat found in foods like avocado, nuts, and vegetable oils, such as canola and olive oils. Meat products contain both saturated and unsaturated fats.

Unsaturated fat is liquid at room temperature.

TRANS FAT: Trans fats are unsaturated fats that are uncommon in nature and created artificially. This type of fat is found in processed foods like cereals, baked goods, fast food, ice cream, and frozen dinners. Anything that contains "partially hydrogenated oil" contains trans fat.

Nutritional authorities, including the U.S. Food and Drug Administration, the European Food Safety Authority, and the UK Scientific Advisory Committee on Nutrition, consider trans fats harmful to our health and recommend reducing the consumption of trans fats to trace amounts.

ORGAN: An organ is made of a group of two or more types of tissue that work together to achieve a specific function in an organism.

While your heart and lungs are organs, skeletal muscle is not an organ because a muscle is just one type of tissue.

GRAM: A gram is a unit of weight in the metric system. One pound is about 454 grams.

KILOGRAM: A kilogram is equal to 1,000 grams, or 2.2 pounds.

MILLIGRAM: A milligram is one thousandth of a gram.

CELSIUS: Celsius is a scale of temperature on which water freezes at 0 degrees and boils at 100 degrees.

In the Fahrenheit scale used in the United States, water freezes at 32 degrees and boils at 212 degrees.

CALORIE: A calorie is a measurement unit of energy potential.

When we talk about the heat output of an organism or the energy value of food, calorie refers to the energy required to raise the temperature of 1 kilogram of water by 1 degree Celsius. This is also known as a *kilocalorie* or *large calorie*.

NUTRIENT: A nutrient is a substance that gives a living body something that it needs to live and grow.

FOOD: Food is material taken into the body to provide it with the nutrients it needs for energy and growth. Food is essentially fuel for the body.

ELEMENT: An element (also called a *chemical element*) is a substance that cannot be broken down into smaller parts by a chemical reaction.

There are more than 100 elements, and they are the primary building blocks of matter.

COMPOUND: A compound is a substance made up of two or more different elements.

MOLECULE: A molecule is the smallest particle of any compound that still exists as that substance. If you were to break it down any further, it would separate into the elements that make it up (meaning it would no longer exist as that original substance).

ACID: An acid is a chemical compound that usually eats away at materials and often tastes sour.

PROTEIN: Proteins are naturally occurring compounds that are used for growth and repair in the body and to build cells and tissues.

AMINO ACID: Amino acids are small units of material that are used to build protein.

GAS: A gas is a substance that is in an air-like form (not solid or liquid).

CARBON: Carbon is a common nonmetallic chemical element found in much of the matter on earth and in all life.

OXYGEN: Oxygen is a colorless, odorless gas and is necessary for most living things to survive.

HYDROGEN: Hydrogen is a colorless, odorless, flammable gas. It is the simplest and most abundant chemical element in the universe.

CARBOHYDRATE: A carbohydrate is a molecule composed of carbon, oxygen, and hydrogen and serves as a source of energy for animals.

DIGESTION: Digestion is the process of breaking down food so that the body can absorb and use it.

ENZYME: An enzyme is a substance produced by organisms that causes specific chemical reactions.

METABOLISM: Metabolism is the term for the series of processes that break down molecules from food to release energy, which is then used to fuel the cells in the body and to create more complex molecules used for building new cells.

Metabolism is necessary for life, and it is how the body creates and maintains the cells that make it up.

ANABOLISM: Anabolism is a metabolic process in which energy is used to make more complex substances (such as tissue) from simpler ones.

This is also known as *constructive metabolism*.

CATABOLISM: Catabolism is the production of energy through the breakdown of complex molecules (such as muscle or fat) into simpler ones.

This is also known as *destructive metabolism*.

Okay, that's it for the first key word list. Simple enough, right?

Take a few minutes to review anything that didn't quite make sense, as the next list is going to build on your understanding of the terms above.

3

WHAT MOST PEOPLE DON'T KNOW ABOUT HEALTH, NUTRITION, AND FITNESS
PART TWO: NUTRITION

There is one remarkable circumstance in our own history which seems to have escaped observation . . . the mischievous effect of the indefinite application of terms.
— NOAH WEBSTER

HEALTHY: Healthy means that the body is in a good physical condition, meaning it has good strength, has high energy levels, and is free from illness or damage.

NOURISH: To nourish is to provide something with the substances needed to grow, live, and be healthy.

NUTRIENT: A nutrient is a substance that provides the nourishment essential for life and growth.

NUTRITION: Nutrition is the process of getting nourishment, especially the process of getting food and nutrients and using them to stay healthy, grow, and build and replace tissues.

MACRONUTRIENT: A macronutrient is any of the nutritional components of the diet required in relatively large amounts.

Specifically, these are protein, carbohydrate, fat, and minerals, such as calcium, zinc, iron, magnesium, and phosphorous.

DIET: 1. A diet is the food and drink that a person usually consumes.

2. A diet is a special course of controlled or restricted intake of food or drink for a particular purpose, such as losing weight, supporting exercise, or medical maintenance.

SUGAR: Sugar is a class of sweet-tasting carbohydrates that comes from various plants, fruits, grains, and other sources.

GLUCOSE: Glucose is a sugar that is an important energy source in living things. Carbohydrates are broken down in the body into glucose, which is the main source of fuel for all cells.

It doesn't matter whether you eat lettuce or candy; both end up as glucose in the body. The only difference is that the lettuce takes a lot longer to break down into glucose than the sugary candy.

FRUCTOSE: Fructose is a sugar found in many plant sources like honey, fruits, flowers, and root vegetables.

SUCROSE: Sucrose is the kind of sugar most commonly called "table sugar" and consists of glucose and fructose.

Sucrose can come from natural sources, such as fruit, but it can be made artificially as well.

GLYCOGEN: Glycogen is a substance found in bodily tissues that acts as a store of carbohydrate.

The body stores glucose in the liver and muscles in the form of glycogen, which can be broken back down into glucose when energy is needed.

BLOOD SUGAR: Your blood sugar level is the amount of glucose in your blood. Glucose is carried in the blood and delivered to cells so that it can be broken down and the energy can be used or stored.

SIMPLE CARBOHYDRATE: A simple carbohydrate is a form of carbohydrate that usually tastes sweet and that the body can break down quickly into glucose.

Examples of simple carbohydrates are the fructose found in fruit, the lactose found in dairy, and the sucrose added to many foods for sweetness.

COMPLEX CARBOHYDRATE: A complex carbohydrate is a carbohydrate made up of a chain of simple carbohydrates linked together. Because of this structure, it takes the body longer to break it down into glucose.

Examples of complex carbohydrates are the sugars found in whole grains, beans, and vegetables.

STARCH: Starch is a complex carbohydrate found naturally in many fruits and vegetables, and it is sometimes added to other foods to thicken them.

Although starch is a complex carbohydrate, some particular foods high in starch break down into glucose quickly, like a simple carbohydrate would.

HORMONE: A hormone is a chemical made in the body that gets transported by the blood or other bodily fluids to cells and organs to cause some action or to have a specific effect.

INSULIN: Insulin is a hormone made in the pancreas that is released into the blood when you eat food. It causes muscles, organs, and fat tissue to take up the nutrients from the food, which are also released into the blood, and either use them or store them as body fat.

INDEX: An index is a system of listing information in an order that allows one to compare it easily to other information.

GLYCEMIC INDEX: The glycemic index (GI) is a scale that measures the effects of different carbohydrates on one's blood sugar level.

Carbohydrates that break down and release glucose into the blood slowly (complex carbs) are low on the glycemic index. Carbohydrates that break down and release glucose into the blood quickly (simple carbs) are high on the index.

Below 55 on the GI is considered low, and above 70 is considered high. Pure glucose is 100 on the GI.

GRAIN: Grains are seeds of different kinds of grasses and are used in many kinds of food.

WHEAT: Wheat is a plant that produces grain.

WHITE BREAD: White bread is bread made from wheat flour that has had parts of the grains removed and has been bleached so it bakes easily and lasts longer.

The process of making white bread removes or kills most of the nutrients from grains, turning the bread into a simpler carbohydrate.

WHOLE GRAIN: Foods containing grains that have not had parts removed are called whole-grain foods.

FIBER: Fiber is a type of carbohydrate found in many types of foods, including fruits, vegetables, legumes, and grains.

FATTY ACIDS: Fatty acids are the molecules that make up fat cells. Some fatty acids are needed to build parts of cells and tissues in the body.

Fatty acids contain twice as many calories per gram as carbohydrates and proteins and are mainly used to store energy in fat cells.

ESSENTIAL FATTY ACIDS: Some fatty acids are called essential fatty acids because they are vital for proper bodily function and must be obtained from food (the body can't synthesize them). Humans have two essential fatty acids: alpha-linolenic acid and linoleic acid.

That's it for list number two. I hope you're finding them helpful and enlightening. I know I did when I first learned all of these words!

Let's wrap up with one final key word list and move on the fun stuff!

4

WHAT MOST PEOPLE DON'T KNOW ABOUT HEALTH, NUTRITION, AND FITNESS
PART THREE: GENERAL HEALTH

Education is the passport to the future, for tomorrow belongs to those who prepare for it today.
— MALCOLM X

SUPPLEMENT: A supplement is a substance added to something to fill a deficiency or to make something more functional or complete.

DIETARY SUPPLEMENT: A dietary (or nutritional) supplement is a product taken to provide the body with nutrients that are not obtained in a large enough quantity in the diet.

VITAMIN: A vitamin is a substance that living organisms need for their cells to function, grow, and develop correctly. The essential vitamins required by the human body must be obtained from the diet, as the body cannot synthesize them in adequate amounts.

MINERAL: A mineral is a substance that contains no carbon (whereas vitamins do) and that forms naturally in the earth. Your body needs minerals for many different physiological functions, including building bones, making hormones, and regulating your heartbeat.

DEHYDRATION: The human body is 75 percent water. Water is lost by sweating, urination, and breathing, and you need to replace it every day.

Dehydration is the state in which the body has replaced too little water for it to properly function. This has various negative side effects like headaches, tiredness, weakness, and, in extreme cases, even death.

NERVE: A nerve is a bundle of tissues in the body that carries electrical messages between the brain, spinal cord, organs, and muscles. These messages give sensations and cause muscles and organs to operate. Nerves are the "communication lines" of the body.

PROCESSED: To process food means to use chemicals or machines to change or preserve it. Many methods of processing food destroy some or most of the vitamins, minerals, and other nutrients that it naturally contains, and often involves the addition of chemicals that can be harmful to the body.

Heavily processed foods often have fewer nutrients but more calories than their less processed counterparts.

ORGANIC: Organic food is free of artificial food additives and often has been raised and made with fewer artificial methods, materials, and conditions, such as chemical ripening, food irradiation, and genetically modified ingredients. Pesticides are allowed as long as they aren't synthetic.

To be certified organic, food products must be grown and manufactured in a manner that adheres to standards set by the governments of the countries they are sold in.

ALL-NATURAL: All-natural foods are often assumed to be foods that are minimally processed or that do not contain any food additives such as hormones, antibiotics, sweeteners, food colors, or flavorings.

That said, while the "all-natural" label implies minimal processing and additives, the lack of standards and regulation means that it is essentially meaningless.

CHOLESTEROL: Cholesterol is a soft, waxy substance found in most body tissues, including the blood and nerves.

Cholesterol is necessary for survival and is used in building the cells and vital hormones in the body, as well as for other important functions. Too much cholesterol in the blood, however, increases the risk of heart attack, stroke, and other disease.[1]

Your body makes some of the cholesterol it needs, and the rest comes from animal products you consume, such as meat, fish, eggs, butter, cheese, and whole milk. Cholesterol is not found in foods made from plants.

BODY MASS INDEX (BMI): The BMI is a scale used for estimating how much people should weigh depending on their height.

The BMI is meant to give a snapshot of the health of large groups of people or whole populations, but when it's used to evaluate an individual, it's often inaccurate because of different body types, like having a thin frame, having a lot of muscle tissue, or being very tall.

BODY FAT PERCENTAGE: Your body fat percentage is a measurement of the fat you have in your body expressed as a percentage of your total body weight. For example, if your body fat percentage is 10 percent, that means that 10 percent of your weight is body fat.

This is a more precise measurement of fat than the BMI as it directly measures the person's fat no matter what that person's body type is or how much weight in muscle that person has, factors that are not taken into account with the BMI.

The amount of fat your body needs to accomplish basic body functions for living is about 3 to 5 percent body fat in men and 8 to 12 percent in women.

BODY COMPOSITION: Body composition is used to describe the percentages of fat, bone, water, and muscle in human bodies.

As you'll learn in this book, weight and BMI aren't nearly as important in gauging our progress as body composition. Our goal isn't to reach a certain number on the scale or a particular BMI reading—it's to achieve a certain type of *look*, and that boils down to a certain amount of muscle with a low body fat percentage or a certain type of *body composition*.

That's it for the key words! Now you know all the basic terminology that will enable you to understand and apply the rest of the information you're going to learn in this book.

Let's carry on!

5

THE 7 BIGGEST MUSCLE-BUILDING MYTHS AND MISTAKES

Just remember, somewhere, a little Chinese girl is warming up with your max.
— JIM CONROY

NINE OUT OF TEN PEOPLE YOU see in the gym don't train correctly. I know that sounds a bit harsh, but it's true, and you'll soon see why.

In many cases, I wouldn't even bother getting out of bed in the morning to do their training routines, which are of the "magazine" variety: lots and lots of sets of isolation exercises with relatively light weights. Even if they're working hard in their training, really pushing themselves to get more and more reps, they're still doing it wrong and will only wind up disappointed in the results. I should know, because I was once one of those guys too.

Most people also compound their training mistakes by eating incorrectly. They're usually eating too much or too little, eating too many low-quality foods, and failing to balance their macronutrients correctly. Proper dieting is much simpler than most people think—it's just a numbers game (and it's not just calories in vs. calories out—that's the foundation, but we need to go a bit deeper to maximize muscle growth and fat loss).

All of these mistakes are why so many people bust their butts only to fail to make any noticeable progress. Case in point: most of the crowd in my gym basically haven't changed one bit in the last couple of years that I've been there. They're still lifting more or less the same weights and look more or less exactly the same as they did when I arrived.

Well, in this chapter, we're going to look at why. Specifically, we're going to go over the seven most common diet and training myths and mistakes that keep people from effectively building muscle and losing fat.

Unless you're brand new to lifting, I can guarantee that you've fallen victim to one or more of these myths and mistakes at some point along the way. I know I did.

Let's get to it.

MYTH & MISTAKE #1
MORE SETS = MORE GROWTH

I used to lift weights for 2 or more hours per day, to the point of complete physical and mental exhaustion. Afterward, all I wanted to do is eat and pass out.

I didn't particularly *like* how tough the routine was, but I used to think this is what it took to build a great physique, so I did it—for years. And I wasn't nearly as ripped as you would have expected given the intensity of my training.

Well, what I later learned is that this type of routine is complete overkill for a natural weightlifter (the guy who originally turned me on to this type of training, it turns out, was on quite a few anabolic drugs).

I learned that doing too many sets and reps for any muscle group per week can lead to *overtraining*, which has a host of negative side effects: impaired muscle growth, general fatigue, lower levels of anabolic hormones, higher levels of catabolic hormones, and in extreme cases, even muscle loss.

Yes, that's right—too much weightlifting every day can cause so much more damage to your muscle fibers than your body can efficiently repair that you actually get smaller and weaker over time.

This is one of the first things about the *Bigger Leaner Stronger* program that is going to surprise you. The workouts are going to call for a lot fewer sets and reps than you're probably expecting. There are no supersets, drop sets, giant sets, or any of the fancy rep schemes typically recommended in other routines.

Instead, you're going to do what most popular mainstream weightlifting programs *never* prescribe: you're going to focus on heavy, compound weightlifting, and you're going to do just enough sets and reps in your workouts to maximize muscle overload and stimulation without going so far as overtraining. This takes no more than 45 to 60 minutes per workout. (Yup, you'll be in and out of the gym in an hour on this program!)

Make no mistake—the workouts won't be *easy*. You're going to push, pull, and squat more weight than you ever have before, and this requires tremendous physical energy and effort.

Nevertheless, if you're currently following one of the many high-rep training programs out there, you're probably going to feel like you're *undertraining* on my program. You're not going to be used to the longer rest periods in between sets and shorter workouts, and you might even feel a bit guilty leaving the gym after less than an hour.

Don't worry—I know exactly how this feels. When I first switched from my old overtraining style to what I teach in this book, I was sure I was going to get weaker and lose muscle.

I didn't though. Since I made the switch, I've gained close to 20 pounds of muscle and more than doubled the weight I can lift across the board.

Follow the program, and you can do the same.

MYTH & MISTAKE #2
YOU HAVE TO "FEEL THE BURN" TO GROW

How many times have you heard training partners yelling for each other to "make it burn" and "squeeze out three more reps"?

Well, "everyone knows" that pumping out reps until the stinging pain is unbearable causes maximum growth, right? "No pain, no gain," right?

Wrong.

This is probably one of the worst muscle-building fallacies out there. Muscle "burn" and pump are *not* paramount in achieving muscle growth.

When your muscles are burning, what you're feeling is a buildup of lactic acid, which continues to accumulate as you contract your muscles again and again.

While lactic acid triggers what's known as the "anabolic cascade," which is a cocktail of growth-inducing hormones, repeatedly elevating lactic acid levels higher and higher doesn't mean you build more and more muscle over time.

Thus, for yet another reason, when guys spend a couple of hours in the gym pounding away with drop sets, burnout sets, supersets, and so forth, they're working very hard for little payoff.

If pump and burn don't drive muscle growth, what does? Well, the short answer is *progressive overload*, which we'll go over in more detail soon.

MYTH & MISTAKE #3
WASTING TIME WITH THE WRONG EXERCISES

Most of what your gym offers in terms of workout machines and contraptions has no place in a proper weightlifting routine.

As the well-known strength coach and author Mark Rippetoe says, if you want to be strong, ditch the machines and pick up a barbell. As you'll see, that's what *Bigger Leaner Stronger* is all about: pushing, pulling, raising, and squatting barbells and dumbbells.

There are studies out there comparing machines and free weights that are often used to disagree with this approach. If you took these studies at face value, you could easily conclude that machines are equally effective as free weights for building muscle and strength and possibly even *better*.

The people who do this are missing a couple of crucial pieces of information:

The subjects in these studies are untrained, and the results seen in untrained subjects simply can't be directly extrapolated to trained subjects.

"Newbie gains" are very real and boil down to the simple fact that your muscles respond exceptionally well to just about any type of training for the first three to six months. Simply put, you can make all kinds of mistakes in the beginning and still make better-than-average progress.

This doesn't last long, though. Once the "magic" runs out, it's gone forever, and what worked for the first few months won't necessarily continue to work.

This is especially true in resistance training. While an untrained subject can make mediocre strength and muscle gains on machines for the first few months, there's no way in *hell* he can build an impressive physique by primarily working on machines.

There is research that proves the opposite: free weights are indeed more effective at building muscle and strength than machines.

A good example is a study conducted by researchers from the University of Saskatchewan, which demonstrated that the free weight squat resulted in 43 percent more leg muscle activation than the Smith machine squat.[1]

Another example is a study conducted by researchers from the University of California that demonstrated that the free weight bench press resulted in greater activation of the upper-body muscles than the Smith machine bench press.[2]

These things shouldn't come as a surprise. For decades, the most impressive bodybuilders have always emphasized free weight training, and I'll bet that the biggest, strongest guys in your gym do the same.

The bottom line is that there's just something special about forcing the body to freely manipulate weight, unaided, against the pull of gravity. Nobody ever built a great chest by just pounding away on the pec deck and machine press: it always took years of pushing around barbells and dumbbells.

Not all free weight exercises are equal, though. The most effective ones are known as *compound exercises*, and they involve and activate multiple muscle groups. Examples of powerful compound exercises are the squat, deadlift, and bench press, which train a lot more than just the legs, back, and chest, respectively.

The opposite of a compound exercise is an *isolation exercise*, which primarily involves and activates just one muscle group. Examples of isolation exercises are the cable fly (which isolates the chest muscles), dumbbell curl (which isolates the biceps), and leg extension (which isolates the quadriceps).

When it comes to building size and strength, numerous scientific studies have confirmed the superiority of compound exercises over isolation exercises.

One such study was conducted at Ball State University in 2000, and it went like this: Two groups of men trained with weights for 10 weeks. The first group did four compound upper-body exercises, while the second group did the same plus bicep curls and triceps extensions (isolation exercises).[3]

After the training period, both groups increased strength and size, but which do you think had bigger arms? The answer is neither. The additional isolation training performed by group two produced no additional effect on arm strength or circumference. The takeaway isn't that you shouldn't directly train your arms, but rather that by overloading your entire body, you cause everything to grow.

Charles Poliquin, trainer to world-class athletes like Olympians and professional sports players, is fond of saying that to gain an inch on your arms, you have to gain 10 pounds of muscle.

His point is that the most effective way to build a big, strong body is with systemic overload, not localized training. If your weightlifting program isn't built around heavy, compound training, you're never going to achieve your genetic potential in terms of overall muscle size and strength.

Now, I'm not saying that all isolation exercises are worthless. Certain isolation exercises, if properly incorporated into a routine, do help with overall development. In fact, they're necessary for fully developing smaller muscles in the body like the shoulders, biceps, and triceps.

So you will find a few isolation exercises in my program, but they are hardly the emphasis.

MYTH & MISTAKE #4
CONSTANTLY CHANGING UP YOUR ROUTINE

Guys who make the mistake of doing lots of ineffective exercises often believe the "muscle confusion" myth, which is the belief that you have to constantly change up your routine to "keep your body guessing" and make gains.

This is complete nonsense. You're in the gym to get bigger and stronger, and that requires four simple things: do the right exercises, lift progressively heavier weights over time, eat correctly, and give your body sufficient rest.

Regularly changing exercises simply isn't necessary because your goals limit the exercises that you should be doing.

You see, if you're looking to build a solid foundation of muscle and strength, you should do the same types of exercises every week, and they will include things like squats, deadlifts, bench presses, dumbbell presses, military presses, and others.

If you do these exercises correctly every week, your strength will skyrocket, and you'll gain muscle faster than you ever imagined possible—without changing a single thing other than the amount of weight on the bar.

Furthermore, constantly changing your routine prevents you from properly evaluating your progress. How can you know whether you're getting stronger if you're doing different exercises and rep ranges every week or two?

You can't, and that's dangerous. That leads to week after week of busting your ass without ever realizing that you aren't progressing at all.

MYTH & MISTAKE #5
LIFTING LIKE AN IDIOT

One of the most painful sights in gyms is the ego lifters spastically throwing around big weights with reckless abandon. I cringe not only out of pity but also out of the anticipation of injuries that could strike at any moment.

While this might sound like another shocking generality, it's nonetheless true. Most guys don't have a clue about proper form on many exercises, and this ignorance stunts their gains; causes unnecessary wear and tear on ligaments, tendons, and joints; and opens the door to debilitating injuries (especially as weights get heavy on the shoulders, elbows, knees, and lower back).

Some of these guys just don't know any better, and some are more interested in looking cool than in making real gains. Others were just taught wrong by, yes, you guessed it, magazines, friends, or trainers.

Well, you're not going to fall into this trap. You're going to do your exercises with perfect form, and while your weights may be lighter than Mr. Huff and Puff, he'll secretly be wondering why you're moving up so quickly in your lifts while he's been stuck for months.

MYTH & MISTAKE #6
LIFTING LIKE A WUSSY

Building a great body is a pain in the butt. It takes considerable time, effort, discipline, and dedication. It doesn't come easy, and anyone who tells you otherwise is either ignorant or lying.

Quite frankly, most guys just train like wussies. They don't want to face up to heavy weights and do the hard work. They seem to believe that just showing up and going through the motions is enough.

Well, it's not. And their bodies, which change little over time, are a testament to that fact.

The truth is these guys are just giving in to one of our most primal instincts. We humans are programmed to avoid pain and discomfort and seek pleasure and ease in life, and in some circumstances, this works out nicely for us. If we let these inclinations color our workouts, however, we're doomed.

If you want to build an impressive physique, you're going to have to work *hard* in the gym. You're going to have to move weights that are just downright intimidating. You're going to have to dig deep to finish that last set. You're going to deal with muscle soreness and other aches.

But you're going to come to love it. You're going to learn that these hardships are just part of the game—the "dues" you have to pay to meet your goals. You're going to look forward to this daily hour of intense, uncomfortable, all-out physical exertion because you know that every workout you finish makes you a little bit stronger, both physically and mentally, and gets you a little bit closer to the "endgame."

MYTH & MISTAKE #7
EATING TO STAY SMALL OR GET FAT

As you've probably heard, your muscles grow *outside* of the gym, when they're provided sufficient rest and proper nutrition.

Well, many guys get it all wrong: they overtrain and then don't eat enough calories or protein in particular (or eat way more food than they should) and eat too much non-nutritious food and wonder why they can't get their bodies to change the way they want.

You see, if you don't eat enough calories and get enough protein every day, you simply *don't grow*. It doesn't matter how hard you lift; if you don't eat enough, you won't gain any muscle to speak of.

On the other hand, if you eat enough protein but too many calories every day, you can gain muscle, but it will be hidden underneath an ugly sheath of unnecessary fat.

If you don't eat enough nutritious foods, you can change your body composition, but eventually you'll develop vitamin and mineral deficiencies that impair both your health and performance, which in turn will limit your gains over time.

When you know how to eat properly, however, you can gain eye-popping amounts of muscle while staying lean, and you can lose layers of fat while maintaining or even increasing your total muscle mass.

THE BOTTOM LINE

You've just learned the path to muscle-building misery: grind away for hours in the gym, do tons of "burnout" sets, do the wrong exercises with bad form, avoid pushing yourself too hard, and eat incorrectly.

These mistakes are responsible for untold amounts of frustration, discouragement, and confusion. They're the prime reasons why guys make little or no gains and quit.

So, if that's how to do it wrong, how do you correctly go about building muscle and losing fat? Continue to find out.

CHAPTER SUMMARY

- More is not always better in weightlifting. Many popular bodybuilder routines result in overtraining for a natural weightlifter.

- As a natural weightlifter, you must emphasize heavy, compound weightlifting if you want to maximize your results. High-rep routines that emphasize isolation exercises are extremely ineffective in the long run.

- Getting a huge pump doesn't stimulate nearly as much muscle growth as you might think.

- You don't have to constantly change up your exercise routine to make gains. Instead, you want to progressively increase your strength on key compound lifts.

- If you want to build an impressive physique, you're going to have to work hard in the gym. Easy workouts don't do much.

- If you chronically undereat, you won't grow any muscle to speak of. If you chronically overeat, you will build muscle but will gain too much body fat.

6

THE 3 SCIENTIFIC LAWS OF MUSCLE GROWTH

Fortunately, there is a solution, and it's not performing multiple sets of whatever cable Kegel exercise is being pushed as 'The Answer.' Just a little hard, smart, basic work.
— JIM WENDLER

THE LAWS OF MUSCLE GROWTH ARE as certain, observable, and irrefutable as those of physics.

When you throw a ball in the air, it comes down. When you take the correct actions inside and outside the gym, your muscles grow. It's that simple, regardless of whether your genetics are "good" or "bad." There's no such thing as the hopeless "hardgainer"—there are only people who don't know and act in accordance with the laws contained in this and the previous chapters.

These principles have been known and followed for decades by people who built some of the greatest physiques we've ever seen, going all the way back to the likes of Steve Reeves and Roy "Reg" Park, and even further back, to the pioneering "father of modern bodybuilding," Eugen Sandow.

Some of these laws will contradict things you've read or heard, but fortunately, they require no leaps of faith or meditation. They are *practical*. Follow them, and you get immediate results.

Once these rules have worked for you, you will know they're true and will never be lured away from them.

THE FIRST LAW OF MUSCLE GROWTH
PROGRESSIVE OVERLOAD OVER ALL

As you know, the "burn" you feel is simply an infusion of lactic acid in the muscle, which is a by-product of muscles burning their energy stores. It does little to induce muscle growth.

A big "pump" is also not a good predictor of future muscle growth. The pump you feel when training is the result of blood being "trapped" in the muscles, and while it's a good psychological boost and studies have shown that it can help with protein synthesis (the process by which cells build proteins), it's not a primary driver of growth.[1]

What drives muscle growth, then?

The answer is known as *progressive tension overload*, which means progressively increasing tension levels in the muscle fibers over time. That is, lifting progressively heavier and heavier weights.

You see, muscles must be given a powerful reason to grow, and nothing is more convincing than subjecting them to more and more mechanical stress and tension.[2]

This makes good intuitive sense—to adapt to handling heavier and heavier weights, the muscles must grow larger—and it's also supported by science.

For example, in a meta-analysis of 140 related studies, researchers from Arizona State University found that a progression in resistance optimizes strength gains and muscle growth.[3] Researchers also found that working in the 4- to 6-rep range (80 percent of one-rep max, or *1RM*) is most effective for those who train regularly.

The conclusion of this research is simple: the best way to build muscle and strength is to focus on heavy weightlifting and increase the weight lifted over time.

Well, that's not just theory—that's fact. And that's what the *Bigger Leaner Stronger* program is all about: lifting heavy weights and doing short, intense sets of relatively low numbers of reps.

Leave the drop sets, giant sets, and supersets prescribed in the magazines to the magazine readers. Those training methods are as ineffective for building muscle as they are grueling. It's a lot of work for little reward.

Instead, from now on, you're going to train differently. You're going to spend more time resting than you're used to, you're going to perform exercises you're probably not used to, and you're going to lift a lot more weight than you thought possible.

But the payoff is huge. You're not only going to come to love your workouts, but you're also going to love how your body changes even more.

THE SECOND LAW OF MUSCLE GROWTH
PROPER REST IS JUST AS IMPORTANT IS PROPER TRAINING

One of the most common problems with the many weightlifting programs out there is they simply have you doing too much, whether in individual workouts or in total weekly training volume.

They play into the common misconception that building muscle is simply a matter of pounding your body into submission through excessive amounts of training. People who have fallen into this bad habit need to realize that if they did less of the *right thing*, they would get *more*.

You see, when you lift weights, you cause tiny tears in the muscle fibers, known as *microtears*, which the body then repairs. This is part of the process by which muscles grow (scientifically termed *hypertrophy*).[4]

One of the things you want to achieve with your workouts is an optimal amount of microtearing in the muscles. Not so much that your body falls behind with repair, as this stunts muscle growth, but not so little that you miss out on potential gains.

While many guys undertrain and thus underdamage their muscles, many more overtrain and overdamage them. That is, the individual workouts they do result in too much microtearing, or they wait too few days before training a muscle group again given the extent of the muscle damage caused in the previous workout.

Studies have shown that, depending on the intensity of your training and your level of fitness, it takes the body two to seven days to fully repair muscles subjected to weight training.[5] Considering the volume and intensity of the *Bigger Leaner Stronger* program, we can safely assume full muscle recovery is going to take four to six days.

THE THIRD LAW OF MUSCLE GROWTH
MUSCLES WILL GROW ONLY IF THEY'RE PROPERLY FED

You could do the perfect workouts and give your muscles the perfect amount of rest, but if you don't eat correctly, you won't grow—*period*. It is that cut and dry.

A proper diet isn't particularly complicated, but it does have several moving parts that you need to know how to coordinate.

Sure, we all know to eat protein, but how much? How many times per day? Which kinds?

What about carbs? Are they good for muscle growth? Which kinds are best? How much? When should you eat them to maximize your gains?

And dietary fats? What role do they play? How much do we need, and what are the best ways to get them?

And last but not least, how many calories should we eat every day and why? When do we adjust this and by how much?

Well, these are all good questions, and in this book, you're going to find definitive answers to all of them and more so that you never make a diet mistake again.

THE BOTTOM LINE

Packing on slabs of rock-solid lean mass is, in essence, just a matter of following these three laws religiously: lift hard and heavy, get sufficient rest, and feed your body correctly. That's how you build a strong, healthy, ripped body, and soon you're going to be on your way, proving it to yourself and others.

So then, let's now flip to the other side of the fitness coin—losing fat—and see what myths, mistakes, and laws await.

CHAPTER SUMMARY

- Progressive overload is the primary driver of muscle growth, not fatigue or pump.

- Working primarily with 80 to 85 percent of your 1RM optimizes strength gains and muscle growth.

- Recovery time is just as important as training time, and studies have shown it takes the body two to seven days to fully repair muscles subjected to weight training.

7

THE 5 BIGGEST FAT LOSS MYTHS AND MISTAKES

The road to nowhere is paved with excuses.
— MARK BELL

FOR THOUSANDS OF YEARS NOW, A lean, muscular body has been the gold standard of the male physique.

It was a hallmark of the ancient heroes and gods, and it has remained a revered quality; it has been idolized in pop culture, achieved by few, but coveted by many.

With obesity rates over 35 percent here in America (and steadily rising), it would appear that getting shredded and becoming one of the "physical elite" must require superhuman genetics or a level of knowledge, discipline, and sacrifice beyond what most people are capable of.

Well, this simply isn't true. The knowledge is easy enough to understand (in fact, you're learning everything you need to know in this book).

Sure, it requires discipline and some "sacrifice" in that no, you probably don't have the metabolism to eat a large pizza every day and have a six pack, but here's the kicker: when you're training and dieting correctly, you'll *enjoy* the lifestyle. You'll look forward to the gym every day. You'll never feel starved, you'll get to eat foods you love, and you won't suffer from overpowering cravings.

When you find this "sweet spot," you'll look and feel better than you ever have before and find it infinitely more pleasurable and valuable than being lazy, fat, and addicted to ice cream and potato chips. When you can get into this "zone," you can do whatever you want with your body. The results are inevitable; it's just a matter of time.

Most people never get there though. They either lack the will or desire to get there (they don't have their "inner game" sorted out), or they lack the know-how required to make it happen, or both.

Well, in this chapter, we're going to address the five most common myths and mistakes of getting ripped. Like the muscle-building fallacies, these errors have permeated the health and fitness space and mucked things up for millions of people.

Let's dispel them once and for all so that they can't block your path to achieving the lean, muscular body that you desire.

MYTH & MISTAKE #1
WATCHING CALORIC INTAKE IS UNNECESSARY

If I had a penny for every person I've spoken with who wanted to lose weight but didn't want to have to count calories…well, you know the rest.

This is about as logical as wanting to drive across the state without paying attention to the gas tank. Could you do it? Maybe. But it's going to be a lot trickier and more stressful than it should be.

Now, I won't be too hard on these people because they often don't even know what a calorie is. They just don't want to be bothered with having to count something or worry about whether they can "afford" one food or another, and I can understand that.

Here's the truth, though: whether you want to call it "counting" calories, meal planning, or something else, to effectively lose fat, you have to regulate your food intake.

You see, the metabolism is an energy system and operates according to the laws of energy. Losing fat requires that you keep your body burning more energy than you're feeding it, and the energy potential of food is measured in calories.

Chances are this isn't news to you, but I want to quickly review the physiology of fat loss just in case you're not convinced that fat loss boils down to the mathematics of energy consumed versus energy burned.

The underlying scientific principle at work is *energy balance*, which refers to the amount of energy you burn every day versus the amount you give your body via food.

According to the laws of physics underlying this principle, if you give your body a bit more energy than it burns every day, a portion of the excess energy is stored as body fat, and thus you gain weight slowly. If you give your body a bit less energy than it burns every day, it will tap into fat stores to get the additional energy it needs, leaving you a bit lighter.

You see, at any given time, your body requires a certain amount of glucose in the blood to stay alive. This is vital fuel that every cell in the body uses to operate, and certain organs like the brain are real glucose hogs.

When you eat food, you give your body a relatively large amount of energy (calories) in a short period. Glucose levels rise far above what is needed to maintain life, and instead of "throwing away" or burning off all excess energy, a portion is stored as body fat for later use.

Scientifically speaking, when your body is absorbing nutrients eaten and storing fat, it's in the "postprandial" state (*post* meaning "after" and *prandial* meaning "having to do with a meal"). This "fed" state is when the body is in "fat storage mode."

Once the body has finished absorbing the glucose and other nutrients from the food (amino acids and fatty acids), it then enters the "postabsorptive" state ("after absorption"), wherein it must turn to its fat stores for energy. This "fasted" state is when the body is in "fat burning mode."

Your body flips between "fed" and "fasted" states every day, storing fat from the food you eat and then burning it once there's nothing left to use from the meals. Here's a simple graph that depicts this cycle:

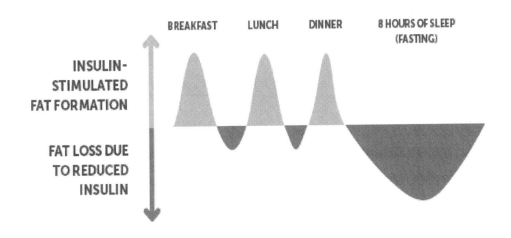

The lighter portions are the periods where your body has excess energy because you ate. The darker portions are the periods when the body has no energy left from food and thus has to burn fat to stay alive. As you can see, we burn quite a bit of fat when we sleep.

If the lighter and darker portions balance out every day—if you store just as much fat as you burn—your weight stays the same. If you store more fat than you burn (by overeating), you get fatter. And if you burn more fat than you store, you get leaner.

This is the fundamental mechanism underlying fat storage and fat loss, and it takes precedence over anything related to insulin or any other hormones or physiological functions.

Simply put, you can't get fatter unless you feed your body more energy than it burns, and you can't get leaner unless you feed it less energy than it burns.

Contrary to (currently) popular belief, it doesn't matter how many carbohydrates you eat or how high your insulin levels are throughout the day. Energy balance is the first law of thermodynamics at work: fat stores can't be increased without the provision of excess energy, nor can they be reduced without the restriction of energy.

That's why research has shown that so long as they're eating less energy than they're burning, people lose fat equally well on high-carbohydrate or low-carbohydrate diets.[1]

The bottom line is that the types of foods you eat have little to do with losing or gaining weight. In this regard, a calorie is a calorie. That isn't to say that you should eat nothing but junk food to lose weight, however. What you eat *does* matter when we're talking about maintaining optimal body composition. If you want to lose fat and not muscle, a calorie is *not* a calorie, but we'll talk more about that later.

So, with that out of the way, let's get back to calorie counting. What people usually dislike most about it isn't the counting but the trying to figure out what to eat while on the run every day or what to buy when rushing through the grocery store.

When you have a 30-minute window for lunch and run to the nearest restaurant, you don't want to have to load an app and try to estimate calories. You want to just order something that sounds healthy and hope for the best.

Unfortunately, these quick, "healthy" meals have hundreds more calories than you might think. Repeat that for dinner, with a few random snacks thrown in for good measure, and you've simply eaten too much to reduce your total fat mass. You'll have stored just as much, if not more, fat as you burned, and your weight will remain the same or go up accordingly.

So the real problem isn't counting calories but failing to make and follow a meal plan that allows you to eat foods you like while ensuring that you burn more fat than you store over time.

Sure, it's easier to just heat up a big plate of leftovers or grab some fast food for lunch and carry on with your day, but that convenience comes with a price: little or no weight loss.

MYTH & MISTAKE #2
DO CARDIO AND YOU'LL LOSE FAT

Every day, I see overweight people grinding away on the cardio machines. And week after week goes by with them looking the same.

They are under the false impression that grinding away on an elliptical machine or stationary bike will somehow flip a magical fat-loss switch in the body. Well, as you now know, that's not how it works.

Cardio can *enhance* fat loss in two ways—burning calories and speeding up your metabolic rate—but that's it.

And since I've brought it up, let's talk briefly about the "metabolic rate." Your body burns a certain number of calories regardless of any physical activity, and this is called your *basal metabolic rate* (BMR). Your *total daily energy expenditure* (TDEE) for a day would be your BMR plus the energy expended during any physical activities.

When your metabolism is said to "speed up" or "slow down," what this means is that your basal metabolic rate has gone up or down. That is, your body is burning more or fewer calories while at rest.

Cardio, especially a variety I recommend called *high-intensity interval cardio* (HIIT), can increase your basal metabolic rate through what's known as the "afterburn effect." While that sounds fancy and is often used in sketchy marketing pitches for sketchy products, it's simple: your body continues burning additional energy *after* you exercise.[2]

But here's the thing with cardio: if you don't also eat correctly, that nightly run or bike ride won't save you.

Let's say you're trying to lose weight and have unwittingly eaten 600 calories more than your body has burned for the day. You go jogging for 30 minutes at night, which burns about 300 calories, with maybe another hundred calories burned from the "afterburn" effect.

You're still 200 calories over your expenditure, and that means no reduction in total fat stores for the day—and maybe even an increase.

You could continue like this for *years* and never get lean; instead, you could slowly get fatter. This is the most common reason why people simply "can't lose weight no matter what they do."

MYTH & MISTAKE #3
CHASING FAD DIETS

The Atkins Diet. The South Beach Diet. The Paleo Diet. The HCG Diet (this one makes me cringe). The Hollywood Diet. The Body Type Diet.

It seems like a new fad diet pops up every month or two. I can't keep up these days.

While not all "latest and greatest" diets are bad (Paleo is unnecessarily restrictive but quite healthy, for example), the sheer abundance of fad diets being touted by ripped models and actors is confusing people as to what the "right way" to lose weight is (and understandably so).

The result is that many people jump from diet to diet, failing to get the results they desire. And they buy into some pretty stupid stuff simply because they don't understand the physiology of the metabolism and of fat loss like you now do. Or they don't want to accept it.

Regardless, the rules are the rules, and no fancy diets or snake oil supplements will help you get around them.

As the old saying goes, the best diet is the one you can follow, and as you'll see, a flexible, balanced approach to eating is by far the most enjoyable and thus the most effective. Once you experience this for yourself, you'll fully realize how asinine many of the fad diets taking gyms by storm are.

MYTH & MISTAKE #4
DOING TONS OF REPS GETS YOU SHREDDED

Many "gurus" recommend that you follow a high-rep, low-weight routine to "shred up," but this is the complete opposite of what you want to do.

The reality is that your body is "primed" for muscle loss when you're in a calorie deficit, and by focusing exclusively on muscle endurance (higher-rep ranges), you'll set yourself up for rapid strength loss, with the potential for significant muscle loss as well.[3]

The key to preserving strength and muscle while losing weight is to lift *heavy* weights. The goal is to continue progressively overloading your muscles, which ensures protein synthesis rates remain elevated enough to prevent muscle loss.[4]

There are fat-loss benefits to heavy weightlifting as well.

A study published by Greek sports scientists found that men who trained with heavy weights (80 to 85 percent of 1RM) increased their metabolic rates over the following three days, burning hundreds more calories than the men who trained with lighter weights (45 to 65 percent of 1RM).[5]

Yes, *hundreds* more calories. That's significant.

And if you want to really score extra calories burned, focus on compound lifts like squats and deadlifts, because these are the types of lifts that burn the most post-workout calories.[6]

The bottom line is getting that shredded look is just a matter of having a fair amount of muscle and a low amount of body fat—and nothing else. There aren't any special exercises that "bring out the striations," and burning your muscles out with tons of reps does nothing to improve your overall look.

MYTH & MISTAKE #5
TRYING TO "SPOT REDUCE" FAT

Pick up just about any fitness magazine, and you'll find workouts for getting a six pack, slimming the thighs, getting rid of love handles, and the like.

I wish it were that simple.

While research has shown that training a muscle results in increased levels of blood flow and lipolysis (the breakdown of fat cells into usable energy) in the area, it's not in a large enough quantity to matter.[7]

The reality is that training the muscles of a certain area of your body burns calories and can result in muscle growth, both of which certainly can aid in fat loss, but it doesn't directly burn the fat covering them to any significant degree.[8]

You see, fat loss occurs in a whole-body fashion. You create the proper internal weight loss environment (a calorie deficit), and your body reduces fat stores all over the body, with certain areas reducing faster than others.

You can do all the crunches you want, but you'll never have a six pack until you've adequately reduced your overall body fat percentage, and that's more a function of proper dieting than anything else.[9]

Ironically, if you want an area of your body to be leaner, training the muscles without also ensuring you're reducing your body fat percentage will only aggravate the problem. The muscles will grow but the layer of fat will remain, which will only result in the area looking bigger and puffier.

I often run into this with women who get into weightlifting without also addressing their body fat percentage. This is why many women believe weightlifting makes them "bulky." They started weightlifting to look lean, toned, and athletic, not to have even more trouble fitting into their clothes.

This is why I often repeat a simple rule of thumb: the more muscle you build, the leaner you have to be to avoid looking big and bulky. A woman who has built an appreciable amount of muscle (one or more years of weightlifting) will want to stay at or under 20 percent body fat to maintain the "athletic" look of toned arms, a tight stomach, shapely legs, a big butt, etc. For us guys, we need to stay at or under 10 percent for the look we're usually after: fully visible abs, small waist, vascularity, "dense"-looking muscles, etc.

Now, we all have our "fat spots" that plague us, and that's just genetics for you. Some guys I know store every last pound in their hips, while others are fortunate to have their fat accumulate more in their chest, shoulders, and arms more so than their waistline.

Rest assured, however, that you can lose as much fat all over your body as you want, and you *can* get as shredded as you want; you'll just have to be patient and let your body lean out in the way it's programmed to.

THE BOTTOM LINE

Like building muscle, many people approach fat loss completely wrong and thus fail to achieve their weight goals.

But, just like building muscle, the laws of healthy fat loss are very simple and incredibly effective. Carry on to learn the laws and how to put them to work for you.

CHAPTER SUMMARY

- The principle of energy balance underlies all weight loss and gain. The types of foods you eat have little to do with losing or gaining weight.

- What you eat *does* matter in terms of body composition, however. If you want to lose fat and not muscle, a calorie isn't a calorie.

- Your body flips between "fed" and "fasted" states every day, storing fat from food you eat and then burning it once there's nothing left to use from the meals.

- If you store just as much fat as you burn every day, your weight stays the same. If you store more fat than you burn (by overeating), you get fatter. And if you burn more fat than you store, you get leaner.

- Doing a bunch of cardio isn't enough to get lean. You simply can't outexercise a poor diet.

- The best diet is the one you can follow. This is why a flexible approach to dieting is the only one that works in the long run.

- The key to preserving strength and thereby muscle while losing weight is to lift *heavy* weights.

- Training the muscles of a certain area of your body burns calories and can result in muscle growth, both of which certainly can aid in fat loss, but it *doesn't* directly burn the fat covering them to any significant degree.

8

THE 4 SCIENTIFIC LAWS OF HEALTHY FAT LOSS

For me, life is continuously being hungry. The meaning of life is not simply to exist, to survive, but to move ahead, to go up, to achieve, to conquer.
— ARNOLD SCHWARZENEGGER

EVOLUTION HAS TAUGHT THE BODY THAT having fat means being able to survive the times when food is scarce. Many thousands of years ago, when our ancestors were roaming the wilderness, they often journeyed for days without food, and their fat stores were all that kept them alive.

Starving, they would finally kill an animal and feast, and their bodies knew to prepare for the next bout of starvation by storing excess energy as fat, as it was literally a matter of life and death.

This genetic programming is still in us. When you restrict your calories for fat-loss purposes, your body reduces its total fat stores to stay alive, but it also slows down its basal metabolic rate to conserve energy.[1]

If you restrict your calories too severely or for too long, this metabolic downregulation, or "metabolic adaptation," as it's often called, can become quite severe, and the basal metabolic rate can plunge to surprisingly low levels.[2]

This mechanism is why "calorie counting" seems to not work for some people. It has nothing to do with hormone problems or eating too many carbs or anything other than the fact that the energy *out* part of the equation is impaired. Their bodies aren't burning nearly as much energy as they should be.

This is only the beginning of the problems with the "crash" approach to dieting, however, that has you enduring severe calorie deficits for extended periods:

- You lose a lot of muscle, which not only leads to the dreaded "skinny fat" look, but it also impairs bone health and increases the overall risk of disease.[3]

- Your testosterone levels plummet and cortisol levels skyrocket, which not only makes you feel horrible but also accelerates muscle loss.[4]

- Your energy levels take a nosedive, you struggle with intense food cravings every day, and you become mentally clouded and even depressed.[5]

Fortunately, you can fix the metabolic adaptation and all the other negative effects of low-calorie dieting by slowly increasing food intake over time and thus bringing your basal metabolic rate back to a healthy level.

But the real goal is to prevent it altogether, and that's what we're going to focus on in this chapter: the laws of healthy fat loss that, when followed, allow for consistent weight reduction without major metabolic slowing or muscle loss.

THE FIRST LAW OF HEALTHY FAT LOSS
EAT LESS ENERGY THAN YOU BURN TO LOSE FAT

As you now know, fat loss is just a science of numbers. No matter what anyone tells you, getting ripped boils down to nothing more than making a simple mathematical formula work for you: energy consumed versus energy expended.

Contrary to much of the mainstream advice these days, it doesn't matter what you eat. If your metabolism is healthy and you set your calorie intake correctly—if you maintain a moderate calorie deficit by eating a bit less energy than you burn every day—you will lose weight.

Don't believe me?

Professor Mark Haub from Kansas State University conducted a weight-loss study on himself in 2010.[6] He started the study at 211 pounds and 33.4 percent body fat (overweight). He calculated that he would need to eat about 1,800 calories per day to lose weight without starving himself.

He followed this protocol for two months and lost 27 pounds, but here's the kicker: while he did have one protein shake and a couple of servings of vegetables each day, two-thirds of his daily calories came from Twinkies, Little Debbies, Doritos, sugary cereals, and Oreos—a "convenience store diet," as he called it. And he not only lost the weight, but his "bad" cholesterol, or LDL, dropped 20 percent and his "good" cholesterol, or HDL, increased 20 percent.

Of course, Haub doesn't recommend this diet, but he did it to prove a point. When it comes to fat loss, calories are king.

This is nothing new in the scientific study of weight loss and energy balance. Metabolic research on human calorie expenditure stretches back nearly a century, and by now, the entire physiology is fully understood.

A fantastic review of the subject can be found in a paper published by researchers at the University of Lausanne, in case you want to dive into the (fairly complicated) details.[7]

As you also know, healthy fat loss *isn't* as simple as drastically cutting your calories and starving yourself. Eventually the muscle loss, metabolic slowdown, and other undesirable effects become too much. Finally, after you can't take the misery anymore, you'll likely go in the other direction, dramatically increasing calorie intake by bingeing and gorging on everything in sight for days or weeks, and wind up back where you began.

In fact, you can end up even worse off. This vicious cycle has been shown to result in rapid fat storage, often beyond prediet body fat levels.[8] In other words, people end up fatter than when they started dieting in the first place.

So the bottom line is this: you will need to watch your calories to effectively lose weight. You'll have to stay disciplined and forego the snacks and goodies not worked into your meal plans. You'll probably have to deal with some hunger now and then.

But, if you do it right, you can get absolutely *shredded* without losing muscle...or even while gaining muscle (yes, this can be done—more on that later).

THE SECOND LAW OF HEALTHY FAT LOSS
USE MACRONUTRIENTS PROPERLY TO OPTIMIZE YOUR BODY COMPOSITION

As I mentioned earlier, while a "calorie is a calorie" for weight-loss purposes alone, a calorie is *not* a calorie when it comes to optimizing body composition. What you eat matters very little if you're just trying to see the number go down on the scale, but it matters very much if you're trying to lose fat and *not* muscle.

If you eat too little protein while restricting calories for weight loss, you'll lose more muscle than you would if you had eaten an adequate amount.[9]

If you eat too few carbohydrates while in a calorie deficit, your training will suffer, your muscle repair will be impaired, and your hormone profile will become more catabolic.[10]

If you eat too little dietary fat, you can experience a significant drop-off in testosterone levels and other undesirable effects.[11]

As you can see, if you want your weight-loss regimen to be maximally effective, you want to restrict your calories but also eat enough protein and carbohydrate to preserve muscle mass and performance and enough dietary fat to maintain healthy hormone levels as well as general health. Adequate dietary fats are necessary to maintain healthy skin and hair, insulate body organs against shock, regulate body temperature, and promote healthy cell function.

While that sounds complicated, it's not. In fact, it's probably the simplest way of going about dieting, and you'll learn all about it later in this book.

THE THIRD LAW OF HEALTHY FAT LOSS
EAT ON A SCHEDULE THAT WORKS BEST FOR YOU

Most meal timing advice calls for eating multiple small meals per day, and the reason often given is that eating like this will speed up your metabolism and thus help you lose weight faster.

It seems to make sense at first. By putting food in our bodies every few hours, it has to constantly work to break it down, which should speed up our metabolism, right?

Well, kind of...but it doesn't help with weight loss.

You see, each type of macronutrient (protein, carbohydrate, and fat) requires varying amounts of energy to break down and process. This is known as the *thermic effect of food* and is the metabolic "boost" that comes with eating.

The magnitude and duration of that boost depends on how much you eat. A small meal causes a small metabolic spike that doesn't last long, whereas a large meal produces a larger spike that lasts longer.

So the question, then, is whether eating more smaller meals per day increases total energy expenditure over a 24-hour period than fewer larger meals?

Well, in an extensive review of literature, scientists at the French National Institute of Health and Medical Research looked at scores of studies comparing the thermic effect of food in a wide variety of eating patterns, ranging from 1 to 17 meals per day.[12]

In terms of 24-hour energy expenditure, they found no difference between nibbling and gorging. Small meals caused small, short metabolic boosts, and large meals caused larger, longer boosts. By the end of each day, they balanced out in terms of total calories burned.

We can also look to a weight-loss study conducted by researchers from the University of Ontario, which split subjects into two dietary groups: three meals per day and three meals plus three snacks per day, with both in a caloric restriction for weight loss.[13] After eight weeks, 16 participants completed the study, and researchers found no significant difference in average weight loss, fat loss, or muscle loss.

So eating more, smaller meals doesn't directly help or hinder fat loss. What about appetite? Can it help there?

A study conducted by scientists at the University of Missouri with 27 overweight/obese men found that after 12 weeks of dieting to lose weight, increasing protein intake improved appetite control, but meal frequency (three vs. six meals per day) had no effect.[14]

Researchers from the University of Kansas investigated the effects of meal frequency and protein intake on perceived appetite, satiety, and hormonal responses in overweight/obese men.[15] They found that higher protein intake led to greater feelings of fullness and that eating six meals resulted in lower daily fullness than three meals.

On the other hand, you can find studies that found participants were less satiated on three meals per day and that increasing meal frequency improved their feelings of fullness and made it easier to stick to their diets.[16]

The bottom line is that many variables are involved with the appetite, including psychological ones, and our hunger patterns are established by our regular meal patterns, so it's usually easiest to work with this, not against it.[17]

This is why clinical evidence shows that both more and fewer meals per day are effective for weight loss and have no inherent drawbacks or advantages in terms of metabolic rate and appetite control.

Let's now talk about a bogeyman that scares dieters everywhere: late-night eating.

Somehow, many people believe that eating too much food later in the day will accelerate fat storage, so they avoid it all costs, preferring to go hungry for hours on end over shifting meals around to better suit their hunger patterns.

Well, as you now know, fat loss and gain depend wholly on energy balance and have nothing to do with meal timing. This means you get to eat as late as you want. This isn't just theory, either—it's been proven in multiple scientific studies.

For example, a study conducted by researchers at the University of Chieti in Italy found that calorie intake in the morning or evening didn't affect weight loss or body composition parameters.[18]

A study performed by researchers at Vanderbilt University demonstrated interesting results: subjects who normally ate breakfast lost more weight by skipping it and eating the majority of calories at dinner, whereas subjects who normally skipped breakfast lost more weight by eating breakfast every day.[19] Researchers chalked this up to greater levels of satiety and thus better dietary compliance.

Another study on the matter, this time from researchers at the of University of São Paulo in Brazil, showed that splitting calories into five equal meals per day eaten between 9 AM and 8 PM, eating all calories in the morning, and eating all calories in the evening didn't affect weight loss parameters or body composition.[20]

I've also put this research to the test many times, both in my own meal planning and with people I help and work with, sometimes jamming large portions of our daily calories into late-night dinners, whether out of necessity or choice.

As expected, it made no difference in our results. So long as you stick to your daily numbers, your body will respond just as it should.

While we're on the subject of late eating, I recommend that you eat 30 to 40 grams of a slow-digesting protein like egg or casein (either from a powder or from a whole-food source like low-fat cottage cheese) thirty minutes before going to bed, as research has shown that this improves muscle recovery due to the increased availability of amino acids for repair while you sleep.[21]

So, the long story short is that you don't need to be a slave to a rigid meal schedule. Eat as frequently or infrequently as you like, because *when* you eat has little bearing on your ability to lose fat. Use meal timing as a tool to make your dieting as enjoyable and convenient as possible. This way, you can stick to your diet, which is what matters in the end.

Now, if you're wondering where to start—with more or fewer meals per day—I recommend that you eat several smaller meals per day (four to six meals per day works well).

In my experience coaching thousands of people, most are like me and prefer the experience of eating more small meals as opposed to fewer large ones. I personally don't like eating between 800 and 1,000 calories to then feel stuffed for several hours. I much prefer a 400-calorie meal that leaves me satisfied for a few hours, followed by another smaller meal of different food.

If you already know that you don't want to or can't eat that frequently, then don't sweat it. Do whatever will work best for you.

THE FOURTH LAW OF HEALTHY FAT LOSS
USE EXERCISE TO PRESERVE MUSCLE AND ACCELERATE FAT LOSS

You can lose weight by restricting calories without exercising, but adding exercise—both resistance and cardiovascular training—comes with some major benefits.

The addition of resistance training to a calorie deficit preserves muscle and BMR, and it provides a substantial "afterburn" effect.[22] Adding cardiovascular training burns more energy and thus more fat.[23]

In my opinion, restricting calories for weight loss without also doing some form of resistance training to preserve muscle is just a mistake. It's going to result in at least mild muscle loss, and this not only isn't good for looks, but it's bad for your health too.

Cardio is negotiable. There's nothing inherently unhealthy or bad about not including it in your weight-loss regimen, but I'll tell you this: you will only get so far with diet and resistance training alone.

If you're planning on getting below 10 percent body fat, I can pretty much guarantee that you're going to need to include some cardio in your routine to get there. Fortunately, however, you won't have to do nearly as much as most people think.

THE BOTTOM LINE

Healthy fat loss depends on these four laws and no others. Drugs and invasive surgeries aside, any and all workable weight loss methods rely on the four simple rules you just learned to achieve results.

Sure, you can get fancy and count "points" instead of calories, restrict your food choices to the point where you simply couldn't overeat if you tried, come up with all kinds of creative low-calorie recipes, use tricks to increase satiety and curb hunger, and so on, but in the end, these laws will either work for or against you and will determine whether you lose weight.

CHAPTER SUMMARY

- When you restrict your calories for fat-loss purposes, your body reduces its total fat stores to stay alive, but it also slows down its basal metabolic rate to conserve energy.

- A calorie is not a calorie when it comes to optimizing body composition. If you want your weight-loss regimen to be maximally effective, you want to eat enough protein and carbohydrate so as to preserve muscle and performance capacity and enough dietary fat so as to maintain general health.

- Increasing or decreasing meal frequency doesn't help or hinder weight loss or muscle growth. Eat on a schedule that works best for you.

- Eating at night doesn't help or hinder weight loss or muscle growth.

- Eating a slow-digesting protein like egg or casein (either from a powder or from a whole-food source like low-fat cottage cheese) 30 minutes before going to bed improves muscle recovery.

- The addition of resistance training to a calorie deficit preserves muscle and BMR, and it provides a substantial "afterburn" effect.

- The addition of cardiovascular training burns more energy and thus more fat.

SECTION II:

INNER GAME

9

THE INNER GAME OF GETTING FIT

Discipline is doing what you hate to do, but nonetheless doing it like you love it.
— MIKE TYSON

WHEN IT COMES TO GETTING FIT, there's something odd about the three-month mark. It's when I see so many people quit.

I've seen it time and time again with dozens of people: they make it to three or four months and, for one reason or another, just disappear. Some got sick and never returned. Others decided to take a week off, and it turned into a permanent break. Others were just plain lazy and started making excuses as to why they didn't care about being in shape anymore.

Most of these people had one thing in common, though: they weren't happy with their gains, and without enough visible results for their efforts, it's understandable that their motivation waned.

Fortunately for you, you're not going to have this problem. If you follow exactly what you learn in this book, you'll make incredible gains and will feel more motivated after three months than you do right now.

Before we get into the nuts and bolts of proper training and diet, however, I want you to know that there are two equally important aspects of achieving the body of your dreams. I call them the "outer" and "inner" games of getting fit.

The outer game is the physical stuff—how to train, eat, rest, and so on—and this is what most trainers, books, and magazines focus on. The inner game, however, is less discussed but equally important. If you don't have this squared away, you'll be in for a rough ride.

The inner game is, of course, the mental side of getting and staying fit, and this is what sets apart the people with great physiques from those with mediocre ones. Building a killer physique is not a matter of jumping on the bandwagon of some new fad workout program for a few months. It's a matter of adopting a disciplined, orderly approach to how you handle your body, and it's quite a lifestyle change for most.

The two biggest inner game barriers are *lack of motivation* and *lack of discipline*, and most people have to wrestle with them at some point, and usually sooner than later.

What I often see is people starting their fitness plans with tanks full of resolve, but within only a few weeks, they're already running low. That new TV show is starting during gym time… That extra hour of sleep would hit the spot… A few days off isn't a big deal… Another cheat meal shouldn't hurt too much…

Giving into these temptations sends you down a slippery slope of getting less than great results, which then leads to wondering why you're even bothering with it all, which naturally leads to quitting. I've seen it over and over and over.

Well, while it's true that some people are just more naturally disciplined than others, anyone can use the simple tricks I'm going to share in this section of the book to help get mentally prepared to win and to stay the course even when tempted to go astray.

10

HOW TO BECOME YOUR OWN MASTER THE SIMPLE SCIENCE OF WILLPOWER AND SELF-CONTROL

Would you have a great empire? Rule over yourself.
— PUBLILIUS SYRUS.

ACCORDING TO A 2010 SURVEY CONDUCTED by the American Psychological Association, the lack of willpower is the number-one obstacle people face in achieving their goals.[1] Many feel guilty about their lack of self-control, like they're letting themselves and others down, and that their lives are, in large part, not under their control. They report feeling like their actions are dictated by emotions, impulses, and cravings and that exerting self-discipline ultimately just leads to exhaustion.

And what about those with higher levels of willpower? Well, they do better in school, earn more money, make better leaders, and are happier, healthier, and less stressed.[2] They have better social and romantic relationships (they can keep their mouths shut), and they even live longer.[3] The bottom line is no matter the circumstances, more willpower trumps less.

Regardless of where we generally fall in the spectrum, we all have willpower challenges to face. Some are biological in nature—the desire to eat greasy, sugary foods that our brains recognize as vital to our survival—and others are more uniquely ours. What we find tempting someone else might find repulsive. Their addictions might be as appealing to us as airline food.

Whatever the details, the machinations are the same. Your excuse for skipping the gym… again…is remarkably similar to the foodie's justification for bingeing…for the third day in a row. How you talk yourself into putting off that important work just one more day is how someone else eases the guilt of giving in to his cravings for a cigarette.

The science is clear: the internal struggle of self-discipline is just part of being human. Why is it such a heavy burden for some people though? Why do they give up so easily on goals, and why do they blissfully indulge in so many self-sabotaging behaviors? And what can be done about it? How can they get themselves and their lives under control?

Well, these are all good questions, and while I definitely don't have all the answers, I'm going to share the research and insights that have helped me understand the nature of the beast and how to tame it.

As you'll see, the self-awareness that comes with gaining a deeper understanding of how we tick is incredibly empowering. By better understanding what makes us likely to lose control, we can skillfully manage our "willpower reserves" and avoid the pitfalls that drain them.

So let's start our little journey with a simple concept: a clear definition of what willpower really is.

I WILL, I WON'T, I WANT

What do we mean when we say someone has or lacks willpower?

We're usually referring to their ability or inability to say no. They're supposed to study for the exam but instead accept the invitation to the movies. They're trying to lose 10 pounds but just couldn't say no to that apple pie. They have trouble saying "I won't."

There are two other aspects to willpower, though: "I will" and "I want."

"I will" power is the other side of the "I won't" coin. It's the ability to do something when you don't want to, like grinding out the workout when you're tired, paying the overdue bill, or burning the midnight oil on that work project.

"I want" is the ability to remember the *why* when temptation strikes—the long-term goal and thing you really want more than the fast food or credit card purchase.

Become the master of your wont's, wills, and wants, and you become the master of your destiny. Procrastination can be licked. Your worst habits can be dismantled and replaced. Whiffs of temptation lose their power over you.

Don't expect these abilities to come easily, though. "Reprogramming" yourself to favor the harder choices is going to be uncomfortable. You might find it overwhelming at first. You're going to be drawn back to what's familiar. Stay the course, however, and the pieces will start falling into place. You'll find it easier and easier to say no to the distractions and yes to the things you need to do without getting frazzled.

So, now that we've established what willpower consists of and what the stakes are, let's move on to the physiology of desire and why it can sometimes make it so hard to resist being "bad."

YOUR BRAIN ON DOPAMINE: WHY THE IDEA OF GIVING IN FEELS SO GOOD

A real willpower challenge isn't a fleeting, "wouldn't that be nice" thought that disappears as quickly as it came. It's more like an all-consuming battle raging inside of you between good and evil, virtue and sin, and yin and yang, and you *feel* it physically.

What's going on?

Well, physiologically speaking, you're experiencing your brain when it's fixated on a promise of reward. Once you catch sight of that cheeseburger, a chemical called *dopamine* gushes through your brain. All of a sudden, all that matters in life in that greasy, delicious pile of meat, cheese, and bun. The dopamine tells your brain that you must consume that sandwich *now*, no matter the cost, or suffer the ghastly consequences.[4]

To make matters even worse, your brain is now anticipating the imminent spike in insulin and energy, so it begins to lower your blood sugar levels. This, in turn, makes you crave the burger even more.[5] And next thing you know, you're in line, anxiously waiting your turn to order one.

You see, once you become aware of an opportunity to score a reward, your brain squirts out dopamine to tell us that this indeed is the droid we're looking for. It plays up the sweet song of immediate gratification and plays down any chatter about long-term consequences.[6]

The chemical isn't engineered to make us feel happy and content, though—its role is to stimulate us to *action*, and it does this by arousing us, sharpening our focus, and revving up our drive us to do something to get our hands on the prize.[7] That's its carrot that it dangles for us. It has a stick too: when dopamine is released, it also triggers the release of stress hormones that make us feel anxious.[8] This is why the more we think about the reward we want, the more important it becomes to us. The more we think we have to get it *now*.

We don't realize, however, that the stress we feel isn't caused by *not having* the apple pie, pair of shoes, or Candy Crush trophy—it's caused by the desire itself. It's dopamine's emotional tool for making sure we obey its commands.

Your brain doesn't give a damn about the bigger picture. It cares nothing about whether you're going to be happy 30 pounds heavier or a thousand dollars poorer. Its job is to identify promises of pleasure and raise red flags, even if pursuing them will entail risky, chaotic behavior and cause more problems than they're worth.

Ironically, the ultimate rewards we're looking for can elude us every time, but the slimmest possibility of payoff and the anxiety of giving up the quest can keep us hooked, even to the point of obsession. And that's why we can find ourselves, just a few days after a guilt-inducing, catastrophic failure of willpower, anxiously chasing the dragon again: scarfing down more artery clogging fare, racking up more credit card debt, and cracking out on more Facebook gaming.

Anything we think will bring pleasure kicks this reward-seeking system into gear: the smell of the cheeseburger, the Black Friday sale, the wink from the girl, or the advertisement for the testosterone booster. Once dopamine has your brain in its grasp, obtaining the desirable object or doing the action that triggered it can become a "do-or-die" proposition.

It's no surprise, then, that eating, smelling, or even just seeing calorie- and sugar-rich foods makes us want to eat everything in sight. There was a time when an insatiable appetite was vital for survival. After fasting for several days, you've finally killed an animal, and you'd better scarf down a huge number of calories to gain the body fat needed to stay alive until the next feast. That was then, however. These days, that instinct is more a liability than a life insurance policy, but it's still there, ready to coax us into getting fatter and fatter.

The dopamine problems don't end here, either. Research shows that the dopamine release triggered by one promise of reward makes us more likely to pursue others. Look at pictures of naked women and you're more likely to make risky financial decisions.[9] Dream about striking it rich, and food can become *really* appetizing.[10]

This is especially problematic in today's modern world, which in many ways is literally engineered to keep us always wanting more. Food companies know how much salt, sugar, and fat to include in recipes to hook us, and they know that a never-ending variety of new flavors and options prevents us from becoming "desensitized" to their brands of reward. Video game makers carefully craft experiences that can elevate dopamine to amphetamine-like levels, which explains a lot of the obsessive-compulsive behavior seen in gaming.[11] Online shopping, constant sexual stimulation in all forms of media, Facebook, and even the aromas pumped into stores, hotels, restaurants, fast food joints, and ice cream parlors all scream "Here's a reward!" to your brain, which wallows in all the dopamine like a pig in—well, you know—and we feel like we have to scratch all of these itches, sooner rather than later.

When we consider how overtargeted and overstimulated our dopamine neurons really are, it's no surprise that the average person is an overweight procrastinator hooked on ice cream, video games, television shows, and social media and that it takes a rather dramatic shift in behavior to escape from these traps.

If we're to succeed in this new world, we must learn to distinguish between the false, distracting, and addicting "rewards" we're enticed with every day, everywhere we go, and the real rewards that give us true fulfillment and that bring meaning to our lives.

THE ARCHENEMY OF WILLPOWER: STRESS

Let's return to the burger shop. Remember? You're still in line, salivating over the several thousand calories of fatty, cheesy bliss that you're about to consume.

Your mind clears for a moment, however, and you remember that you're on a diet. Losing the weight matters too. You want to be fit, healthy, and happy. You swore on everything sacred you would see it through this time.

When viewed in that context, the food you're about to eat poses a sort of *threat* to you, and your brain has a protocol for dealing with threats as well: fight or flight. Stress levels rise, but there's nothing to kill or escape from because there's a catch: this isn't a real threat. The cheeseburger can't force itself down your throat and join its friends lining your belly. It needs your cooperation. In this way, *you're* the threat.

In short, we need protection from ourselves, not from the diabolical ground beef patties, and that's what self-control is for. It's for relaxing the muscles, slowing the heart rate, elongating the breaths, and buying some time to think about what we really want to do next, whereas fight or flight is for speeding us up to react as quickly as possible.

You see, research has conclusively proven that nothing undermines willpower like *stress*—and not just the stress we feel when our brains are bathed in dopamine, but the stress of everyday living.[12] The more stress we feel, the more likely we are to overeat, overspend, and do the many other things we regret shortly thereafter.

A good way to measure stress levels in your body is by looking at something called *heart rate variability*, which is how much your heartbeat speeds up and slows down as you breathe. The more stressed you are, the less variability there is in your heartbeat—the more it gets "stuck" at a faster rate.

Research shows that people who are less stressed—whose heart rate has a desirable amount of variability—display remarkably better self-control than those with less variability.[13] They're more likely to resist temptations and less likely to experience depression and give up on difficult work, and generally just deal with stressful situations better.[14]

Anything that causes stress, whether mental or physical, drains our "reserve" of willpower and reduces our capacity for self-control. Thus, as a corollary, anything we can do to reduce stress in our lives and improve mood—both acutely and chronically—improves our self-control.

Now, what do many people turn to for consolation when they're stressed? Research shows they chase "feel good chemicals," of course, through food, alcohol, video games, television, shopping, and so forth.[15] Ironically, the same people using these strategies also rate them as ineffective for reducing stress levels, and research shows that certain activities like watching TV and drinking alcohol can increase, not decrease, stress.[16] Indulging often just leads to guilt, followed by more indulging, followed by more guilt, and so it goes.

Comfort food is often used to cope with stress, as sugary fare that spikes blood sugar levels is the standard go-to when we're feeling overwhelmed. While this may give us temporary emotional reprieve, it comes with a price higher than just the calorie count. The rush of glucose and energy is soon followed by a crash, which, like stress, is a precursor to willpower failures.[17] Research shows that when blood sugar levels are low, we're more likely to give up on difficult tasks, vent our anger, stereotype others, and even refuse to donate to charity.[18]

This is one of the many reasons why it's smarter to get the majority of your daily carbohydrates from complex, slower-burning foods that keep energy levels steady. We'll talk about this more in a later chapter.

So, with comfort foods, alcohol, video games, shopping, and television off the list as a way of coping with stress, what should we do instead? Well, an effective way to recover from the stresses of the "daily grind" is to simply relax. If you want to see this in action, the next time you face a willpower challenge, deliberately slow your breathing down to about 10 to 15 seconds per breath, or four to six breaths per minute. An easy way to do this is to exhale through your mouth slowly and fully with your lips pursed as if you were blowing lightly through a straw. Research shows that simply slowing down your breathing like this increases heart rate variability and helps you better resist the effects of stress and strengthen your willpower.[19]

While that's a nifty little trick for staying strong in the face of a momentary temptation or challenge, it's important that you remember to take some time to relax every day, as research shows that this not only reduces stress hormones and increases your willpower but preserves your health as well.[20] Don't confuse "relaxation" with "indulgent and inactive," though. A bottle of wine and a *24* marathon isn't going to help you.

Instead, you want to engage in activities that elicit a specific type of physiological response: your heart rate slows, your blood pressure drops, your muscles relax, and your mind stops analyzing and planning. Everything just slows down. Research has shown that there are various ways to enter this state, such as going for a walk outside, reading, drinking a cup of tea, listening to soothing music, doing yoga, lying down and focusing on breathing and relaxing your muscles, and even gardening.[21]

Another important part of keeping stress levels low is getting adequate sleep. If you sleep too little too regularly, you'll find yourself more susceptible to stress and temptation and lacking the "energy reserve" needed to keep your good habits in play and your bad habits in check. In fact, research shows that sleep deprivation causes symptoms similar to ADHD: distractibility, forgetfulness, impulsivity, poor planning, and hyperactivity.[22] These are hardly the types of behavior conducive to good self-control.

Reducing your consumption of pessimistic, fear-mongering media can reduce stress levels as well. Research has shown that exposing yourself to a constant barrage of bad news, scare tactics, and morbid reminders of our mortality increases the likelihood of overeating, overspending, and other willpower failures.[23]

If you really want to "stress-proof" yourself and build up your willpower reserve, however, you want to start exercising. Research shows that regular exercise reduces cravings for both food and drugs, increases heart rate variability, makes us more resistant to stress and depression, and even optimizes overall brain function.[24]

The bottom line is that nothing seems to improve self-control in all aspects of our lives like exercise.[25] Its effects are immediate, and it doesn't even take a lot to reap its willpower benefits: research shows that even *five minutes* of low-intensity exercise outdoors is enough to improve your mental state.[26] If you want a willpower "quick fix," exercise is it.

So the next time you're feeling too tired or short on time to work out, remember the bigger picture—every workout you do replenishes your willpower and energy. Think of it as your "secret weapon" for staying on top of your game.

DON'T CARE HOW, I JUST WANT IT NOW

I want the works
I want the whole works
Presents and prizes and sweets and surprises
Of all shapes and sizes
And now
Don't care how
I want it now
Don't care how
I want it now

Those words were sung by Veruca in *Willy Wonka and the Chocolate Factory*, and many people sing along every day, regardless of whether they realize it.

The problem is that when we think about rewards, the longer we have to wait, the less desirable they become. Psychologists call this "delay discounting," and it explains why in the moment of having to make a decision regarding an immediate reward versus a future one, one bird—or Big Mac—in the hand can be worth an inordinately large number of other things in the bush.

Whatever we can get *right now* tends to appear decidedly more valuable than whatever we have to wait for. This is why credit card companies make so much money, why fast food joints are far more profitable than gyms, and why people make some really poor life choices.

While we're all susceptible to these types of behaviors, some people discount future rewards more than others. And the more someone engages in this behavior, the worse his self-control is and the more likely he is to behave impulsively and even have problems with addiction.[27]

What this boils down to is how much discomfort can you endure now to achieve a long-term goal? How well can you ignore immediate rewards and keep your eye on the bigger prize on the horizon?

Fortunately, regardless of how infatuated we currently are with immediate gratification, we can favorably change our discount rates by simply changing how we view the nature of today's and tomorrow's rewards.

For example, if I gave you a $200 check postdated a couple of months from now and then tried to buy it back for $100 today, would you accept the deal? Probably not. What if I gave you $100 now and tried to buy it back with the $200 postdated check? Would you make that deal? Again, probably not. Why is that? Simple: we don't want to lose something we have, even if we're going to gain something of greater value later. It's just human nature, and it's why we tend to gravitate toward choosing smaller, immediate rewards over larger, delayed ones. When you're hovering over it, a doughnut now sure feels a lot more desirable than some weight loss later.

We can use this psychological quirk to help us pursue long-term goals instead of sabotage them.

When you face a willpower challenge, if you think about the future reward first and how giving in now sacrifices progress toward or some part of it, research shows that you'll be less likely to discount the future and indulge.[28] When you face the delicious prospect of bingeing on pizza, think first about how eating it gives up progress toward your long-term goal of the ideal weight or body composition, and it'll suddenly become much less appealing.

Are you really willing to give up a week's worth of progress toward the body you've always desired for one measly binge meal?

LET'S ALL GET FAT AND JUMP OFF BRIDGES

How many times have you heard how few people exercise and eat enough fruits and vegetables, choosing to binge on TV and sugar- and fat-laden foods instead?

These types of statistics are supposed to "scare us straight," but to those addicted to reruns and junk food, the data is music to their ears. It reminds them of the comforting reality that they're not alone—that everyone else is just like them. And if everyone is doing it, how wrong can it really be?

You may not be one of those people, but don't think you're immune to the underlying psychological mechanisms. It's comforting to think that we singularly chart our own course in our lives, uninfluenced by how other people think and act, but it's simply not true. Extensive psychological and marketing research has shown that what others do—and even what we *think* they do—has a marked effect on our choices and behaviors, especially when the people we're observing are close to us.[29]

In the world of marketing, this effect is known as "social proof," and it's a well-established principle used in myriad ways to influence us to buy. When we're not sure how to think or act, we tend to look at how other people think and act and follow along, even if subconsciously. Whenever we justify behaviors as acceptable because of all the other people doing it too or because of how "normal" it is, we're appealing to social proof. We can pick up anything from temporary solutions to long-term habits this way, and both people we know and even people we see in movies can influence us.[30]

For example, having obese friends and family members dramatically increases your risk of becoming obese as well.[31] The more a student believes that other students cheat on tests, the more likely he is to cheat (even if he's wrong in his estimates),[32] and the more people believe others underreport income on their taxes, the more like they are to cheat the IRS too.[33]

Research has demonstrated the contagious nature of habits and mind-sets with many other behaviors, including drinking, smoking, using drugs, not getting enough sleep, and even feeling lonely and depressed.[34] Because these things are able to spread from person to person to person, whom we keep as company has a much larger influence on our lives that most of us think.

Even if drinking, smoking, or even binge eating isn't your thing, seeing others indulge in these activities can still influence you and encourage you to give in to your impulses as well.[35] Seeing someone overspend might subconsciously justify your overeating. Hearing about someone skipping class might make you feel okay about skipping your workout.

The silver lining, however, is that good behaviors and moods are contagious as well. If we hang around people who are generally goal-driven and happy with high levels of self-control, we too can "catch" these traits.[36] Simply *thinking* about people with high levels of self-control—self-control role models, if you will—has been shown to increase willpower.[37]

So, if you're struggling with sticking to your diet or exercise routine, you can make it easier on yourself by joining forces with someone else who is on the same path and thinking about how others have successfully dealt with these issues. You don't even have to physically make the journey together; regular e-mail check-ins can be enough to feed, and feed on, each other's success.

It may also be wise to limit your exposure to instances of people failing your willpower challenges—overeating and poo-pooing exercise, for example—as merely seeing others giving in can pique your appetite and help you find reasons to skip a workout too.

That said, seeing others lose control doesn't *have* to weaken your resolve. In fact, it can strengthen it if you're mentally prepared to view such displays of self-indulgence as threats to your long-term goals, not tempting invitations.[38]

You can "vaccinate" yourself against these threats by simply spending a few minutes every day reviewing your goals and how you might be tempted to go astray. Imagine how the situation will play out. How will you be enticed? What specific actions or willpower strategies will you use to escape the trap? What will it feel like to succeed and stay strong? Research shows that reflecting on these things will strengthen your will and help you turn away from immediate gratification when necessary.[39]

USING THE "GOOD" TO JUSTIFY THE "BAD"

Have you ever told yourself that you were "good" when you did what you needed to do or didn't give in to temptation but "bad" when you procrastinated or lost a battle with your impulses?

Have you ever used "good" behavior as permission to be "bad?"

Chances are you answered yes and yes, and that's fine. You have firsthand experience with the trap that psychologists call *moral licensing*, which is an insidious destroyer of willpower.

You see, when we assign moral values to our actions, they become fodder for our desire to simply feel good (enough) about ourselves, even when we are sabotaging our long-term goals or harming others. By being "good," we reckon, we "earn" the "right" to be a little (or a lot) "bad." For example, if you do your workout, stick to your diet for a day, and pat yourself on the back for how "good" you were, you might find yourself overeating tomorrow but feeling virtuous, guilt-free, and in control.

Interestingly, "good" behaviors that people use to justify the "bad" don't even have to be related. Shoppers who pass up something desired are more likely to feel justified in indulging in tempting food.[40] When reminded of their virtue, people donate less to charity.[41] Hell, research shows that when people merely *think* about doing something good, it increases the likelihood of immoral or indulgent behavior.[42] And in an even stranger feat of mental acrobatics, when some people imagine what they *could* have done but didn't, they feel virtuous. They *could have* eaten the entire cheesecake but only had one slice. They *could* have skipped four workouts but only skipped three. They *could have* bought the $2,000 suit but opted for the $700 one instead.

Just to illustrate how absurd moral licensing can get, can you figure out why, after adding healthier items to its menus, McDonald's began selling more Big Macs than ever? Yup—the mere *opportunity* to eat healthily subtly gave people some of the satisfaction of actually doing it, which in turn permitted them to choose the immediate gratification of a cheeseburger.[43]

As you can see, once we go searching for moral permission to stray from our goals, it's not hard to drum up some virtue so we can get the green light. For some people, ordering a healthy main dish leads to higher-calorie beverages, sides, and desserts.[44] People who buy chocolate and donate it to charity are likely to "reward" their benevolence with some chocolate of their own.[45] Organic Oreos are perceived to be lower in calories and more suitable for daily consumption than regular Oreos.[46]

The great irony of all of this is that, in the end, all of these "licensed" bad behaviors simply prevent people from achieving what really matters—a fit body, a long life, a balanced budget, a completed project shipped out the door, and so forth. They're tricking themselves into believing that squandering their health, finances, time, opportunities, and relationships are "treats"—that self-sabotage is a reward to be cherished. Who are these people kidding? Only themselves.

The moral of this section is that we simply can't trust our feelings to guide our actions. If we wander through life chasing "good feelings," we'll figure out plenty of ways to not feel bad about every "little" bout of procrastination, overeating, overspending, and what have you, and, one day we'll wonder why the hell we're so fat, broke, lazy, and ignorant.

Escaping from this trap requires that we first stop moralizing our behaviors—that we stop using vague feelings of "right" and "wrong" and "good" and "bad" to guide our immediate actions. Instead, we need to remember *why* we've committed to doing the "hard" things like exercising, following a budget, working overtime, and so on.

In terms of diet and exercise, you need to look at both of these things as independent steps necessary to achieving the body you desire, not as "good" behaviors that you can "cash in" for indulgences. Successfully sticking to your workout routine doesn't "buy" the right to cheat on your diet.

Remember that the goal isn't a good workout or day of proper eating: it's a radically transformed physique. There are bigger reasons why you're doing all of this, including fitness, health, happiness, confidence, and all the rest. And doing things like bingeing on pizza and skipping workouts aren't little "oopsies" that you can erase with justifications. They're *threats* to those overarching goals.

Whenever you're struggling with a willpower challenge, review your whys. What will you get in the end by staying strong? What's the big payoff? Who else will benefit from it? What will your life be like when these things are a reality? Are you willing to delay gratification to get there? To experience some discomfort in the present to have that future?

"OH WHAT THE HELL, I'M A LAZY IDIOT ANYWAY!"

What do people tend to do after a minor lapse in a willpower challenge like following a diet? Do they cut their losses, get back on track, and move on? Or do they figure what the hell, the whole gig is blown, and just go all-in on the buffet?

Unfortunately, the latter is far more common. For many, the vicious cycle of indulge, regret, and seriously indulge—called the "what-the-hell effect" by psychologists—feels inevitable and inescapable.[47] The handful of chips becomes the whole bag. The two little bites of chocolate are followed by a lot more. The glass of wine is the prelude to the bottle…or two.

Whenever people confront a setback and say to themselves, "I've already messed it up, so what the hell, I might as well have some fun," they've committed themselves to the downward spiral of the what-the-hell effect. They give in and feel bad. Then, to feel better, they turn to what started the whole mess, which in turn triggers even worse feelings of shame and guilt, which leads to even bigger failures, and on and on it goes.

Well, you're going to make some mistakes along the way. You're going to eat too much at the party or skip a workout that you could have made. As good as I am about keeping all my plates spinning, I slip up sometimes too. There's nothing wrong with us—we're just human like everyone else. What we do next is what really matters.

What we definitely *don't* want to do is get really down on ourselves when we do mess up. Launching into a tirade of self-criticism will only increase feelings of guilt and shame, which will increase the likelihood of us turning to whatever will make us feel good (back to the cookie jar we go).[48] The tougher, stricter, and more abusive we get with ourselves, the worse we are in the end.

Instead, we should show ourselves the same compassion and forgiveness that we would show a friend. This probably sounds counterintuitive to you. Wouldn't this likely excuse us to continue the unwanted behavior? Research says no—several studies show that being kind to oneself in times of stress and failure is associated with better willpower and self-control.[49] Self-compassion helps us accept responsibility for our actions and move forward, having learned a lesson.

Pride is another effective weapon that we can use to overcome our willpower challenges. Research shows that imagining how proud you will be once you've accomplished your goals, who you'll tell, and what their reactions will be can increase your willpower and make you more likely to do what it takes to make those goals a reality.[50] Anticipating the shame and disapproval from others that comes with failure can also help you stay strong in the face of temptation, but it isn't as powerful in this regard as pride.[51]

THE CRYSTAL BALL OF DELUSION

One of our favorite ways to abandon our self-control is to justify our sins of the present with planned virtues of the future. For example, research shows that simply planning on exercising later can increase the likelihood of cheating on a diet.[52]

This type of thinking not only reeks of moral licensing, but it also introduces another critical flaw into the mix: the assumption that we'll somehow make different decisions in the future than we do today. Today I will eat twice the dessert, but tomorrow I will stick to my diet. Today I will skip my workout, but tomorrow I'll double up. Today I will binge on my favorite TV shows, but I won't watch anymore for the rest of the week.

We simply give our future selves too much credit, counting on them to be able to do whatever we can't bring ourselves to do now. We're too quick to assume that we'll be more enthusiastic, energetic, willful, diligent, motivated, brave, morally strong…insert virtues ad nauseam…in a couple of days, weeks, or months.

Such optimism would be okay if we knew we could actually follow through on it all. But we both know that's not how it goes. When the future finally arrives, that noble, idealized version of ourselves is nowhere to be found, and the demands we face aren't nearly as easy as we told ourselves they would be. What to do, then? Put it all off again, of course, hoping that our savior will rescue us next time.

This type of thinking simply burdens our future selves with an impossible load of tasks and responsibilities.

As you make your way on the *Bigger Leaner Stronger* program, be on the lookout for the lure of future virtue justifying today's vice. Avoid the trap of viewing Future You as some abstract entity whose emotions and desires will be different than Present You's. Realize that, when tomorrow comes, the chances of actually following through on what you didn't do earlier are slim. More often than not, you're going to find yourself in the exact same state of mind as previously, and you're going to sell yourself a little further down the river.

As you get better at this, you'll be improving what scientists call your "future self-continuity," which is your ability to connect future consequences with present actions.[53] High future-self continuity will not only help you get into shape, but it will also improve many other areas of your life as well.

You can also use a couple of mental exercises to build your future self-continuity. Research shows that just thinking about the future—not even the rewards, per se—can strengthen willpower. Thus, by imagining the future, doing what you need to do or refraining from doing what you shouldn't do, you can increase the likelihood of your following through.[54] For example, if you're struggling with starting a diet, just imagining shopping and eating differently is enough to make it more "real" and appealing.

Another exercise is writing a letter to your Future Self about what you think he'll be like, what your hopes for him are, what you're doing for him now that will pay off later, what he might say about your Present Self, and even what the consequences of your present willpower failures will turn into down the line. FutureMe.org offers a cool little tool for this that allows you to write an e-mail to yourself and choose a future date on which it will be delivered.

The final exercise is similar to the others and entails imagining your Future Self in vivid detail, which has been shown to increase self-control.[55] Explore the consequences of current behaviors, good and bad. What will your Future Self look like if you don't commit to changing your ways? What are the likely physical, mental, and emotional consequences? Disease, regret, shame, ugliness, depression, and loneliness? Don't hold back. And what if you do change? How will your life look then? How will you look and feel? Will you be proud and thankful? Again, explore the possibilities.

DON'T FIGHT THE URGE—RIDE THE WAVE

You've just sat down on the couch after a long, tiring day, and your mind begins to wander. Suddenly, a pint of ice cream materializes, and your taste buds snap to attention. No, you think, anything but ice cream. Do *not* think of ice cream!

The commands don't work, though. The harder you try to banish the visions of creamy, fluffy clouds of delight, the more the thought dominates your consciousness and salivary glands. Finally, the only way to make it stop is to spoon the stuff down your gullet.

Ironically, however, the experience rarely lives up to the expectations.

The problem with this scenario isn't the spark of imagination that started it but rather the forceful attempt at suppressing it. Research shows that a willingness to think thoughts and feel feelings without having to act on them is an effective method of dealing with a wide variety of challenges, such as mood disorders, food cravings, and addiction.[56] On the other hand, trying to suppress negative thoughts and feelings, like self-criticism, worries, sadness, or cravings, can lead to greater feelings of inadequacy, anxiety, depression, and even overeating.[57]

So, when you have disturbing thoughts, face them calmly instead of trying to sweep them under the mental rug. You don't have to *believe* them or contemplate their meaning; you just have to accept that they're there and be aware of them. Don't read into them—just play them down. They're not that important and will fade.

This is particularly relevant to dieting, as research shows that thought suppression is very poor dietary strategy. The more you suppress thoughts about food, the more likely you are to struggle with cravings and binge eating.[58] When cravings hit, instead of trying to distract or argue with yourself, notice and accept the feelings. Realize that while you may not always be able to control where your mind wanders, you can *always* control your actions. And before you act on the desires, remember your goal and why you committed to abstaining in the first place. Ride out the wave of desire until it finally crashes and dissolves.

Researchers from the University of Washington called this "surfing the urge" and found that it helped smokers cut back on daily cigarette smoking.[59] It helped them learn how to handle their feelings internally instead of turning to something external for support.

A simple rule of thumb for putting this into use is to wait 10 minutes before acting on a craving or other impulsive urge to do something you know you shouldn't. This not only gives you time to pause and reflect on the matter, but it also takes away the power of immediate gratification and future discounting. By pushing the reward just 10 minutes into the future, you can take away its most effective weapon against your willpower.

If you're facing an "I will" challenge—if you're dreading something you know you need to do—then commit to do it for 10 minutes and *then* decide whether to continue. Chances are, you'll find that once you're in motion, you'll want to keep going.

WHEN THE GOING GETS TOUGH, THE TOUGH GET GOING

It's six o'clock, and you've just finished your work for the day. You're feeling drained. Fires were fought, meetings endured, and bosses placated. You're shuffling toward your car, and a sense of dread washes over you as you realize you're supposed to head to the gym now to train legs. Ugh.

Before you know it, your mind is racing with reasons to just go home. It'll be a terrible workout anyway. The gym is really full on Mondays. You can make it up next week. You don't skip as much as your friends. The onslaught quickly breaks through your weakened defenses, and you're on to the next decision: order pizza for dinner or cook a healthy meal? If you order now, you could pick it up on the way home…

This experience is all too familiar for many people. They use anything they can—tiredness, soreness, fatigue, or depression—as excuses to skip workouts, cheat on diets, lash out at loved ones, and put off work that's long overdue. Being "exhausted" is just an easy way for them to feel okay about their failures.

Well, just as elite athletes are able to push themselves far beyond the first feelings of physical fatigue—the point where "normal" people give up, figuring they've reached their limits—we too must learn to push past the barrier of mental and emotional fatigue that can convince us to stray from our routines and goals.

This isn't as hard as it might sound, either. Research shows that people who simply don't believe that using self-control results in mental fatigue or a weakening of the "willpower muscle" don't experience the same gradual deterioration in the strength of their willpower seen in those who do.[60]

So, in a very real sense, you're as tough as you think you are, and you can exert as much self-control as you think you can. The next time you feel "too tired" to say "I will" or "I won't," toughen up and push past it. Challenge yourself to go beyond that point, into discomfort, and you'll likely find you can without consequences.

USE IT OR LOSE IT—HOW TO TRAIN YOUR WILLPOWER

Modern life bombards us with willpower challenges that require us to call on our self-control mechanisms to successfully avoid distractions and do the things we need to do and not do what we shouldn't.

The problem with this is research shows that we can, at some point, "run out" of self-control juice, leaving us susceptible to temptation.[61] Scientists have observed that, regardless of the types of tasks performed, people's self-control is at its highest in the morning and that it steadily declines as the day wears on.[62] Resisting sweets, fighting emotional impulses, keeping distractions at bay, compelling yourself to do difficult tasks, or even making trivial purchase decisions all seem to pull from the same willpower reserve.[63]

These findings have given rise to the "willpower as a muscle" metaphor: it only has so much strength, and every time you "flex" it, it becomes a little bit weaker. The positive side of the metaphor, however, is that you can train your "willpower muscle" like a physical one and make it stronger and more resistant to fatigue.

Research backs this up too. We can increase our overall willpower by performing regular, small acts of self-control like eating fewer sweets, tracking spending, correcting our posture, refraining from swearing, squeezing a handgrip every day, and using our nondominant hand for various tasks.[64]

What we're really training when we do these "trivial" things is what psychologists call the "pause-and-plan response," which involves pausing before we act, noticing what we're about to do, and choosing differently instead.[65]

We can use this research to build our own "willpower workouts" that train our self-control. For example, you can build your "I won't" power by refraining from slouching when you sit, committing to not eating a junk food indulgence every day, or not swearing. You can build your "I will" power by committing to some new daily habit like doing five minutes of breathing exercises, going for a walk outside, doing 20 push-ups after waking up, finding something that needs cleaning in your house and cleaning it, or tracking something in your life that you don't usually pay attention to, such as how many calories you take in and expend daily, how much coffee you drink, or how much time you spend surfing the Internet.

You might be surprised by how far these "little" self-control exercises can go in increasing your ability to make bigger changes in your life, such as adopting a new, healthier lifestyle.

Another highly effective way to train your willpower is to use a strategy called "precommitment," which entails taking action now to strengthen your position and commitment to a behavior and ward off any underhanded attempts at sabotage from Future You.[66] For many people, the best way to beat temptation is to simply avoid facing it in the first place.

For example, if you have trouble with procrastinating on the Internet instead of working, you can download a program called *Freedom* (www.macfreedom.com) that turns off your Internet for a set period of time. *Anti-Social* (www.anti-social.cc) blocks social networks and e-mail. If sticking to a diet is your struggle, you could precommit by throwing out every bit of tempting junk food in the house and not buying it again, bringing a healthy lunch to work every day that you've prepared, or joining a "Diet Bet" at www.dietbetter.com. If you want to ensure you do your workouts, you could pay for an annual membership at your gym instead of going month to month.

Another good tool for precommitment is the website Stickk (www.stickk.com), which was created by Yale economist Ian Aryes. The site allows you to set a goal and time frame, put money on the line, decide what happens with the money if you fail (it goes to charity, for example, or even to an organization you *don't* like, which can be a stronger incentive), designate a "referee" who will monitor your progress and confirm the truthfulness of your reports, and invite supporters to cheer you on.

In short, anything you can do to show that you mean business and to make it difficult and uncomfortable to change your mind and give up is going to help you keep your impulses and feelings at bay and thus keep you on course.

NOTHING FAILS LIKE SUCCESS

Once we've decided on a goal, what do we crave most? *Progress*, of course. We want to see positive change and forward movement to give us the energy to push even harder. But that's not how it necessarily goes.

It turns out that progress comes with a risk: complacency. Research has shown that some people use progress toward a goal as an excuse to let off the gas and indulge in some self-sabotage.[67]

When we make progress, we can be lulled by feelings of accomplishment and entitlement. As with moral licensing, we can feel that our one step forward has earned us the privilege of taking two steps back.

Instead of patting ourselves on the back and pondering all the progress we've made, which increases the likelihood that we will act contrary to it, we should view our successes as evidence of how important our goals are to us, or of how *committed* we are to seeing the process through to the end.[68]

That is, we should look for a reason to keep going, not to slow down and take in the scenery.

THE BOTTOM LINE

Human nature is full of paradoxes, and the subject of self-control is no exception. We're drawn to both delayed and immediate gratification in the forms of long-term goals and temporary jolts of pleasure. We're inherently susceptible to temptation but have the power to resist. We're constantly juggling feelings of stress, anxiety, fear, and sadness intermingled with calm, hopefulness, and excitement.

While I don't think we can fundamentally change ourselves through the strengthening of our willpower, we can certainly improve our ability to meet the demands of daily living with more mindfulness, effectiveness, and confidence.

CHAPTER SUMMARY

INTRODUCTION

- Those with higher levels of willpower? Well, they do better in school, earn more money, make better leaders, and are happier, healthier, and less stressed. They have better social and romantic relationships (they can keep their mouths shut), and they even live longer.

- Your excuse for skipping the gym…again…is remarkably similar to the foodie's justification for bingeing…for the third day in a row. How you talk yourself into putting off that important work just one more day is how someone else eases the guilt of giving in to his cravings for a cigarette.

I WILL, I WON'T, I WANT

- Most people think of willpower as the ability to say "I won't," but there are two other aspects to it as well.

- "I will" power is the other side of the "I won't" coin. It's the ability to do something when you don't want to, like grinding out the workout when you're tired, paying the overdue bill, or burning the midnight oil on that work project.

- "I want" is the ability to remember the why when temptation strikes—the long-term goal and thing you really want more than the fast food or credit card purchase.

YOUR BRAIN ON DOPAMINE: WHY THE IDEA OF GIVING IN FEELS SO GOOD

- Once you become aware of an opportunity to score a reward, your brain squirts out dopamine to tell us that this indeed is the droid we're looking for. It plays up the sweet song of immediate gratification and plays down any chatter about long-term consequences.

- When dopamine is released, it also triggers the release of stress hormones that make us feel anxious. This is why the more we think about the reward we want, the more important it becomes to us. The more we think we have to get it *now*.

- Ironically, the ultimate rewards we're looking for can elude us every time, but the slimmest possibility of payoff and the anxiety of giving up the quest can keep us hooked, even to the point of obsession.

- Research shows that the dopamine release triggered by one promise of reward makes us more likely to pursue others. Look at pictures of naked women and you're more likely to make risky financial decisions. Dream about striking it rich, and food can become *really* appetizing.

- If we're to succeed in this new world, we must learn to distinguish between the false, distracting, and addicting "rewards" we're enticed with every day, everywhere we go, and the real rewards that give us true fulfillment and that bring meaning to our lives.

THE ARCHENEMY OF WILLPOWER: STRESS

- Self-control is for relaxing the muscles, slowing the heart rate, elongating the breaths, and buying some time to think about what we really want to do next, whereas fight or flight is for speeding us up to react as quickly as possible.

- Research has conclusively proven that nothing undermines willpower like *stress*— and not just the stress we feel when our brains are bathed in dopamine, but the stress of everyday living. The more stress we feel, the more likely we are to overeat, overspend, and do the many other things we regret shortly thereafter.

- Anything that causes stress, whether mental or physical, drains our "reserve" of willpower and reduces our capacity for self-control. Thus, as a corollary, anything we can do to reduce stress in our lives and improve mood—both acutely and chronically—improves our self-control.

- An effective way to recover from the stresses of the "daily grind" is to simply relax. If you want to see this in action, the next time you face a willpower challenge, deliberately slow your breathing down to about 10 to 15 seconds per breath, or four to six breaths per minute.

- Research has shown that there are various ways to enter this state of relaxation, such as going for a walk outside, reading, drinking a cup of tea, listening to soothing music, doing yoga, lying down and focusing on breathing and relaxing your muscles, and even gardening.

- If you sleep too little too regularly, you'll find yourself more susceptible to stress and temptation and lacking the "energy reserve" needed to keep your good habits in play and your bad habits in check.

- Research has shown that exposing yourself to a constant barrage of bad news, scare tactics, and morbid reminders of our mortality increases the likelihood of overeating, overspending, and other willpower failures.

- Research shows that regular exercise reduces cravings for both food and drugs, increases heart rate variability, makes us more resistant to stress and depression, and even optimizes overall brain function.

I DON'T CARE HOW, I WANT IT NOW

- When we think about rewards, the longer we have to wait, the less desirable they become. Psychologists call this "delay discounting," and the more someone engages in this behavior, the worse his self-control is and the more likely he is to behave impulsively and even have problems with addiction.

- When you face a willpower challenge, if you think about the future reward first and how giving in now sacrifices progress toward or some part of it, research shows that you'll be less likely to discount the future and indulge.

LET'S ALL GET FAT AND JUMP OFF BRIDGES

- Extensive psychological and marketing research has shown that what others do— and even what we *think* they do—has a marked effect on our choices and behaviors, especially when the people we're observing are close to us.

- When we're not sure how to think or act, we tend to look at how other people think and act and follow along, even if subconsciously. We can pick up anything from temporary solutions to long-term habits this way, and both people we know and even people we see in movies can influence us.

- Research has demonstrated the contagious nature of habits and mind-sets with many other behaviors, including drinking, smoking, using drugs, not getting enough sleep, and even feeling lonely and depressed.

- Good behaviors and moods are contagious as well. If we hang around or even *think about* people who are generally goal-driven and happy with high levels of self-control, we too can "catch" these traits.

- If you're struggling with sticking to your diet or exercise routine, you can make it easier on yourself by joining forces with someone else who is on the same path and thinking about how others have successfully dealt with these issues.

- Research shows that reflecting on your goals and how you might be tempted to go astray will strengthen your will and help you turn away from immediate gratification when necessary.

USING THE "GOOD" TO JUSTIFY THE "BAD"

- You see, when we assign moral values to our actions, they become fodder for our desire to simply feel good (enough) about ourselves, even when we are sabotaging our long-term goals or harming others. By being "good," we reckon, we "earn" the "right" to be a little (or a lot) "bad."

- If we wander through life chasing "good feelings," we'll figure out plenty of ways to not feel bad about every "little" bout of procrastination, overeating, overspending, and what have you, and, one day we'll wonder why the hell we're so fat, broke, lazy, and ignorant.

- Escaping from this trap requires that we first stop moralizing our behaviors— that we stop using vague feelings of "right" and "wrong" and "good" and "bad" to guide our immediate actions. Instead, we need to remember *why* we've committed to doing the "hard" things like exercising, following a budget, working overtime, and so on.

- Whenever you're struggling with a willpower challenge, review your whys.

"OH WHAT THE HELL, I'M A LAZY IDIOT ANWAY!"

- Whenever people confront a setback and say to themselves, "I've already messed it up, so what the hell, I might as well have some fun," they've committed themselves to the downward spiral of the what-the-hell effect.

- What we definitely *don't* want to do is get really down on ourselves when we do mess up. The tougher, stricter, and more abusive we get with ourselves, the worse we are in the end.

- Instead, we should show ourselves the same compassion and forgiveness that we would show a friend. Several studies show that being kind to oneself in times of stress and failure is associated with better willpower and self-control.

- Research shows that imagining how proud you will be once you've accomplished your goals, who you'll tell, and what their reactions will be can increase your willpower and make you more likely to do what it takes to make those goals a reality.

- Anticipating the shame and disapproval from others that comes with failure can also help you stay strong in the face of temptation, but it isn't as powerful in this regard as pride.

THE CRYSTAL BALL OF DELUSION

- One of our favorite ways to abandon our self-control is to justify our sins of the present with planned virtues of the future.

- We're too quick to assume that we'll be more enthusiastic, energetic, willful, diligent, motivated, brave, morally strong…insert virtues ad nauseam…in a couple of days, weeks, or months.

- Research shows that just thinking about the future—not even the rewards, per se—can strengthen willpower. For example, if you're struggling with starting a diet, just imagining shopping and eating differently is enough to make it more "real" and appealing.

- Another exercise is writing a letter to your Future Self about what you think he'll be like, what your hopes for him are, what you're doing for him now that will pay off later, what he might say about your Present Self, and even what the consequences of your present willpower failures will turn into down the line.

- The final exercise is similar to the others and entails imagining your Future Self in vivid detail, which has been shown to increase self-control.

DON'T FIGHT THE URGE—RIDE THE WAVE

- Research shows that a willingness to think thoughts and feel feelings without having to act on them is an effective method of dealing with a wide variety of challenges, such as mood disorders, food cravings, and addiction.

- Trying to suppress negative thoughts and feelings, like self-criticism, worries, sadness, or cravings, can lead to greater feelings of inadequacy, anxiety, depression, and even overeating.

- When cravings hit, instead of trying to distract or argue with yourself, notice and accept the feelings. Realize that while you may not always be able to control where your mind wanders, you can *always* control your actions.

- A simple rule of thumb for putting this into use is to wait 10 minutes before acting on a craving or other impulsive urge to do something you know you shouldn't.

WHEN THE GOING GETS TOUGH, THE TOUGH GET GOING

- Research shows that people who simply don't believe that using self-control results in mental fatigue or a weakening of the "willpower muscle" don't experience the same gradual deterioration in the strength of their willpower seen in those who do.

- The next time you feel "too tired" to say "I will" or "I won't," toughen up and push past it. Challenge yourself to go beyond that point, into discomfort, and you'll likely find you can without consequences.

USE IT OR LOSE IT—HOW TO TRAIN YOUR WILLPOWER

- Research shows that we can, at some point, "run out" of self-control juice, leaving us susceptible to temptation. Resisting sweets, fighting emotional impulses, keeping distractions at bay, compelling yourself to do difficult tasks, or even making trivial purchase decisions all seem to pull from the same willpower reserve.

- We can increase our overall willpower by performing regular, small acts of self-control like eating fewer sweets, tracking spending, correcting our posture, refraining from swearing, squeezing a handgrip every day, and using our nondominant hand for various tasks.

- Another highly effective way to train your willpower is to use a strategy called "precommitment," which entails taking action now to strengthen your position and commitment to a behavior and ward off any underhanded attempts at sabotage from Future You.

NOTHING FAILS LIKE SUCCESS

- Research has shown that some people use progress toward a goal as an excuse to let off the gas and indulge in some self-sabotage.

- Instead of patting ourselves on the back and pondering all the progress we've made, which increases the likelihood that we will act contrary to it, we should view our successes as evidence of how important our goals are to us, or of how *committed* we are to seeing the process through to the end.

11

THE SIMPLE WAY TO SET HEALTH AND FITNESS GOALS THAT WILL MOTIVATE YOU

I'm not the kind of guy who tries to run between the drops. Sometimes you gotta get a little wet to reach your destination.
— ERIK FRANKHOUSER

NOW THAT YOU'VE GOTTEN A CRASH course on willpower and self-control and what it really takes to commit to a long-term change, let's take a few minutes to set up a powerful set of goals that will serve as "why reminders" when temptations strike.

People with vague, unrealistic, or uninspiring health or fitness goals (or none at all) are always the first to quit. They're easy to spot too. They show up randomly and seem to sleepwalk through their workouts, wandering from machine to machine, monotonously going through the motions without even breaking a sweat.

Week after week, they complain about how hard it is to gain or lose weight, and they get nowhere. Months can go by without a single noticeable change, if they make it that long.

Well, let me assure you that people who have the type of body that you aspire to have specific, realistic health and fitness goals and are driven by them, progressing slowly but surely every day. When they meet one goal, they set another goal to stay motivated. This is what we're going to work out for you in this chapter.

Now, different people have different reasons for training. Some just like the game of pushing their bodies past their limits. Others want to look good to impress the opposite (or same) sex. Others still want to increase their self-confidence or improve their overall health and just feel good.

All of these things are good reasons to be fit. Sure, I could give you a nice list of benefits of being in great shape, such as looking great, feeling great, having high energy levels, living longer, being resistant to sickness and disease, and so on, but the important thing is that you work out specifically what fires *you* up about it.

We might as well start with what people usually consider more important: the visual. There's nothing to be ashamed of here. Every person I know who has built an awesome physique was motivated by the looks they wanted as much as anything else, if not more.

Of course, there are the over-the-top narcissists who chase "aesthetics" with little regard for their health, and this often leads to drug use and other harmful habits, but there's nothing wrong with a bit of vanity. Let's face it: looking awesome just makes you feel good.

I value my health highly and am not solely driven by how I look in the mirror, but I would be lying if I said I don't care as much about looks as I do the many other benefits of regular exercise. I want to smile when I look in the mirror like everyone else.

That's me, though. Let's take a deeper look at what is going to drive *you*.

WHAT DOES YOUR IDEAL BODY LOOK LIKE?

The first step in establishing your goals is to determine what your ideal body looks like—not just in your head, but in reality. You need to find pictures of exactly what you want to look like and save them for motivation.

It might seem silly for you to search on the Internet for pictures of jacked guys, but it's important that you have an exact visual image of how you want your body to look. Throwing around words like "ripped" and "six pack" to describe your goal isn't nearly as motivating as looking at pictures of real bodies that you're working toward.

Unless your goal is to look like a top-tier physique competitor or a hulking, professional bodybuilder, which requires an absurd amount of drug use to achieve, this book is going to give you everything you need to get there.

But I doubt that's your goal. Most guys just want to be muscular and lean, and *everyone* can accomplish that by dedicating themselves to it and following the right game plan.

A good place to look for ideal body shots is BodyBuilding.com's BodySpace. I'm also building a little collection of my inspiration on Pinterest, which you can find at http://www.pinterest.com/mikebls.

So, take a break and go find some pictures of how you want to look!

WHAT WOULD YOUR IDEAL STATE OF HEALTH BE LIKE?

Now that you've worked out what you want to look like, let's take a look at the health aspect.

Even if looking a certain way is your primary motivation for working out, you'll soon learn that the health benefits are just as motivating. You're going to feel better physically, you're going to have higher energy levels, you're going to get stronger, you're going to be more mentally alert, you're going to have a stronger sex drive, and more. In short, your entire life might just change.

Thus, I recommend that you also work out a health goal that you find motivating. Mine is along these lines: to have a vital, energetic, strong, and disease-free body that lives long and allows me to stay active and enjoy my life to the fullest.

For me, that's just as motivating as looking great. I want to live a long, productive life, feel good, watch my kids grow up, and never suffer from debilitating diseases.

I'm sure your health interests are along the same lines, but feel free to work out your individual goals in whatever words best communicate to you and write them down.

WHY DO YOU WANT TO ACHIEVE THESE GOALS?

All right, now that you've worked out what you want to look like and what level of health you want, the next question is *why*.

What are the reasons for achieving those goals? This is completely personal, so write whatever is most motivating to you.

Why do you want to achieve your ideal body? Maybe you want to boost your confidence? Play sports better? Get better at physically taxing hobbies of yours? Get more attention from girls or guys? Feel the satisfaction of overcoming physical barriers? Participate in physical activities with your kids? Hell, beat your friends in arm-wrestling matches?

Whatever your reasons, just write them all down.

And why do you want to achieve your health goal? Does a certain disease run in your family and you want to make sure you never suffer from it? Do you want to be able to stay active well into your retirement years? Slow down the processes of aging and retain a youthful vitality? Just have a body that works the way it's supposed to?

Again, give this some thought and write everything down.

You know you've got it right when you feel pumped up—when you want to get into action and start making these things a reality.

Keep your write-up in a safe place and refer back to it regularly. It's a great way to stay excited and on track.

THE BOTTOM LINE

By doing these three simple steps, you'll have created a powerful "motivation sheet" that will always point you in the right direction.

When you feel tired and are dreading the gym, you can just look at that sheet, and you'll probably change your mind. When you're out with friends, watching them stuff themselves silly while you're eating a moderate, well-balanced meal, you'll know exactly why you're doing it.

This is the simple yet powerful formula that I've used to keep myself continually motivated to train and diet for years. My goals have changed over time, but I've always ensured that I knew where I was going and why. Chances are you will greatly benefit by doing the same.

CHAPTER SUMMARY

- Building a killer physique is not a matter of jumping on the bandwagon of some new fad workout program for a few months—it's a matter of adopting a disciplined, orderly approach to how you handle your body.

- Anyone who has the type of body that you aspire to has specific, realistic health and fitness goals and is driven by them, progressing slowly but surely every day.

- The first step of establishing your goals is to determine what your ideal body would look like. Find pictures of exactly what you want to look like and save them for future reference.

- Work out a health goal that you find motivating as well.

- What are the reasons for achieving those goals? You know you've got it right when you feel pumped up—when you want to get into action and start making these things a reality.

- Keep your write-up in a safe place and refer back to it regularly. It's a great way to stay excited and on track.

SECTION III:

NUTRITION & DIET

12

GOING BEYOND "CLEAN EATING" THE DEFINITIVE GUIDE TO EFFECTIVE NUTRITION

There's more to life than training, but training is what puts more in your life.
— BROOKS KUBIK I WON'T BOTHER REPEATING a cliché about how important nutrition is when it comes to building muscle and losing fat.

Some people say it's 70 percent of the game, while others say it's 80 or even 90 percent. Well, I say it's 100 percent. And lifting heavy, overloading your muscles…that's also 100 percent of the game. Being properly hydrated is also 100 percent. Having the right attitude is 100 percent too. (Yeah, we're at 400 percent so far…)

My point is this: the building blocks of a great body are more like pillars than puzzle pieces. Weaken one enough, and the whole structure collapses.

You can't build any appreciable amount of muscle if you don't train correctly. Your muscles won't grow if you don't give your body proper nutritional support. Performance and thus muscle growth is stunted by dehydration. Your gains will be lackluster if you don't train with the right attitude.

That's why I want you to have an "all or nothing" attitude about achieving your fitness goals. I want you to be 100 percent about each aspect of the *Bigger Leaner Stronger* program and achieve 100 percent of the potential results. Let the weak and undisciplined give only 60 percent in their training, 30 percent in their diet, or 40 percent in their attitude. They're going to make you look like a god.

So, then, let's now talk about this vital—and confusing for many—pillar of muscle growth… *nutrition.*

Your diet either works for or against you, multiplying or dividing your training results. Think of the nutritional aspect of the game as a series of tollbooths along the highway of muscle growth. If you don't stop and pay each one, you don't get to go any further. It's that simple.

Contrary to what you're constantly told in the magazines, there's a lot more to proper nutrition than slamming down buckets of protein powder every week and loading up on the latest, greatest "advanced muscle-building" supplements that clutter the shelves of your local supplement store.

Contrary to what "leading health experts" claim these days, it has much less to do with "clean eating" than you probably think. It's also much more than eating a couple of good meals per day with some snacks here and there so you don't get hungry.

Proper nutrition boils down to just two things:

1. Supplying your body with the nutrients needed to efficiently recover from your workouts.

2. Manipulating your energy intake to lose, maintain, or gain weight as desired.

It's that simple. When you know how to accomplish these two targets, you can change your body composition with ease while also being incredibly flexible with your diet.

You can eat plenty of carbohydrates and do great (in fact I'm going to *recommend* this). You can eat grains and even sugar every day and get shredded (gasp!). You can eat on just about any schedule you like. You can eat large or small meals. The list goes on.

What you can't do, however, is supply your body with inadequate nutrients or get the energy balance wrong for your goals. Do either of those things, and you'll flounder no matter what else you do.

Now, there are seven aspects of nutrition that are of primary concern when trying to build muscle and lose fat and stay healthy. They are calories, protein, carbohydrates, fats, water, vitamins and minerals, and fiber.

As you know, a calorie is a measurement of potential energy in a food, whether it comes from protein, carbohydrate, or fat.

Protein, carbohydrates, and fats are macronutrients, and how you structure these in your diet is vitally important to your overall results.

Many people are surprised to learn how important drinking enough water is and how much better their bodies feel and perform when they're properly hydrated.

Then there are vitamins and minerals, known as "micronutrients," that are essential for your body to efficiently perform the many different physiological processes connected with building muscle and losing fat.

Last but not least is fiber, which is an indigestible type of carbohydrate found in many types of foods, including fruits, vegetables, legumes, and grains. Fiber is vital for overall health.

Let's dive into each of these subjects separately.

CALORIES

You already know the role that calories play in determining the body's energy balance and how this determines fat loss and fat gain. In this section, I want to touch on a few other calorie-related things that you should know.

Regardless of the source, 1 gram of protein contains 4 calories, 1 gram of carbohydrate contains 4 calories as well, and 1 gram of fat contains 9 calories.

Yes, a gram of carbohydrate found in lettuce contains the same amount of energy as a gram of carbohydrate found in a Snickers bar. This is why so many people fail to lose weight by simply "eating clean"—they give their bodies an abundance of micronutrients through eating a bunch of nutritious foods, which is great, but they also give it too many calories, which means no weight loss.

Another big mistake people often make is they overestimate the number of calories they burn every day and accidentally overeat.

Quite a few factors determine the total energy your body burns every day, such as body size, total lean mass, body temperature, the thermic effect of foods, stimulants such as caffeine, and the types and amounts of physical activity.

Later in the book, when we break down how to diet properly, I'm going to give you simple dietary formulas for losing fat, building muscle, and maintaining weight that use macronutrient targets. I do, however, want you to know how to calculate approximately how many calories your body burns every day (your TDEE), as you may need to tweak the formulas I give later to your circumstances.

We must first calculate our BMR, which is easily accomplished by using the Katch McArdle formula. Here's how it works:

$$BMR = 370 + (21.6 * LBM)$$

LBM refers to *lean body mass*, and it's in kilograms for this calculation. In case you're not familiar with it, lean body mass refers to the nonfat components of the human body.

You calculate LBM by subtracting your body fat weight from your total body weight, giving you the weight of everything but your body fat. Here's how it looks:

$$LBM = (1 - BF\% \text{ expressed as decimal numeral}) * \text{total body weight}$$

For instance, I'm currently 186 pounds at about 6 percent body fat, so my LBM is calculated like this:

$$1 - 0.06 = 0.94$$
$$0.94 * 186 = 175 \text{ lbs. (LBM)}$$

There are 2.2 pounds in a kilogram, so here is the formula to calculate my BMR:

$$175 / 2.2 = 80 \text{ kg}$$
$$370 + (21.6 * 80) = 2,100 \text{ calories per day}$$

Once you know your BMR, you can calculate your TDEE by multiplying it as follows:

- by 1.2 if you exercise 1 to 3 hours per week,

- by 1.35 if you exercise 4 to 6 hours per week, or

- by 1.5 if you exercise vigorously for 6 or more hours per week.

The resulting number will be a fairly accurate measurement of the total energy your body burns every day.

Some people prefer to start with BMR and then add calories burned through physical activity, as determined by estimations or an activity tracker, but I find this an unnecessary complication. When we look at the bigger picture, the TDEE calculation method works just as well, and it makes meal planning easy as we can just stick to the same numbers every day.

In case you're wondering why those multipliers are lower than the standard Katch McArdle multipliers and other similar models elsewhere on the Internet, it's simply because the standard Katch McArdle multipliers are too high. Unless you have an abnormally fast metabolism, standard multipliers will overshoot your actual TDEE and cause you to fail to lose weight or gain weight too quickly, depending on what you're trying to accomplish.

Now, if math isn't your strong suit and you're a little confused, don't worry. You don't have to even calculate your BMR or TDEE, as I'm going to make dieting simple for you by providing easy macronutrient formulas to follow based on your weight and approximate body fat percentage and goals.

I just wanted you to know how to calculate these things as many people hear about them but don't know what they are or how to properly calculate them.

PROTEIN

A high-protein diet is absolutely vital for building muscle and preserving it when you're dieting for fat loss. A low-protein diet is absolutely good for nothing. End of story.

One of the easiest ways to get stuck in a rut is to simply not pay attention to how much protein you eat on a day-to-day basis or miss meals and figure it's no big deal.

You see, when you eat food with protein, your body breaks it down into a pool of amino acids, which it can then use to build muscle tissue (among other things). If your diet contains too little protein, your body can become deficient in these essential amino acids, and thus its ability to build and repair muscle tissue becomes impaired.

This is true regardless of whether you exercise. The basic processes whereby cells die and are replaced require these essential amino acids.

Regular exercise, and weightlifting in particular, increases your body's need for essential amino acids and thus protein. Your body must repair the damage you're causing to muscle fibers, and that requires a lot of "building blocks." This is why research has shown that athletes need to eat a high-protein diet to maximize performance.[1]

How much protein is enough, you wonder? Let's find out.

THE PROTEIN NEEDS OF ATHLETES

According to the Institute of Medicine, 10 to 35 percent of our daily calories should come from protein.[2]

That's not helpful for us, though, because 10 to 35 percent is quite a range to choose from. Even if we go with 35 percent, if our daily calorie intake is too low, we won't get enough protein, and if it's too high, we'll get more than we need.

So, to find a more definitive answer, let's look at some of the clinical research available on the matter, starting with research conducted by scientists at McMaster University.

According to their work, protein intake of 1.3 to 1.8 grams per kilogram of body weight (0.6 to 0.8 grams per pound of body weight) is adequate for stimulating maximal protein synthesis.[3] They note, however, that more protein might be needed in the case of frequent and/or high-intensity training and in the case of dieting to lose fat (restricting calories).

A widely cited study conducted by researchers from the University of Western Ontario concluded the same: 1.6 to 1.8 grams per kilogram of body weight might be enough for athletes, but higher intakes may also be warranted depending on a variety of factors, including energy intake; carbohydrate availability; exercise intensity, duration, and type; dietary protein quality; training history; gender; age; timing of nutrient intake; and more.[4]

As you can see, the topic is complex, and there may not be a "one-size-fits-all" solution. That said, the anecdotal evidence of "gym lore" can lend some insight here, and it agrees with the above findings.

- One gram of protein per pound of body weight (2.2 grams per kilogram of body weight) per day has been a bodybuilding rule of thumb for decades.

- Higher levels of protein intake, usually in the range of 1.2 to 1.5 grams per pound of body weight (2.6 to 3.3 grams per kilogram of body weight) per day, are commonly recommended when dieting to lose fat.

If those numbers sound high to you, consider these findings from research published in 2013 by researchers from the Auckland University of Technology:

"Protein needs for energy-restricted resistance-trained athletes are likely 2.3-3.1g/kg of FFM [1 - 1.4 grams per pound of fat free mass] scaled upwards with severity of caloric restriction and leanness." [5]

Fat-free mass, by the way, refers to the nonfat components of the human body, such as skeletal muscle, bone, and water. Technically, fat-free mass differs from lean body mass because there is some essential fat in the marrow of your bones and internal organs. Thus, lean body mass includes a small percentage of essential fat. Practically speaking, however, we can treat them the same and calculate fat-free mass in the same way as we calculated lean body mass.

In my case, my fat-free mass is currently 175 pounds. So, according to the research cited above, if I were to restrict my calories for fat-loss purposes, I should eat anywhere from 175 to 245 grams of protein per day.

Well, I've found this to be true, not only with my body but also with the thousands of people I've worked with. As you get leaner, keeping your protein intake high becomes very important. If it drops too low (below 1 gram per pound of body weight, in my experience), the loss of strength and muscle is noticeably accelerated.

So that's it for the amount of protein you should eat. And again, don't worry about trying to remember everything I talked about here, as I'm going to give you some simple dietary guidelines to follow when it comes time to create your meal plan. At this point, all you need to do is understand the research and reasoning behind the guidelines.

With that out of the way, let's now move on to the best types of protein for our purposes.

THE BEST SOURCES OF PROTEIN

There are two main sources of protein: whole-food protein and supplement protein. Whole-food protein is, as you guessed, protein that comes from natural food sources, such as beef, chicken, fish, plants, and the like.

As you can imagine, not all protein is metabolized in the same way. Different proteins digest at different speeds, and some are better used by the body than others. For example, beef protein is digested quickly, and 70 to 80 percent of what's eaten is used by the body.[6] On the other hand, the protein found in eggs is digested much more slowly than beef, but the body uses it even more efficiently.[7]

The general rule of protein intake is that you want to stick to proteins that are easily digested and that supply plentiful amounts of the essential amino acids required by the body. To determine what these proteins are, we can turn to the Protein Digestibility Corrected Amino Acid Score (PDCAA) of various types of protein, which assigns ratings on a scale from 0 to 1 to indicate the overall quality of the food (with 0 being the worst and 1 being the best possible score).

While I could give you a big table with the PDCAA scores of various proteins, I'm going to just keep it simple: your best choices are meat, dairy products, and eggs; second to those are certain plant sources like legumes, nuts, and high-protein vegetables such as peas, broccoli, and spinach.[8]

Protein from meat is particularly helpful when you're weightlifting, as research has demonstrated that eating meats increases testosterone levels and is more effective for building muscle than vegetarian sources.[9] One study conducted by researchers at the University of Arkansas had two groups of men aged 51 to 69, all comparable in health and body composition, follow a weightlifting program for 12 weeks. One group followed a meat-free lactoovovegetarian diet (wherein meat is avoided but eggs and dairy are eaten) and the other ate a meat-containing omnivorous diet. By the end of the program, all had progressed about equally in strength, but only the meat eaters enjoyed significant muscle growth and fat loss.[10]

"Meat" doesn't only mean red meat, by the way. Fish, chicken, turkey, pork, buffalo, and so on all qualify as "meat" in this sense.

You'll also want to stick mainly to lean varieties and cuts of meats, as fattier meats are hard to fit into a proper meal plan. It's generally good advice to limit your saturated fat intake and get a good amount of your dietary fat from unsaturated sources.

If you're a vegetarian, while it's true that you would do better if you ate meat, don't despair: you can still do well on the program so long as you eat enough protein every day and stick to high-quality sources.

And while we're on the subject of high-quality vegetarian proteins, let's address the claim that as a vegetarian or vegan eater, you must carefully combine your proteins to ensure your body gets all of the amino acids it needs to build and repair its tissues.

This theory and the faulty research it was based on was thoroughly debunked as a myth by the Massachusetts Institute of Technology, yet it still hangs around.[11] While it's true that some sources of vegetable protein are *lower* in certain amino acids than other forms of protein, there is no scientific evidence to prove that they lack them altogether.

Let's now talk about protein supplements. These are powdered or liquid foods that contain protein from various sources, with the four most popular sources being whey, casein, egg, and soy, as well as plant-based supplements made from various foods such as quinoa, brown rice, peas, hemp, and even fruit.

While you don't *need* protein supplements to build muscle and get fit, it can be impractical to try to get all the protein you need from whole foods. Protein powder is convenient and, in some cases, it offers some unique benefits.

Let's take a closer look at each type of protein supplement and see what the research says about their value in our quest to get fit.

Whey Protein Powder

Whey protein is by far the most popular type of protein supplement on the market today. You get a lot of protein per dollar spent, it tastes good, and its amino acid profile is particularly suited to muscle building.

What is it, though?

Well, whey is a semi-clear, liquid by-product of cheese production. After curdling and straining milk, whey is left over. It used to be thrown away as waste, but scientists discovered that it's a complete protein. It is abundant in *leucine*, which is an essential amino acid that plays a key role in initiating protein synthesis.[12]

When the world of sports nutrition caught on to this research, the whey protein supplement was born.

You can take whey protein anytime, but it's particularly effective as a post-workout source of protein because it's rapidly digested, which causes a dramatic spike in amino acids in the blood (especially in leucine).[13] This, in turn, stimulates more immediate muscle growth than slower-burning proteins.[14]

So whey is an all-around good choice for protein powder for men and women.

I should mention, however, that even if you're not lactose intolerant, you can still have problems digesting one of the types of protein found in cow's milk.[15] This is why some people don't do well with highly refined forms of whey, such as isolate or hydrolysate, which have virtually all lactose removed.

If whey bothers your stomach, try a nondairy alternative and you will be fine. My favorite nondairy protein is egg protein powder, but there are vegan options that work as well.

Casein Protein Powder

Casein protein is probably second in popularity behind whey, and it's also a protein found in milk. The curds that form as milk coagulates, such as the chunks in cottage cheese, are casein.

Casein protein is digested more slowly than whey, causing a smaller spike in amino acids in the blood but a steadier release over the course of several hours.[16]

There's an ongoing debate about whether supplementing with whey is better than casein for building muscle or vice versa, but here's what most reputable experts agree on:

- Due to its rapid digestion and abundance of leucine, a 30 to 40 gram serving of whey is probably your best choice for post-workout protein.

- Due to its slow release of amino acids, casein is a great "general use" protein supplement.

- While it may or may not be as optimal as whey for post-workout protein (the jury is still out on this), there is a growing body of evidence indicating that, when supplementing with powders, a slow-burning protein is the best overall choice for building muscle.[17]

- Casein is a good protein to have before you go to bed, which can help with muscle recovery.[18]

Personally, I use whey in my post-workout meal and then have a scoop or two of egg protein (which is slow burning) throughout the day to help hit my numbers. The reason I don't use casein is that my stomach starts to bother me if I eat too much dairy.

Egg Protein Powder

Many people don't even know that you can buy egg protein in a powder form. You can, and it has three primary benefits:

- It's used well by the body (it has a perfect PDCAA score of 1). Its exact score varies based on the research, but it's always at the top of the list.

- According to animal research, egg protein is similar to whey in its ability to stimulate muscle growth.[19]

- Egg protein is digested even more slowly than casein, which, as you know, means it results in a longer release of amino acids into the blood, and this may be particularly conducive to overall muscle growth.[20]

- Because egg protein powders are made from the egg whites only, they have no fat and very little carbohydrate.

The bottom line is that egg protein is just a great all-around choice. It's what I personally use for any supplementation outside of pre- and post-workout needs.

Soy Protein Powder

Soy protein is a mixed bag.

While research has shown it's an all-around effective source of protein for building muscle, it's also a source of ongoing controversy for men.[21]

According to some research, regular intake of soy foods has feminizing effects in men due to estrogen-like molecules found in soybeans called *isoflavones*.

For instance, a study conducted by Harvard University researchers analyzed the semen of 99 men and compared it against their soy and isoflavone intake during the three previous months.[22] What they found is that both isoflavone and soy intake were associated with a reduction in sperm count. Men in the highest intake category of soy foods had, on average, 41 million sperm per milliliter fewer than men who did not eat soy foods.

On the other hand, a study conducted by scientists from the University of Guelph had 32 men eat low or high levels of isoflavones from soy protein for 57 days and found that it didn't affect semen quality.[23] Furthermore, literature reviews like those conducted by researchers from Loma Linda University and St. Catherine University suggest that neither soy food nor isoflavones alter male hormone levels.[24]

What gives, then?

Well, there isn't a simple answer just yet, but we do know that soy's effects in the body can vary depending on the presence or absence of certain intestinal bacteria. These bacteria, which are present in 30 to 50 percent of people, metabolize an isoflavone in soy called *daidzein* into an estrogen-like hormone called *equol*.[25]

In a study published in 2011, researchers at Peking University found that when men with the equol-producing bacteria ate high amounts of soy food for three days, their testosterone levels dropped while their estrogen levels rose.[26] These effects were not seen in women, regardless of equol production or lack thereof.

Related to this is a study conducted with women by scientists at Sungkyunkwan University, which found that in a high-estrogen environment, isoflavones suppressed estrogen production, and in a low-estrogen environment, they increased estrogen production.[27]

Research has also shown that soy protein contains substances that inhibit the digestion of protein molecules and the absorption of other nutrients as well as several known allergens.[28]

While there is research that indicates soy might have special benefits for women, such as reducing the risk of heart disease and breast cancer, other research casts doubt on these findings.[29] And to the contrary, studies have shown that soy can even stimulate the growth of cancer cells.[30]

Yet another issue that we have to deal with when we eat soy is the fact that the vast majority of soybeans grown in the United States are genetically modified (91 percent, according to government data[31]).

The subject of genetically modified foods is incredibly heated and too complex to fully address in this book, but the safest bet at the moment is to avoid genetically modified foods as much as possible until more research is done on the potential long-term health effects in humans.

So, all things considered, I think you understand why I generally recommend for men to avoid soy if at all possible. There are just too many unknowns for my liking.

Other Plant-Based Protein Powders

While soy is the most popular plant-based protein powder on the shelves, you'll often find rice, hemp, and pea protein powders as well. Here's how they stack up:

With a middling PDCAA score of 0.47, rice protein isn't too exciting. When you combine it with pea protein, however, it gets a lot better because of pea's better PDCAA score of 0.69 and high amount of leucine.[32]

In fact, a rice and pea blend is often called "vegan's whey" because its amino acid profile is similar to that of whey protein.

Hemp protein is the poorest choice of the three options. While it has a great micronutrient profile, including omega-3 and omega-6 fatty acids, hemp is only about 30 to 50 percent protein by weight, whereas other options discussed in this chapter are 90 to 100 percent. Furthermore, the protein it does contain isn't nearly as digestible as rice or pea protein, let alone animal products like whey, casein, or egg protein.[33] Hemp should be viewed more as a whole food and not a pure protein supplement.

So, that's all you need to know about what types of protein to eat. Let's move on to a question I'm often asked: how much protein can you eat and efficiently absorb in one meal?

THE "PROTEIN ABSORPTION" MYTH

A quick Google search on protein absorption numbers will yield all kinds of opinions and numbers. A recommendation commonly thrown around by "experts" is to limit your intake to no more than 30 to 40 grams of protein per meal, as any more will be discarded by the body.

This type of "one-size-fits-all" advice smacks of nonsense.

I highly doubt an NFL linebacker's body deals with protein intake in exactly the same way as a 120-pound weakling's. Protein needs due to lifestyle and lean mass should influence the matter of protein metabolism, right?

Additionally, if it were true that a person can only absorb a relatively small amount of protein in one meal, then "super-dosing" daily protein needs into two to three meals would result in protein deficiencies. This assumption begs the question of how the human species survived the hunter-gatherer days when we experienced regular feasts and famines, but the body *is* incredibly adaptive.

To better evaluate the issue at hand, let's look at what happens when you eat protein.

First, your stomach uses its acid and enzymes to break the protein down into its building blocks, amino acids. These amino acids are transported into the bloodstream by special cells that line the intestines and are then delivered to various parts of the body. Your body only has so many transporter cells, which limits the amount of amino acids that can be infused into your blood every hour.

This is what we're talking about with "protein absorption," by the way: how quickly our bodies can absorb the amino acids into our bloodstreams.

As you know, the human body absorbs different proteins at different rates. According to one review, whey clocks in at 8 to 10 grams absorbed per hour, casein at 6.1, soy at 3.9, and egg at 1.3.[34] These numbers aren't completely accurate due to the complexities involved in measuring protein absorption, but they lend insight nonetheless: certain proteins are absorbed slowly, whereas others can be absorbed quickly.

Another fact relevant to the current discussion is that food substances don't move uniformly through the digestive tract, and they don't leave sections in the same order that they arrived in.

For instance, the presence of protein in the stomach stimulates the production of a hormone that delays "gastric emptying" (the emptying of the food from the stomach) and that slows down intestinal contractions.[35]

This causes food to move more slowly through the small intestines, where nutrients are absorbed, and this is how your body buys the time it needs to absorb the protein you eat. Carbohydrates and fats can move through and be fully absorbed while your body is still working on the protein.

Once the amino acids make it into the bloodstream, your body does various things with them, such as grow and repair tissues, and it can also temporarily store (up to about 24 hours or so) excess amino acids in muscle for future needs.[36] If amino acids are still in the blood after doing all of the above, your body can break them down into fuel for your brain and other cells.

Now, how does all that relate to strict claims about how much protein can be absorbed in one meal? Well, such claims are usually based on one of two things:

An ignorance of how food moves through the digestive system.

Some people believe that all foods move through the small intestines in 2 to 3 hours and thus also believe that even if you ate even the type of protein that can be absorbed the quickest—at a rate of 8 to 10 grams per hour—you could only absorb 25 to 30 grams of it before it passes to the large intestine to be disposed of. According to this line of thinking, slower-digesting proteins result in even fewer grams absorbed into the bloodstream.

Well, as we now know, your body is smarter than that, and it regulates the speed at which protein moves through the small intestines to ensure it can absorb all of the available amino acids.

References to studies relating to the anabolic response to protein consumption.

A study commonly cited in connection with protein absorption showed that 20 grams of post-workout protein stimulated maximum muscle protein synthesis in young men.[37] That is, eating more than 20 grams of protein after working out did nothing additional in terms of stimulating more muscle growth.

The most obvious flaw in this argument is you can't use studies on the anabolic response to protein consumption to extrapolate ideas about how much we can absorb in one sitting. Acute anabolic responses to eating protein just don't give us the whole picture.

Absorption relates to the availability of amino acids over extended periods of time, which prevents muscle breakdown and provides raw materials for growth. And, as we now know, our body doesn't just throw away all of the amino acids it can't immediately use: it can store them for later needs.

Further supporting this position is a study conducted by researchers at the Human Nutrition Research Center.[38] It had 16 young women eat 79 percent of their daily protein (about 54 grams) in one meal or four meals over the course of 14 days. Researchers found no difference between the groups in terms of protein synthesis or degradation.

Furthermore, if we look at the amount of protein used in the above study relative to body weight, it comes out to about 1.17 grams per kilogram. Apply that to a man weighing 80 kilograms (176 pounds), and you get about 94 grams of protein in one sitting. While this isn't definitive scientific proof, it's food for thought.

Research on the style of dieting known as *intermittent fasting* is also relevant. This style of dieting has people fasting for extended periods, followed by anywhere from 2- to 8-hour "feeding windows." One study on this method of meal timing found that eating the entire days' worth of protein in a four-hour window (followed by 20 hours of fasting) didn't have a negative impact on muscle preservation.[39]

So, as you can see, it's hard to put an accurate cap on how much protein your body can absorb in one meal. It's definitely a hell of a lot more than the 20 to 30 grams that some people claim.

All that said, however, it turns out that eating smaller amounts of protein more frequently may be superior to larger amounts in fewer meals…

THE "PROTEIN FREQUENCY" DEBATE

Another aspect of protein intake that is a subject of much opinion and debate is how frequently you should eat it.

For decades now, it's been fairly standard advice to eat protein every 2 to 3 hours to maximize muscle growth, but as you're beginning to see, the progressive march of scientific research is sending many of the old sacred cows of fitness to the slaughterhouse. Is this "protein every few hours" animal another whose time has come?

Well, what we *do* know is you don't *have* to eat protein every couple of hours to build muscle and strength or avoid "going catabolic." Reaching your daily protein requirement is crucial, but the feeding schedule isn't.[40]

That said, research has demonstrated that how frequently we eat protein *can* influence whole-body protein synthesis rates (and thus overall muscle growth). Specifically, researchers at the University of Illinois found that when healthy adults split up their protein intake (about 100 grams) equally into three daily meals (30 to 33 grams at breakfast, lunch, and dinner), 24-hour muscle protein synthesis rates were higher than when intake was skewed toward dinner (11 grams at breakfast, 16 at lunch, and 64 at dinner).[41]

This isn't surprising when we consider the fact that research has also shown that eating about 30 to 40 grams of protein in a meal maximally stimulates protein synthesis rates.[42] If we eat less, the resulting protein synthesis rates are lower; and if we eat more, they don't rise (we can't double protein synthesis rates by eating 60 grams of protein).

Thus, if you ate small amounts of protein—10 to 20 grams, let's say—a few times per day, each meal would fail to stimulate as much protein synthesis as possible. If you then followed these meals with a large amount of protein, you would stimulate maximal protein synthesis but not so much that you "made up for" the protein synthesis that you missed out on throughout the day due to the inadequate earlier meals.

If, on the other hand, you ate 30 to 40 grams of protein in each of the meals instead, they would each cause the maximum amount of potential protein synthesis, which means that by the end of the day, your body would have created more muscle proteins than in the previous example.

So, considering everything we now know about protein absorption and frequency research, I think we can derive some simple rules of thumb:

- Eating protein more frequently is likely superior to less frequently.
- Each protein feeding should contain at least 30 to 40 grams of protein.
- Feedings can contain quite a bit more protein if necessary to hit daily targets.

For example, here's how my daily protein intake generally looks:

Pre-workout: 30 grams of protein
Post-workout: 50 to 60 grams of protein
Lunch: 40 grams of protein
Afternoon snack: 30 to 40 grams of protein
Dinner: 30 to 40 grams of protein
Before bed: 30 grams of protein

Well, that covers everything you need to know about protein. If you're reeling a bit because of the sheer amount of information you've just jammed into your brain, feel free to review the section again and it'll sink in.

CARBOHYDRATE

I feel bad for the carbohydrate these days. It's misunderstood, maligned, and feared…and all without good reason.

Thanks to the scores of bogus diet "experts" out there and their many books, DVDs, blogs, and so forth, many people equate eating carbs with getting fat.

Well, while eating *too much* carbohydrate can make you fat (just as eating too much protein or fat can), carbs are hardly your enemy. Ironically, carbohydrate (in all forms) isn't stored as body fat as efficiently as dietary fat is.[43] Yes, strictly speaking, olive oil is more fattening than table sugar.

The reality is carbohydrates actually play an essential role in not only muscle growth but also in overall body function. For instance, when you eat carbs, some of the glucose released into the blood turns into glycogen and is then stored in the liver and muscles. When you lift weights, you rapidly drain your muscles' glycogen stores, and you replenish those stores when you eat carbohydrates.[44] By doing this and keeping your muscles "full" of glycogen, you improve performance and reduce exercise-induced muscle breakdown.[45]

But before we get into the other benefits of eating carbs, let's take a more in-depth look at the carbohydrate molecule itself and how it works in the body, and let's dispel some nasty myths that have dieters shaking in their boots when they consider eating a dessert.

There are three forms of carbohydrate:

- monosaccharides,
- oligosaccharides, and
- polysaccharides.

Let's look at each separately.

Monosaccharides

Monosaccharides are often called simple carbohydrates because they have a simple structure. *Mono* means one and *saccharide* means sugar. So, one sugar.

The monosaccharides are…

- glucose,
- fructose, and
- galactose.

Glucose is a type of sugar also known as blood sugar, which is found in our blood and produced from the food we eat (most dietary carbohydrates contain glucose, either as the sole form of sugar or combined with the other two simple sugars given above). When people talk about "blood sugar levels," they're talking about the amount of glucose floating around in the blood.

Fructose is a type of sugar naturally found in fruit and also found in processed products like sucrose (table sugar) and high fructose corn syrup (HFCS), both of which are about 50 percent fructose and 50 percent glucose. Fructose is converted into glucose by the liver and then released into the blood for use.

Galactose is a type of sugar found in dairy products, and it's metabolized similarly to fructose.

Oligosaccharides

Oligosaccharides are molecules that contain several monosaccharides linked together in chain-like structures. *Oligos* is Greek for "a few," so *oligosaccharides* means "a few sugars."

Oligosaccharides are one of the components of fiber found in plants. Our bodies are able to partially break down oligosaccharides into glucose (leaving the fibrous, indigestible parts behind to do good things in our guts).[46]

Many vegetables also contain *fructo-oligosaccharides*, which are short chains of fructose molecules. The body metabolizes these accordingly (it breaks the chains, and then it converts the individual fructose molecules into glucose for use).

Another common form of oligosaccharide that we eat is *raffinose*, which consists of a chain of galactose, glucose, and fructose (called a *trisaccharide*), that can be found in whole grains and in vegetables including beans, cabbage, Brussels sprouts, broccoli, and asparagus, other vegetables, and whole grains.

Galactooligosaccharides round out the list of oligosaccharides and are short chains of galactose molecules. These are indigestible but play a role in stimulating healthy bacteria growth in the gut.[47]

POLYSACCHARIDES

Polysaccharides are long chains of monosaccharides, usually containing 10 or more monosaccharide units. *Poly* is Greek for "many" and accordingly, these molecules consist of many sugars.

Starch (the energy stores of plants) and cellulose (a natural fiber found in many plants) are two examples of polysaccharides that we often eat. Our bodies are able to easily break starches down into glucose, but not cellulose: it passes through our digestive system intact (making it a source of dietary fiber).

THERE'S A PATTERN HERE...THEY ALL END UP AS GLUCOSE

As you've probably noticed, all forms of carbohydrate we eat are either metabolized into glucose or are left indigested, serving as dietary fiber.

Our body can't distinguish between the natural sugar found in fruit, honey, or milk and the processed sugar found in a Snickers bar. They're all digested in the same way: they're broken down into monosaccharides, which are then turned into glucose, which is then shipped off to the brain, muscles, and organs for use.

Yes, in the end, the candy bar turns into glucose just like the cup of peas. Sure, the candy bar turns into glucose *faster*, but that's the only difference (carbohydrate-wise). The candy bar has a bunch of monosaccharides that are quickly metabolized, whereas the peas have a bunch of oligosaccharides that take longer to break down.

Now, I'm not saying peas are "the same as" candy bars, so dump the veggies and bring on the chocolate. Obviously, peas are more nutritious than Snickers bars, but there's more to this story.

Chemically speaking, simple carbohydrates like the sugar and HFCS found in processed foods are pretty simple. Table sugar, or sucrose, is a disaccharide (two sugars) consisting of one part fructose and one part glucose. Sucrose occurs in natural foods like pineapples, sweet potatoes, beets, sugarcane, and even walnuts, pecans, and cashews. It's also added to foods to make them sweeter.

HFCS is chemically similar, usually consisting of about 55 percent fructose and 45 percent glucose. It isn't found in nature (it's artificially produced) and the only difference between it and sucrose is the fructose and glucose aren't chemically bonded, which means the body has to do even less work to metabolize it into glucose.[48]

Now, when viewed that way, neither seems all that nefarious. The sucrose found in a pineapple is no different chemically than the sucrose in our favorite type of dessert. And HFCS is chemically similar to sucrose.

What's the big deal, then? Why are we told that eating the sucrose in a pineapple is okay but the chemically identical sucrose in the chocolate bar or some other form of simple carbohydrate is disastrous? Why is HFCS often vilified as the ultimate metabolic miscreant when it's pretty dang similar to sucrose?

Well, while it's true that some people's bodies do better with carbohydrates (all forms) than others, it's simply not true that sucrose, HFCS, or other simple forms of carbohydrate are *especially* fattening.

As you now know, these two molecules just aren't that special. They are just a source of glucose for the body like any other carbohydrate.

Don't believe me? Well, let's look at some research.

In one study, researchers from the Sugar Bureau in the UK (tasked with researching all forms of sugars, not with convincing us to eat a bunch of sucrose or HFCS) set out to determine whether there should be a guideline for daily sugar consumption.[49] They found that increased sugar intake was associated with *leanness*, not obesity, and concluded that there simply wasn't enough evidence to warrant a quantitative guideline for sugar consumption.

Another study, conducted by researchers at the University of Hawaii, extensively reviewed sugar-related literature.[50] Here's a quote from the paper:

"It is important to state at the outset that there is no direct connection between added sugars intake and obesity unless excessive consumption of sugar-containing beverages and foods leads to energy imbalance and the resultant weight gain."

Overconsumption and *energy imbalance* are the keys here.

You see, it's a known fact that over the past couple of decades, Americans have increased the number of calories they eat every day, and much of this increase is in the form of carbohydrates, primarily from soft drinks.[51]

This is where we get to the actual problem with sugar and HFCS intake and getting and staying fat: the more you eat foods with added sugars, the easier it is to overeat.

This is especially true of liquid carbohydrates, including beverages with added sugar.[52] If you love caloric beverages, you'll probably stay fat forever. You can drink 1,000 calories and be hungry an hour later, whereas eating 1,000 calories of high-quality food, including a good portion of protein and fiber, will probably keep you full for five to six hours.

And what about HFCS? What does the literature reveal about this sucrose-like molecule? More of the same, of course.

Here's a quote from an extensive review of HFCS literature published in 2008:

"Sucrose, HFCS, invert sugar, honey, and many fruits and juices deliver the same sugars in the same ratios to the same tissues within the same time frame to the same metabolic pathways. Thus…it makes essentially no metabolic difference which one is used." [53]

Here's one from an HFCS literature review conducted by researchers from the University of Maryland and published in 2007:

"Based on the currently available evidence, the expert panel concluded that HFCS does not appear to contribute to overweight and obesity any differently than do other energy sources." [54]

And yet another from yet another literature review published in 2008:

"The data presented indicated that HFCS is very similar to sucrose, being about 55 percent fructose and 45 percent glucose, and thus, not surprisingly, few metabolic differences were found comparing HFCS and sucrose. That said, HFCS does contribute to added sugars and calories, and those concerned with managing their weight should be concerned about calories from beverages and other foods, regardless of HFCS content." [55]

The bottom line is that HFCS is just another simple sugar, and as far as we can currently tell, it can only harm us when overconsumed.

Now, at this point, you're probably thinking that you have carte blanche to eat as much sugar and as many simple carbohydrates as you want. While doing so may not be as harmful as you're told, there's more to consider.

When Eating Too Many Simple Sugars Can Become a Problem

A high, long-term intake of simple carbohydrates (disaccharides like sucrose and HFCS) has been associated with an increased risk of heart disease and Type 2 diabetes. [56]

Many "experts" will use a factoid like that as definitive evidence that simple carbohydrates ruin our health, but this is misleading. There's more to the story.

One is the fact that the effects of these simple carbohydrates vary greatly among individuals depending on how fat and active they are. [57] Overweight, sedentary bodies don't deal with simple sugars nearly as well as lean, physically active ones do. [58]

Furthermore, when you mix carbohydrates (all forms) with other forms, the insulin response is mitigated. [59] That is, eating a couple of tablespoons of sucrose on an empty stomach causes a larger insulin reaction in the body than eating a couple of tablespoons of sucrose as a part of a mixed meal (contained in a dessert eaten after dinner, for example).

That said, even as part of a mixed meal, simple carbohydrates still do elevate insulin levels higher than more complex forms of carbohydrates, such as the polysaccharides found in vegetables. [60]

From this, we can derive a sensible recommendation: if you're overweight and don't exercise, you shouldn't eat a bunch of simple carbohydrates every day. This makes intuitive sense: carbohydrate is primarily energetic, and as a sedentary individual, your body doesn't need an abundance of food energy.

On the other hand, if you exercise regularly and aren't overweight, your body can deal with simple carbohydrates just fine. You're not going to get diabetes or ruin your heart by having a bit of sucrose every day.

One other health-related concern is the fact that eating a lot of foods with added sugars can reduce the amount of micronutrients your body gets and thus cause deficiencies. [61] This is because many foods with added sugars just don't have much in the way of essential vitamins and minerals.

The solution here is obvious, though: get the majority of your daily calories from nutrient-dense foods, and you'll be fine.

Personally, many of the carbohydrates I eat every day are of the "complex" variety found in fruits, vegetables, legumes, and certain grains and seeds like whole wheat, brown rice, and quinoa. This not only provides me plenty of micronutrients, but I also find my energy levels are stabler than if I eat a bunch of simple carbohydrates.

I do, however, include some sort of small dessert every day. Some days it's a bit of chocolate, and others it's a few spoons of ice cream or something else tasty. I'll usually have a larger dessert once per week with my "cheat meal" as well, which we'll talk more about later in the book.

When you break it all down, though, I never get more than 10 percent of my weekly calories from added sugars, and considering how much micronutrient-dense food I eat and how much I exercise, this low level of sugar intake will *never* cause me any problems.[62]

So all forms of carbohydrate eventually turn into glucose, with the main difference between simple and complex sugars being the speed with which this occurs. As a general rule of thumb, you want to get the majority of your carbs from complex, slower-burning sources.

How can we know which carbs are metabolized slowly and which are broken down quickly? We can use the glycemic index.

How to Use the Glycemic Index

The glycemic index (GI) is a numeric system that ranks how quickly the body converts carbohydrates into glucose. Carbs are ranked on a scale of 0 to 100 depending on how they affect blood sugar levels once eaten.

A GI rating of 55 and under is considered low on the index, while a rating of 56 to 69 is medium, and a rating of 70 or above is high.

Simple carbohydrates are converted into glucose quickly and thus have high GI ratings. Examples of simple carbohydrates and their corresponding GI ratings are sucrose (65), white bread (71), white rice (89), and white potato (82).

Complex carbohydrates are converted into glucose more slowly and thus have lower GI ratings. Examples of complex carbohydrates and their corresponding GI ratings are apples (39), black beans (30), peanuts (7), and whole-grain pasta (42).

As I said earlier, you'll probably notice better all-around energy levels by getting the majority of your carbs from complex, lower-GI foods. These foods are often more nutritious as well.

You see, if you look at the GI ratings of various carbohydrates, you'll quickly notice that most nutritious, unprocessed sources of carbohydrate are naturally low on the GI. The majority of high-GI foods are junk like white bread, breakfast cereals, pretzels and chips, candy, soda, and so forth that are quite low in nutrients and often filled with chemicals and other additives that are best avoided.

If you got the majority of your carbs from these low-quality types of foods, your body composition may not be noticeably affected but your health would be—you would likely develop micronutrient deficiencies over time and suffer from various nagging health issues.

So, to repeat, my recommendation is simple: get the majority of your daily carbohydrates from nutritious, unprocessed foods, which will incidentally be lower on the GI, but don't be afraid to include a few higher-GI foods that you like.

Now, as you can probably tell, I'm not anti-carb, which might strike you as a bit odd. It seems like every guru and his mother is jumping on the low-carb bandwagon these days, and everywhere you look, there's another book or news story about why low-carb is the way of the future.

Well, I'm in the *opposite* camp.

I'm going to recommend that you eat a healthy number of carbs every day—even when you want to maximize fat loss. And I have good data and reasons to back this up.

If that sounds blasphemous to you, I understand. There's a *lot* of misinformation out there about carbs and how they affect the body, and it usually begins with the claim that the spike of insulin production makes us fat and ruins our health.

This scientifically debunked myth is little more than the perversion of basic physiology to convince you of a bogeyman that doesn't exist.

Insulin Isn't the Enemy—It's Actually Your Friend

As you know, when you eat food, your pancreas releases insulin into the blood, and its job is to shuttle the nutrients from the food into cells for use. As this occurs, insulin levels gradually drop until finally all nutrients are out of the blood, and insulin levels then remain steady at a low, "baseline" level and the pancreas waits for us to eat food again and repeat the process.

Generally speaking, carbohydrates cause a larger insulin spike than protein or dietary fat, which is why "insulin haters" say they're so harmful.

Why is insulin so viciously attacked by mainstream diet "gurus," though? It plays a vital physiological role in our bodies—a role that we simply couldn't live without. Why are we told that it makes us fat and sick?

The answer relates to one of insulin's functions that influences fat storage. Specifically, it inhibits the metabolic breakdown of fat cells for energy and stimulates the creation of body fat.[63] That is, insulin tells the body to stop burning its fat stores and instead absorb some of the fatty acids and glucose in the blood and turn them into more body fat.

When explained like that, insulin becomes an easy target and scapegoat and shows why carbohydrates are often pilloried right next to it. The "logic" goes like this:

High-carb diet = high insulin levels = burn less fat and store more = get fatter and fatter.

And then, as a corollary:

Low-carb diet = low insulin levels = burn more fat and store less = stay lean.

At first glance, these statements sound plausible. Simple explanations are popular, and "going low-carb" sounds like an easy way to get the bodies we desire without having to fuss over numbers.

Well, while it's true that insulin causes fat cells to absorb fatty acids and glucose and thus expand, that physiological mechanism isn't what causes you to get fatter over time—overeating does.

Remember that the overriding factor in weight loss or gain is *energy balance*. No hormone can magically produce the surplus of energy required to "fill up" fat cells and make our waistlines grow. Only you can provide this by regularly feeding your body more energy than it burns.

Another little fact that those with a phobia of carbs and insulin like to ignore is that the body doesn't need high levels of insulin to store dietary fat as body fat thanks to an enzyme called *acylation stimulating protein*.[64]

This is why you can't just eat as much dietary fat as you want and lose weight. And it's why research has shown that separating carbs and fats doesn't affect weight loss (eating carbs and fats together or separately doesn't change anything).[65]

Now, chances are this is news to you and you're not sure what to think. Every month, some new article blows up all over the Internet extolling the almost magical fat-loss powers of low-carb dieting, usually referencing one study or another to back up its claims. It all seems very convincing.

Well, there are about 20 studies that low-carb proponents bandy about as definitive proof of the superiority of low-carb dieting for weight loss. If you simply read the abstracts of some of these studies, low-carb dieting definitely seems more effective:

"Compared with a low-fat diet, a low-carbohydrate diet program had better participant retention and greater weight loss. During active weight loss, serum triglyceride levels decreased more and high-density lipoprotein cholesterol level increased more with the low-carbohydrate diet than with the low-fat diet." [66]

"This study shows a clear benefit of a VLCK [very-low-carbohydrate ketogenic] over LF [low-fat] diet for short-term body weight and fat loss, especially in men. A preferential loss of fat in the trunk region with a VLCK diet is novel and potentially clinically significant but requires further validation. These data provide additional support for the concept of metabolic advantage with diets representing extremes in macronutrient distribution." [67]

"Severely obese subjects with a high prevalence of diabetes or the metabolic syndrome lost more weight during six months on a carbohydrate-restricted diet than on a calorie- and fat-restricted diet, with a relative improvement in insulin sensitivity and triglyceride levels, even after adjustment for the amount of weight lost." [68]

Well, this type of glib "abstract surfing" is what many low-carbers base their theories and beliefs on, but there's a *big* problem with many of these studies, and it has to do with protein intake.

The problem is the low-carb diets in these studies *invariably* contained more protein than the low-fat diets. Yes, one for one...without fail.

What we're looking at in these studies is a high-protein, low-carbohydrate diet vs. a low-protein, high-fat diet, and the former wins every time. But we can't ignore the high-protein part and say it's more effective because of the low-carb element.

In fact, better designed and executed studies prove the opposite: that when protein intake is high, low-carb dieting offers no special weight loss benefits. But we'll get to that in a minute.

Why is protein intake so important when restricting our calories for fat loss? You already know the answer: because it's vital for preserving lean mass, both with sedentary people and especially with athletes.[69]

If you don't eat enough protein when dieting to lose weight, you can lose quite a bit of muscle,[70] and this in turn hampers your weight loss in several ways:

1. It causes your basal metabolic rate to drop.[71]
2. It reduces the number of calories you burn in your workouts.[72]
3. It impairs the metabolism of glucose and lipids.[73]

As you can see, when you want to lose fat, your number-one goal is to *preserve lean mass*, and eating an adequate amount of protein every day is vital to achieve this goal.

Now, let's turn our attention back to the "low-carb dieting is better" studies mentioned earlier. In many cases, the low-fat groups were given less protein than even the recommended daily intake (RDI) of 0.8 grams per kilogram of body weight, which is just woefully inadequate for weight-loss purposes. Research has shown that even doubling or tripling those RDI levels of protein intake isn't enough to fully prevent the loss of lean mass while restricting calories for fat loss.[74]

So, what happens in terms of weight loss when you keep protein intake high and compare high and low levels of carbohydrate intake? Is there even any research available to show us?

Yup.

I know of four studies that meet these criteria, and gee whiz look at that…when protein intake is high and matched among low-carb and high-carb dieters, there is no significant difference in weight loss.[75]

Here are snippets from each study. I recommend that you read the entire papers if you'd like to get the details or assess the overall quality of the research:

"KLC [ketogenic low-carbohydrate] and NLC [non-ketogenic low-carbohydrate] diets were equally effective in reducing body weight and insulin resistance, but the KLC diet was associated with several adverse metabolic and emotional effects. The use of ketogenic diets for weight loss is not warranted."[76]

(In case you're wondering, the "NLC" diet mentioned above wasn't particularly low-carb—subjects got 40 percent of their daily calories from carbohydrates.)

"Reduced-calorie diets result in clinically meaningful weight loss regardless of which macronutrients they emphasize."[77]

"The objective of this research was to evaluate the effect of low-fat or low-carbohydrate diet counseling on weight loss, body composition, and changes in metabolic indexes in overweight postmenopausal breast cancer survivors.

…

"Weight loss averaged 6.1 (± 4.8 kg) at 24 wk and was not significantly different by diet group; loss of lean mass was also demonstrated."[78]

"Weight loss was similar in LF [low-fat] (100+/-4 to 96.1+/-4 kg; P<0.001) and LC [low-carb] (95.4+/-4 to 89.7+/-4 kg; P<0.001) diets."[79]

So long as you maintain a proper calorie deficit and keep your protein intake high, you're going to maximize fat loss while preserving as much lean mass as possible. Going low-carb as well won't help you lose more weight.

Now, with all that out of the way, let's take a look at the benefits of eating adequate amounts of carbohydrate, starting with insulin's role in supporting muscle growth.

You see, insulin doesn't directly induce protein synthesis like amino acids do, but it *does* have anti-catabolic properties.[80] What that means is when insulin levels are elevated, the rate at which muscle proteins are broken down decreases. This, in turn, creates a more anabolic environment in which muscles can grow larger more quickly.[81]

That sounds good in theory, right? But does it pan out in clinical research? Yup. Several studies conclusively show that high-carbohydrate diets are superior to low-carbohydrate varieties for building muscle and strength.

For example, researchers at Ball State University found that low muscle glycogen levels (which are inevitable with low-carbohydrate dieting) impair post-workout cell signaling related to muscle growth.[82]

A study conducted by researchers at the University of North Carolina found that when combined with daily exercise, a low-carbohydrate diet increased resting cortisol levels and decreased free testosterone levels.[83] (*Cortisol*, by the way, is a hormone that breaks tissues, including muscle, down. In terms of maximizing muscle growth, you want low resting cortisol levels and high free testosterone levels.)

These studies help explain the findings of a study conducted by researchers at the University of Rhode Island that looked at how low- and high-carbohydrate intakes affected exercise-induced muscle damage, strength recovery, and whole-body protein metabolism after a strenuous workout.[84]

The results showed the subjects on the low-carbohydrate diet (which wasn't all that low—about 226 grams per day, versus 353 grams per day for the high-carbohydrate group) lost more strength, recovered more slowly, and showed lower levels of protein synthesis.

Similar results were demonstrated by a study conducted by researchers at McMaster University, which compared high- and low-carbohydrate dieting with subjects performing daily leg workouts.[85] They found that those on the low-carbohydrate diet experienced higher rates of protein breakdown and lower rates of protein synthesis, resulting in less overall muscle growth than their higher-carbohydrate counterparts.

So, for all of these reasons, *Bigger Leaner Stronger* doesn't involve any form of low-carb dieting. Instead, you'll eat quite a few grams of delicious carbohydrates per day, and that's going to help you get big, lean, and strong.

DIETARY FAT

Dietary fat is the densest energy source available to your body, with each gram of fat containing more than twice the calories of a gram of carbohydrate or protein (9 versus 4, respectively).

Healthy fats, such as those found in meat, dairy, olive oil, avocados, and various seeds and nuts, help your body absorb the other nutrients that you give it, nourish the nervous system, maintain cell structures, regulate hormone levels, and more.

Chemically speaking, dietary fat is composed of chains of carbon atoms that can be anywhere from 2 to 22 atoms in length. Most of the dietary fat found in the American diet is of the "long-chain" variety, with 13 to 21 carbons per molecule.

If the carbon atoms are bound together in a certain way, the result is the unsaturated form of fat, which is liquid at room temperature and found in high amounts in foods like fish, oils, and nuts.

If there are no such bonds between the carbon atoms, the result is the saturated form of fat that is solid at room temperature and found in high amounts in dairy products. While meats are generally thought of as rich in saturated fat (and red meat in particular), they contain about as much unsaturated fat as saturated.

It's also commonly believed that eating saturated fat increases your risk of heart disease. However, a panel of scientists from the University of Cambridge and Medical Research Council, University of Oxford, Imperial College London, University of Bristol, Erasmus University Medical Centre and Harvard School of Public Health recently analyzed 72 studies and more than 1 million subjects and showed this to be untrue.[86]

While we now know that saturated fat isn't the danger we once thought it was, we don't quite know what the optimal daily intake should be either. The most recent report of dietary guidelines published by the USDA (2010) maintains the 2002 recommendation that we get less than 10 percent of our daily calories from saturated fat.[87]

But researchers point out that this recommendation is based on flawed research linking saturated fat intake with heart disease, so there's a good chance this restriction will be modified in future guidelines. Until then, I recommend that you loosely follow the USDA's recommendation.

The type of fat that you want to avoid at all costs is *trans fat*. In case you don't remember, trans fat is a form of unsaturated fat not commonly found in nature. Trans fat is created artificially and added to food primarily to increase shelf life, and it's bad news. Research has associated trans fat intake with a variety of health problems: heart disease, insulin resistance, systemic inflammation, female infertility, diabetes, and more.[88] There's a reason why the Institute of Medicine recommends that our trans fat intake be "as low as possible."[89]

Many cheap, packaged foods contain trans fat, such as microwavable popcorn, yogurt, and peanut butter. So do frozen foods such as pizza, packaged pastries, cakes, and the like, and fried foods are often cooked in trans fat. Any food that contains hydrogenated oil or partially hydrogenated oil contains trans fats.

Unfortunately, avoiding trans fats isn't as simple as finding foods with labels claiming them to be trans fat free. To meet the FDA's definition of "zero grams trans fat per serving," food doesn't have to contain no trans fats—it must simply contain less than 1 gram per tablespoon, or up to 7 percent by weight, or less than 0.5 grams per serving. So, if a bag of cookies contains 0.49 grams of trans fat per serving, the manufacturer can claim it's trans fat free on the packaging.

The best way to avoid trans fats is to shun the types of foods that commonly contain them, regardless of what the nutrition facts panel says.

So, to recap, you can be quite flexible in how you get your dietary fats: dairy, meat, eggs, oils, nuts, and fish are all healthy sources. You don't have to fret over your saturated fat intake, but you should strive to get plenty of unsaturated fats in your diet as well and should eat as little trans fat as possible (I eat absolutely none).

WATER

The human body is about 60 percent water in adult males and about 70 percent in adult females. Muscles themselves are about 70 percent water.

That alone tells you how important staying hydrated is to maintaining optimal levels of health and body function. Your body's ability to digest, transport, and absorb nutrients from food depends upon proper fluid intake, and staying hydrated helps prevent injuries in the gym by cushioning joints and other soft-tissue areas.

As you can see, when your body is dehydrated, just about every physiological process is negatively affected.

To avoid dehydration, the Institute of Medicine reported in 2004 that women should consume about 91 ounces of water—or three-quarters of a gallon—per day, and men should consume about 125 ounces per day (a gallon is 128 ounces).[90]

Now, keep in mind that those numbers include the water found in food, which accounts for about 20 percent of the water in the average person's diet.

I've been drinking 1 to 2 gallons of water per day for years now, which is more than the Institute of Medicine's baseline recommendation, but I sweat a fair amount when I exercise and I live in Florida, which means even more fluid loss through sweating.

Make sure the water you drink every day is filtered and not straight from the tap. While some people assume that tap water is clean enough to drink regularly, research has shown that it is becoming more and more contaminated with all kinds of pollutants, including bacteria, pharmaceuticals, heavy metals, and various types of poisonous chemicals.[91]

Many people are already aware of this and stick to bottled water, but this isn't a great solution. Not only is it expensive, but research has also shown that bottled water is chock full of chemicals. One study examined 18 different bottled waters from 13 different companies and found more than *24,000* chemicals present, including endocrine disruptors.[92]

Martin Wagner, a scientist at Goethe University Frankfurt's Department of Aquatic Ecotoxicology, had this to say:

"Bottled water had a higher contamination of chemicals than glass bottles. There are many compounds in bottled water that we don't want to have there. Part is leaching from the plastic bottles, lids or contamination of the well." [93]

This is why I recommend investing in an effective water filtration device and why I stick to filtered water myself.

What you want to achieve with water filtration is low levels of dissolved solids in the water, as measured by an inexpensive testing device that gives a "parts per million" reading. The closer to 0, the better. (Tap water generally tests at anywhere from 200 to 700 PPM of dissolved solids.)

You can find a link to the testing device I use in the kitchen recommendations of the bonus report at the end of the book, along with my preferred filtration products.

VITAMINS AND MINERALS

Many people aren't aware of the physiological role and importance of vitamins and minerals.

Guys will rush to their local supplement stores to buy the latest super-advanced, muscle-maximizing pills and powders containing proprietary blends of fancy-sounding junk ingredients, but few of them will invest money in healthier foods or a multivitamin.

Well, the fact is that your body needs a wide variety of vitamins and minerals to perform the millions of physiological processes that keep you alive and well. This is a basic building block of optimal health and performance, just like protein, carbohydrates, fats, and water. Neglecting the nutritional aspect of dieting will, in time, severely compromise both your overall health and your performance capacity.

Ideally, we'd get all of the vitamins and minerals we need from the food we eat, but this is easier said than done. First there's the issue of the ever-declining quality of soil and food (even in the world of organic), which makes it harder to get adequate nutrition from our diets.[84] And then there's the fact that maintaining optimal levels of vitamin and mineral intake requires a bit of planned dietary diversity, which can be done but can also be time consuming.[95]

Personally, I prefer a simpler approach. I make sure the majority of my calories come from nutrient-dense foods, such as the following:

- avocados;

- greens (chard, collard greens, kale, mustard greens, and spinach);

- bell peppers;

- Brussels sprouts;

- mushrooms;

- baked potatoes;

- sweet potatoes;

- berries;

- low-fat yogurt;

- eggs;

- seeds (flax, pumpkin, sesame, and sunflower);

- beans (garbanzo, kidney, navy, and pinto);

- lentils and peas;

- almonds, cashews, and peanuts;

- whole grains, such as barley, oats, quinoa, and brown rice;

- salmon, halibut, cod, scallops, shrimp, and tuna;

- lean beef, lamb, and venison; and

- chicken and turkey.

I also supplement with a good multivitamin to fill any holes left by my diet and ensure my body gets all the micronutrients it needs.

Eating plenty of nutritious foods and supplementing with a good multivitamin takes care of all of your micronutrient needs, but I want to take a minute to discuss two minerals in particular that usually need some special attention in most people's diets: sodium and potassium.

Balancing Your Sodium and Potassium Levels

The Institute of Medicine recommends 1,500 milligrams of sodium per day as the adequate intake level for most adults and an upper limit of 2,300 milligrams per day.

Most people eat a lot more than this, however. According to the Centers for Disease Control, the average American over age two eats 3,436 milligrams of sodium per day.[96] Chronic high sodium intake not only promotes excessive water retention (making you look fatter), but it can also raise blood pressure and increase the risk of heart disease.[97]

Overconsumption of sodium is surprisingly easy too. A teaspoon of table salt contains a whopping *2,300 milligrams* of sodium. Yup, you read that right: one teaspoon of table salt per day provides you with the recommended upper limit of sodium!

Thus, I recommend that you keep an eye on your sodium intake and keep it around the Institute of Medicine's adequate intake level. I do this by just salting one meal per day (dinner).

You also want to ensure your body gets enough potassium as well, as it helps balance fluid levels in the cells (sodium sucks water in, and potassium pumps it out). According to the Institute of Medicine, we should consume sodium and potassium at about a 1:2 ratio, with 4,700 milligrams per day as the adequate intake of potassium for adults.[98]

There are many natural sources of potassium, such as all meats and fish; vegetables like broccoli, peas, tomatoes, sweet potatoes, and beans; fruits like bananas, dried apricots, avocado, and kiwi; dairy products; and nuts. You can also buy potassium tablets that you can supplement with, if necessary.

FIBER

Fiber comes in two forms: *soluble* and *insoluble*.

Soluble fiber dissolves in water and tends to slow the movement of food through the digestive system. Research has shown that soluble fiber is metabolized by bacteria in the colon, and hence it has little effect on stool weight.[99] However, it can increase fecal output by stimulating the growth of healthy bacteria and fatty acids, and it is an important source of fuel for the colon.[100]

Common sources of soluble fiber are beans and peas; oats; certain fruits like plums, bananas, and apples; certain vegetables like broccoli, sweet potatoes, and carrots; and certain nuts, with almonds being the highest in dietary fiber.

Unlike soluble fiber, insoluble fiber doesn't dissolve in water and does contribute to stool weight.[101] It bangs against the walls of the intestines, causing damage, but research has shown that this damage and the resulting repair and cellular regeneration are healthy processes.[102]

Common sources of insoluble fiber are whole-grain foods like brown rice, barley, and wheat bran; beans; certain vegetables like peas, green beans, and cauliflower; avocado; and the skins of some fruits like plums, grapes, kiwis, and tomatoes.

The importance of getting adequate fiber has been known for a long time. The ancient Greek physician Hippocrates, who famously said "let food be thy medicine, and medicine be thy food," recommended whole-grain breads to improve bowel movements.

Ensuring our fiber intake is adequate is much more important than just taking good poops though…

Fiber Intake and Cancer

A study conducted by researchers at the Institute of Social and Preventive Medicine in Switzerland found that the fiber in whole grains was associated with a reduced risk of mouth and throat cancer.[103] Refined grains had no such association because the fiber is removed during processing.

According to research conducted by scientists at Imperial College, getting adequate fiber every day may also reduce the risk of breast cancer.[104]

Fiber Intake and Heart Disease

Heart disease is the leading cause of death in the United States.[105]

This type of disease is caused by a buildup of cholesterol in the blood vessels that feed the heart (arteries), which makes them hard and narrow. This is known as *atherosclerosis*, and a total blockage of an artery produces a heart attack.

A pooled analysis conducted by researchers at the University of Minnesota analyzed the data from 10 studies to investigate the association between fiber intake and heart disease.[106] Researchers found that each 10-gram increase in daily fiber intake was associated with a 14 percent decrease in risk of all heart disease and a 27 percent decrease in risk of death from such disease.

Research conducted by scientists from Harvard University supports these findings.[107] After following 43,757 men for six years, these researchers found that as fiber intake increased, the risk of heart disease decreased.

Further research from Harvard University demonstrated that soluble fiber decreases total and LDL (bad) cholesterol levels, which helps protect against heart disease.[108]

Fiber Intake and Metabolic Syndrome

Metabolic syndrome is a combination of disorders including high blood pressure, high insulin levels, obesity (with excessive weight in the abdomen area), high levels of triglycerides (particles in the body that carry fats), and low HDL (good) cholesterol levels. Among its many obvious dangers, metabolic syndrome markedly increases the risk of heart disease and diabetes.[109]

Research conducted by scientists at Tufts University demonstrated that increasing whole grain intake reduced the risk of developing this syndrome.[110] It was found that the fiber and magnesium in the whole grains were primarily, but not wholly, responsible for these benefits.

Fiber's ability to help preserve metabolic health isn't surprising, as studies have shown that it improves blood sugar control, reduces blood pressure, decreases cholesterol levels, and can prevent weight gain and promote weight loss.[111]

Fiber Intake and Type 2 Diabetes

Type 2 diabetes is characterized by chronically high blood sugar levels and is caused by an inability to produce enough insulin to lower blood sugar levels or by cells being unable to use insulin properly.

Studies have shown that fiber reduces the risk of developing type 2 diabetes because it improves your body's ability to use insulin and regulate blood sugar levels.[112]

On the other hand, a diet low in fiber and high in simple carbohydrates has been shown to increase the risk of developing type 2 diabetes and heart disease.[113]

FIBER INTAKE AND DIVERTICULITIS

Diverticulitis is an intestinal inflammation and is one of the most common colon disorders in the Western world. It's quite painful and especially prevalent in those over 45 years of age.

Researchers at Harvard University conducted a study that followed 43,881 men, and they found that eating adequate fiber—insoluble fiber in particular—was associated with a 40 percent reduction in the risk of diverticulitis.[114]

HOW MUCH FIBER DO YOU NEED EVERY DAY?

The evidence is pretty clear: eat enough fiber, and you're more likely to live a long, healthy life.[115]

According to the Institute of Medicine, children and adults should consume 14 grams of fiber for every 1,000 calories of food eaten.[116]

Here are some easy ways to make sure you hit your daily requirement:

- Eat whole fruits instead of drinking juices.

- Choose whole-grain breads, rice, cereals, and pasta over processed forms.

- Eat raw vegetables as snacks instead of chips, crackers, or energy bars.

- Include legumes in your diet (a tasty way to do this is to cook some international dishes that use a lot of whole grains and legumes, such as Indian or Middle Eastern food).

If you'd like to see the fiber content of a wide variety of common foods, Harvard University created a handy chart that you can find here: http://bit.ly/hvd-fiber.

SUBTRACTING FIBER FROM YOUR DAILY CARBOHYDRATE INTAKE

Chances are you've heard that fiber is calorie-free and thus can be subtracted from your total daily carbohydrate intake to "free up" room for more yummy carbs.

Unfortunately, it's not that simple.

Only *insoluble* fiber can't be processed by your body and goes right through you. *Soluble* fiber turns into a fatty acid in the gut and contains somewhere between 2 and 4 calories per gram (scientists aren't sure yet).[117]

If you wanted to, you could sit down and work out how many grams of *insoluble* fiber you're eating every day and subtract that number from your daily carbohydrate intake, but in my opinion, it's not worth the trouble to find out that you can take a few extra bites of food every day.

This is also a good place to quickly address the concept of "net" or "active" or "impact" carbs, as these terms are commonly used marketing ploys to convince people they can eat all kinds of foods without having them count.

For example, a protein bar might proclaim only 4 grams of "net carbs," but when you check the nutrition facts panel, it lists 25 grams of carbohydrate and all the calories. What's up with that?

Well, the problem is that there is no legal definition for these marketing terms, and the FDA doesn't evaluate any claims using them. What most manufacturers do is take the total number of carbohydrates a product contains and subtract fiber and sugar alcohols and list that number as the net, active, or impact number.

This is misleading because most sugar alcohols contain calories (although less than the standard 4 calories per gram found in other forms of sugar), and as you now know, every gram of soluble fiber contains calories as well that can't be subtracted.

You can eat these foods if you'd like, but just count all the carbs and calories listed on the nutrition facts panel and ignore the marketing buzzwords.

THE BOTTOM LINE

You may find this chapter a bit hard to swallow (no pun intended). Some people have a hard time changing their eating habits, but the benefits of following my dietary advice far outweigh the negatives.

1. If this is a completely new way of eating for you, I guarantee you'll feel better than you have in a *long* time. You won't have energy highs and lows or feel lethargic or mentally foggy from micronutrient deficiencies or the overconsumption of simple sugars.

2. The types of proteins, carbs, and fats that you eat can have a significant impact on how you look. Eat poorly, and you can easily wind up bloated and puffy. Eat well, and you can look noticeably leaner.

3. You'll enjoy "bad" food so much more when you eat less of it. Pizza tastes so much better when you haven't had it in a week.

4. On the flip side, the more you eat nutritious foods, the more you'll come to enjoy them—I promise! Even if they don't taste too good to you at first, just groove in the routine, and soon you'll look forward to your whole grains and fruit instead of doughnuts and candy.

CHAPTER SUMMARY

INTRODUCTION

- The nutritional aspect of fitness is incredibly powerful, and it either works for or against you, multiplying or dividing your results.

- Proper nutrition boils down to supplying your body with the nutrients needed to efficiently recover from your workouts and manipulating energy intake to lose, maintain, or gain weight as desired.

- Regardless of the sources foodwise, 1 gram of protein contains 4 calories, 1 gram of carbohydrates contains 4 calories as well, and 1 gram of fat contains 9 calories.

- Many factors determine the total amount of energy that your body burns every day, such as body size, total lean mass, body temperature, the thermic effect of foods (the amount of energy it "costs" to process food for use and storage), stimulants such as caffeine, and the level of physical activity.

PROTEIN

- A high-protein diet is absolutely vital for building muscle and preserving it when you're dieting for fat loss.

- Regular exercise, and weightlifting in particular, increases your body's need for essential amino acids and thus protein.

- Your best choices are meat, dairy products, and eggs, and second to those are certain plant sources like legumes, nuts, and high-protein vegetables like peas, broccoli, and spinach.

- Protein from meat is particularly helpful when you're weightlifting, as research has demonstrated that eating meat increases testosterone levels and is more effective for building muscle than vegetarian sources.

- If you're vegetarian, while it's true that you would do better if you ate meat, don't despair—you can still do well on the program so long as you eat enough protein every day and stick to high-quality sources.

- It's hard to put an accurate cap on how much protein your body can absorb in one meal. It's definitely a hell of a lot more than the 20 to 30 grams that some people claim.

- Eating protein more frequently is likely superior to less frequently; each protein feeding should contain at least 30 to 40 grams of protein, and feedings can contain quite a bit more protein if necessary to hit daily targets.

- Whey protein can be taken anytime, but it's particularly effective as a post-workout source of protein because it's rapidly digested, which causes a dramatic spike in amino acids in the blood (especially in leucine).

CARBOHYDRATE

- Carbohydrates (in all forms) aren't stored as body fat as efficiently as dietary fats are.

- Carbohydrates play an essential role in not only muscle growth but also in overall body function.

- Monosaccharides are often called simple carbohydrates because they have a simple structure.

- Oligosaccharides are molecules that contain several monosaccharides linked together in chain-like structures.

- Polysaccharides are long chains of monosaccharides, usually containing 10 or more monosaccharide units.

- All forms of carbohydrate we eat are either metabolized into glucose or are left indigested, serving as dietary fiber.

- High, long-term intake of simple carbohydrates (disaccharides like sucrose and HFCS) has been associated with an increased risk of heart disease and Type 2 diabetes.

- Overweight, sedentary bodies don't deal with simple sugars nearly as well as lean, physically active ones do.

- If you exercise regularly and aren't overweight, your body can likely deal with simple carbohydrates just fine.

- Eating a lot of foods with added sugars can reduce the amount of micronutrients your body gets and thus cause deficiencies.

- The glycemic index (GI) is a numeric system of ranking how quickly carbohydrates are converted into glucose in the body. A GI rating of 55 and under is considered "low GI," 56 to 69 is medium, and 70 and above is high on the index.

- Get the majority of your daily carbohydrates from nutritious, unprocessed foods, which will incidentally be lower on the GI, but don't be afraid to include a few higher-GI foods that you like.

- Insulin tells the body to stop burning its fat stores and instead absorb some of the fatty acids and glucose in the blood and turn them into more body fat…but that's not what causes you to get fatter over time—overeating does.

- When protein intake is high and matched among low-carb and high-carb dieters, there is no significant difference in weight loss.

- When insulin levels are elevated, the rate at which muscle proteins are broken down decreases. This, in turn, creates a more anabolic environment in which muscles can grow larger more quickly.

DIETARY FAT

- Dietary fat is the densest energy source available to your body, with each gram of fat containing over twice the calories of a gram of carbohydrate or protein.

- Healthy fats, such as those found in meat, dairy, olive oil, avocados, and various seeds and nuts, help your body absorb the other nutrients that you give it, nourish the nervous system, help maintain cell structures, regulate hormone levels, and more.

- While we now know that saturated fat isn't the danger we once thought it was, we don't quite know what the optimal daily intake should be either. The most recent report of dietary guidelines published by the USDA (2010) maintains the 2002 recommendation that we get less than 10 percent of our daily calories from saturated fat.

- Research has associated trans fat intake with a variety of health problems: heart disease, insulin resistance, systemic inflammation, female infertility, diabetes, and more.

- The best way to avoid trans fats is to shun the types of foods that commonly contain them, regardless of what the nutrition facts panel says.

WATER

- When your body is dehydrated, just about every physiological process is negatively affected.

- The Institute of Medicine reported in 2004 that women should consume about 91 ounces of water—or three-quarters of a gallon—per day, and men should consume about 125 ounces per day (a gallon is 128 ounces).

- Make sure the water you drink every day is filtered and not straight from the tap.

VITAMINS AND MINERALS

- Your body needs a wide variety of vitamins and minerals to perform the millions of physiological processes that keep you alive and well.

- Ideally, we'd get all of the vitamins and minerals we need from the food we eat, but this is easier said than done.

- Get the majority of your calories from nutrient-dense foods.

- The Institute of Medicine recommends 1,500 milligrams of sodium per day as the adequate intake level for most adults and an upper limit of 2,300 milligrams per day. A teaspoon of table salt contains a whopping 2,300 milligrams of sodium.

- According to the Institute of Medicine, we should be consuming sodium and potassium at about a 1:2 ratio, with 4,700 milligrams per day as the adequate intake of potassium for adults.

FIBER

- The evidence is pretty clear: eat enough fiber and you're more likely to live a long, healthy life.

- According to the Institute of Medicine, children and adults should consume 14 grams of fiber for every 1,000 calories of food eaten.

- Only *insoluble* fiber can't be processed by your body and goes right through you. *Soluble* fiber turns into a fatty acid in the gut and contains somewhere between 2 to 4 calories per gram.

- Play it safe with food products that promote "net," "active," or "impact" carbs and just count all the carbs listed on the nutrition facts panel.

13

HOW TO MAXIMIZE YOUR GAINS WITH PRE- AND POST-WORKOUT NUTRITION

Most champions are built by punch-the-clock workouts rather than extraordinary efforts.
— DAN JOHN

AS YOU KNOW, WHEN YOU EAT generally doesn't matter. So long as you hit your daily numbers, you can lose fat and build muscle with ease.

That said, there are two meals that do matter: pre- and post-workout meals.

THE PRE-WORKOUT MEAL

Like most aspects of bodybuilding, the subject of pre-workout nutrition is riddled with contradictions.

Does pre-workout nutrition even matter? Should you eat protein before you train? Carbohydrates? Fats? If so, what types and amounts of food are best? Or will eating before training have no appreciable effect on your performance or results?

Well, let's get to the bottom of these questions and come to some definitive, science-based conclusions as to what's what with pre-workout nutrition.

Pre-Workout Protein

Some people say eating protein before you work out doesn't matter, and they'll often cite a study or two to back up their claims.[1] On the other hand, you can find scientific evidence that pre-workout protein *does* enhance post-workout muscle growth.[2]

What gives?

Well, a big "invisible" piece of this puzzle has to do with when study subjects had last eaten protein before eating their pre-workout meals.

You see, when you eat food, it takes your body several hours to fully absorb the nutrients contained within.[3] The larger the meal, the longer it takes (research shows that absorption can take anywhere from 2 to 6 or more hours).

This means that if you had eaten a sizable amount of protein an hour or two prior to working out, your plasma (blood) amino acid levels would be quite high come workout time, and protein synthesis rates would be maximally elevated. In this case, it's unlikely that more protein before training would make much of a difference in terms of helping you build more muscle because your body is already in an anabolic state.

On the other hand, if it had been several hours since you last ate protein, and especially if the amount you ate was small (less than 20 grams), your plasma amino acid levels would likely be low come workout time, and protein synthesis rates would be lower than they could be.

In this case, research shows that pre-workout protein likely *will* help you build more muscle because it spikes plasma amino acid levels (and thus protein synthesis rates) before training.[4]

Most people train early in the morning or several hours after lunch (after work or before dinner), and this is why I generally recommend 30 to 40 grams of protein about 30 minutes before training.

If, however, you train within 1 to 2 hours of eating at least that much protein, you can probably skip the pre-workout protein and not miss out on any extra potential muscle growth.

Regarding the best types of pre-workout protein, we know that the faster a protein is digested and the more leucine it has, the more short-term muscle growth it stimulates.[5] And while any form of pre-workout protein will elevate plasma amino acid levels, you'll get the quickest and greatest elevation from a faster-digesting form like whey protein, which is also high in leucine.[6]

Pre-Workout Carbohydrate

Fortunately for us, the research on eating carbohydrates before a workout is much more straightforward: it improves performance, period.[7]

Specifically, eating carbohydrates 15 to 30 minutes before exercise will provide your muscles with additional fuel for your workouts, but it will not directly stimulate additional muscle growth.[8]

I say *directly stimulate* because while eating carbohydrates before a workout doesn't affect protein synthesis rates, it can help you push more weight and reps in your workouts, thus indirectly helping you build more muscle over time.

So, if eating pre-workout carbs is good, what types are best?

Again, the research is pretty straightforward: low-glycemic carbohydrates are best for prolonged (2 or more hours) endurance exercise, and high-glycemic carbohydrates are best for shorter, more intense workouts.[9]

In terms of *what* to eat, I don't like pre-workout carbohydrate supplements. They're little more than overhyped, overpriced tubs of simple sugars like dextrose and maltodextrin. Don't buy into the marketing BS. There's nothing inherently special about these types of molecules other than that they're easy to digest.

Instead, I much prefer getting my pre-workout carbohydrates from food. My favorite sources are rice milk (tastes great with whey protein!) and bananas, but other popular nutritious choices are instant oatmeal, dates and figs, melon, white potato, white rice, raisins, and sweet potato.

In terms of numbers and timing, I recommend eating 40 to 50 grams of carbohydrates 30 minutes before you train to feel a noticeable improvement in your performance.

PRE-WORKOUT DIETARY FAT

Some people claim that by eating dietary fat before a workout, you can reduce carbohydrate utilization during exercise and thereby improve performance. Research has proven otherwise, however.

A study conducted by researchers at Ball State University demonstrated that increased dietary fat intake 24 hours before exercise (cycling, in this case) reduced time-trial performance compared with a high-carbohydrate diet.[10]

A study conducted by researchers from the Australian Institute of Sport demonstrated that even when your body becomes "fat adapted" and uses carbohydrates more sparingly while exercising, performance doesn't improve.[11]

Here's how researchers at Deakin University summarized their 2004 review of pre-workout fat intake literature:

"Thus, it would appear that while such a strategy can have a marked effect on exercise metabolism (i.e. reduced carbohydrate utilization), there is no beneficial effect on exercise performance."[12]

So, feel free to have dietary fat before you work out, but don't expect anything special to come out of it.

That's it for pre-workout nutrition: 30 to 40 grams of protein (and whey is best), and 40 to 50 grams of carbohydrate 30 minutes before training is all you need.

THE POST-WORKOUT MEAL

The post-workout meal is part of the "bodybuilding canon," so to speak.

If you've been lifting for any period of time, you've heard the story: if you don't eat protein and/or carbs after training, you'll either impair muscle growth or miss out on an opportunity to accelerate it.

It's also often claimed that there is a post-workout "anabolic window" of time in which you must eat your food. If you miss this window, so the story goes, you either lose or miss out on additional gains.

Well, the truth is although these dogmas are overstated, there is some truth to them.

You see, when you work out, you start a process whereby muscle proteins are broken down (technically known as *proteolysis*). This effect is mild while you're training, but it rapidly accelerates thereafter.[13] If you're training in a fasted state, proteolysis is even greater, especially at three or more hours after training.[14]

Now, muscle breakdown isn't inherently bad, but when it exceeds the body's ability to synthesize new proteins, the net result is muscle loss. Conversely, when the body synthesizes more protein molecules than it loses, the net result is muscle growth.

The goals of post-workout nutrition are minimizing post-workout muscle breakdown and maximizing protein synthesis. And similar to pre-workout nutrition, you achieve these effects by eating protein and carbohydrate after training.

Post-Workout Protein

Eating protein after a workout stimulates protein synthesis, which halts muscle breakdown and initiates muscle growth.

A study conducted by researchers at the University of Texas makes the importance of this clear.[15] Researchers had subjects perform heavy leg-resistance training followed by the slow (over the course of several hours) ingestion of a placebo, a mixture of essential and nonessential amino acids, or a mixture of just essential amino acids.

The result was the group that drank the placebo showed a negative muscle protein balance several hours after their workouts (that is, they were losing muscle), whereas the groups that ingested the amino acid mixtures showed a positive balance (they were building muscle).

We also know that post-workout protein stimulates more protein synthesis than protein eaten at rest. This was demonstrated by a study conducted by researchers at the Shriners Burns Institute.[16] They took six normal, untrained men and intravenously infused them with a balanced amino acid mixture both at rest and after a leg workout. The post-workout infusion resulted in 30 to 100 percent more protein synthesis than the at-rest infusion.

While these may seem like minor benefits, they add up over time. The more time your body spends building up proteins instead of breaking them down, the more muscle you gain as a result. Over the course of months or years, small protein synthetic advantages accrued every day can add up to several pounds of additional muscle mass.

That isn't just theory, either. Clinical research indicates that protein ingested within 1 to 2 hours of finishing a workout can indeed increase overall muscle growth over time.

For example, a study conducted by researchers from Bispebjerg Hospital had 13 untrained elderly men follow a 12-week resistance training program.[17] One group received an oral protein/carbohydrate supplement immediately post-workout, while the other received the same supplement two hours following the exercise.

The result: the post-workout ingestion group built more muscle than the two-hours-later ingestion group.

A well-designed and well-executed study conducted by scientists at Victoria University is also worth reviewing.[18] It was conducted with 23 recreational bodybuilders who followed an intense weightlifting program for 10 weeks and were divided into two groups:

1. a group that ate a protein and carbohydrate meal immediately before and after training and

2. a group that ate the same meals in the morning and evening, at least five hours outside the workouts.

After 10 weeks, researchers found that the first group (pre- and post-workout consumption) built significantly more muscle than the second group (morning and evening consumption).

So…if post-workout protein is good, the obvious question is how much should you eat?

Well, earlier in the book, I mentioned a study commonly cited in connection with post-workout protein recommendations that demonstrated that 20 grams of post-workout protein stimulates maximum muscle protein synthesis in young men.[19] That is, eating more than 20 grams of protein after working out did nothing more in terms of stimulating additional muscle growth.

We can't assume that this 20-gram number applies to everyone, however, because protein metabolism is affected by several things:

How much muscle you have.

The more you have, the more amino acids your body needs to maintain your musculature, and the more places your body can store surpluses.

How active you are.

The more you move around, the more protein your body needs.[20]

How old you are.

The older you get, the more protein your body needs to maintain its muscle.[21]

Your hormones.

Elevated levels of growth hormone and insulin-like growth factor 1 (IGF-1) stimulate muscle synthesis.[22] If your body has high levels of these anabolic hormones, it will use protein better than someone who has low levels.

On the other hand, elevated levels of cortisol reduce protein synthesis and accelerate the process whereby the body breaks down amino acids into glucose (*gluconeogenesis*), thereby reducing the amount available for tissue generation and repair. Some people have chronically elevated cortisol levels, and this impairs protein metabolism.[23]

So, while 20 grams of protein might be enough to stimulate maximal muscle growth in certain people under certain conditions, it won't be enough for everyone. Some people will need more to reach the same level of synthesis, and others will be able to benefit from more protein (it will result in more protein synthesis).

And this is why I recommend that you eat the familiar number of 30 to 40 grams of protein in your post-workout meal. The protein I use, which you can find in the bonus report, also contains additional leucine, which has been shown to further increase muscle protein synthesis over just whey protein alone.[24]

Post-Workout Carbohydrate

The most common reason we're told to eat carbs after training is to spike insulin levels, which is supposed to kick muscle growth into overdrive. This isn't entirely accurate because, as you now know, insulin doesn't tell your muscles to grow—it only has anti-catabolic properties.[25]

What *is* true, however, is that a post-workout insulin spike decreases the rate of protein breakdown that occurs after exercise.[26] And as muscle growth is nothing more than protein synthesis rates exceeding protein breakdown rates, anything that increases the former and decreases the latter improves this "equation" in our favor.

A good example of this at work is a study conducted by researchers from McMaster University that compared the effects of high- and low-carbohydrate dieting with subjects engaging in regular exercise.[27] Researchers found that subjects following the low-carb diet had increased protein breakdown rates and reduced protein synthesis rates, resulting in less overall muscle growth.

These insulin-dependent benefits level off around 15 to 30 microns per liter, or about three to four times the normal fasting insulin levels.[28] "Spiking" insulin levels higher than this doesn't deliver more "protein sparing" effects.

And it turns out that you don't even need to eat carbs to reach such a level: you can do it with protein alone. One study showed that the insulin response to the ingestion of 45 grams of whey protein peaked at about 40 minutes, and these levels were sustained for about 2 hours.[29]

If you include carbs with your post-workout meal, however, insulin levels will rise faster and remain elevated longer. One study showed that the ingestion of a mixed meal containing 75 grams carbs, 37 grams protein, and 17 grams fat resulted in an elevation of insulin levels for more than five hours.[30] (At the five-hour mark, when researchers stopped testing, insulin levels were still double the fasting level.)

So, two reasons to include carbs in your post-workout meal are to quickly raise insulin levels and keep them elevated for longer periods of time.

Another reason relates to glycogen. If you're weightlifting regularly, keeping your muscles as full of glycogen as you can is important. It improves performance, and research has shown that when muscle glycogen levels are low, exercise-induced muscle breakdown is accelerated.[31]

Anaerobic exercise like weightlifting and high-intensity interval cardio cause marked reductions in muscle glycogen stores, and when your body is in this post-workout glycogen-depleted state, its ability to use carbohydrates to replenish glycogen stores is greatly increased.[32] In this state, your muscles can "supercompensate" with glycogen, meaning they can store more than they had before the depletion.

This "supercompensation" likely won't affect your workout performance unless you engage in multiple bouts of intense exercise in the same day. So long as you eat enough carbs throughout the day, your body will eventually fill its glycogen stores back up.

That said, the post-workout depleted state *does* create a nice "carb sink," which you can use to enjoy a large number of carbs with little to no fat storage (as the body will not store carbohydrates as fat until glycogen stores are replenished).[33]

In terms of how much carbohydrate to eat in your post-workout meal, a good rule of thumb is about 1 gram per kilogram of body weight.

And in terms of when to eat the carbs, the general recommendation is "immediately after exercise." Research also shows that eating about half of the 1 gram per kilogram amount 2 hours later can help further replenish glycogen stores, but this is optional as the effects aren't nearly as pronounced as the initial post-workout meal.[34] I recommend that you include this second post-workout meal if it fits your meal planning needs but don't if it doesn't.

WHAT ABOUT CARDIO WORKOUTS?

All the above advice is for weightlifting workouts. As far as cardio workouts go, it's smart to have some protein before to counteract any potential muscle loss, but otherwise, you don't need to do anything special.

If you need to perform well (sports, for instance), then including carbs in your pre-workout meal is a good idea as well.

Post-workout protein or carbs would only be needed if the cardio were particularly long and intense (longer than 1 hour, with a fair amount of sprinting).

CHAPTER SUMMARY

- Eating protein before working out, and especially a quickly digested protein high in leucine like whey, can help you build more muscle over time. I recommend 30 to 40 grams of protein 30 minutes before training.

- Eating carbohydrate before working out, and especially a quickly digested form, will improve your performance. I recommend 40 to 50 grams of carbs 30 minutes before training.

- Eating dietary fat before working out provides no benefits.

- The goals of post-workout nutrition are minimizing post-workout muscle breakdown and maximizing protein synthesis. And similar to pre-workout nutrition, you achieve these effects by eating protein and carbohydrate after training.

- Eating protein after working out, and especially a quickly digested protein high in leucine like whey, can help you build more muscle over time. I recommend eating at least 30 to 40 grams of protein in your post-workout meal.

- Eating carbohydrate after working out, and especially a quickly digested form, raises insulin levels faster and keeps them elevated longer, which in turn keeps muscle breakdown rates low. I recommend 1 gram of carbohydrate per kilogram of body weight in your post-workout meal, which you should eat immediately after exercise.

- Research also shows that eating about half of the 1 gram of carbohydrate per kilogram amount 2 hours later can help further replenish glycogen stores, but this is optional as the effects aren't nearly as pronounced as the initial post-workout meal.

- It's smart to have some protein before a cardio workout to counteract any potential muscle loss. Post-workout protein or carbs would only be needed if the cardio were particularly long and intense (longer than 1 hour, with a fair amount of sprinting).

14

BUILD THE BODY YOU WANT EATING THE FOODS YOU LOVE
THE BIGGER LEANER STRONGER "DIET"

You are right to be wary. There is much bullshit. Be wary of me too, because I may be wrong. Make up your own mind after you evaluate all the evidence and the logic.
— MARK RIPPETOE

IN THIS CHAPTER, WE'RE GOING TO take everything you've learned about proper nutrition and turn it into a simple, easy-to-follow diet plan.

Specifically, we're going to learn how to create three types of meal plans: one for "cutting," one for "bulking," and one for "maintaining."

Cutting is "fitness speak" for feeding your body less energy than it burns every day to maximize fat loss while minimizing muscle loss.

Bulking refers to feeding your body slightly more energy than it burns every day so as to maximize muscle growth. You also gain body fat while bulking.

Maintaining refers to feeding your body the energy it burns every day, which enables you to make slow muscle gains without adding any fat.

Most people have heard how energy balance relates to fat loss, but few know how it also relates to muscle growth.

For example, did you know that restricting calories hinders your body's ability to build muscle, while eating a slight surplus of calories maximizes it?

Every day, our muscle cells go through a natural process whereby degraded cells are eliminated and new cells are created to take their place. Under normal health and dietary circumstances, muscle tissue is fairly stable, and the cycle of cellular degradation and regeneration remains balanced.[1] That is, the average person doesn't lose or gain muscle at an accelerated rate; his or her lean mass more or less remains level. (Well, unless we train our muscles, we slowly lose lean mass as we age, but you get the point.[2])

When we engage in resistance training, we damage the cells in our muscle fibers, and this signals the body to accelerate the normal rate of protein synthesis to repair the large number of damaged cells.[3]

When you restrict your calories, however, your anabolic hormone levels drop, and your body's ability to synthesize proteins becomes impaired.[4] That is, a calorie deficit blunts your body's ability to fully repair the damage you cause to your muscles through exercise. This is why it's also easier to overtrain when you're in a calorie deficit.

This is why you generally can't build muscle efficiently while restricting calories for fat loss—something often referred to as "body recomposition" and often pitched as the new school of bodybuilding.

The people selling the body recomp will usually say that bulking and cutting doesn't work or is old hat and that anyone and everyone can get big and lean simultaneously by following some fancy type of diet or exercise routine.

Well, they're lying.

The only people who can effectively (and naturally) build muscle and lose fat simultaneously are newbies who have a fair amount of fat to lose and people who used to be in great shape and are now getting back at it ("muscle memory" allows you to rapidly regain muscle you once had).[5]

If you're an experienced weightlifter who has already built a fair amount of muscle, however, you won't be able to build any appreciable amount of muscle while restricting your calories for fat loss. No matter what type of diet or training protocol you use. Period. Your goal while cutting is to *preserve* muscle, not gain it.

The "big secret" of experienced, accomplished weightlifters who are able to build muscle and strength while getting lean is…drugs. Lots and lots of drugs.

So, don't become one of the many guys who spin their wheels for years chasing the "recomp," jumping from one fad workout and diet to next, with little to show for it in the end.

What does that leave, though? If we can't recomp our way into the ideal physique, how do we get there?

By bulking and cutting. *Properly.*

You see, there's validity in some of the popular critiques of this approach. It's true that many of the bulking programs you can find on the Internet are flawed in various ways, namely improper training that doesn't result in much muscle growth, excessive overeating that results in rapid fat storage, and improper cutting that burns away too much muscle.

These programs result in cycles of bulking and cutting that go like this: gain some muscle and a bunch of fat while bulking, strip away fat and muscle while cutting, look exactly the same as the starting point.

This is incredibly common and frustrating, and it gives bulking and cutting a bad name. It's not inevitable, though—it's simply the result of bulking and cutting *incorrectly.* If you know what you're doing, however, you can build significant amounts of muscle while bulking without adding thick layers of fat and retain *all* of your muscle while cutting, shedding only the excess pounds.

Proper bulking starts with understanding that when you raise your calorie intake and take your body out of a deficit, your anabolic hormone levels rise, and your body's ability to synthesize proteins is restored to normal levels.

This is why bulking involves eating slightly more energy than you're burning but *not* eating everything under the sun, moon, and stars, which leads to excessive fat storage. This not only makes you look like a big, bloated mess, but it also makes it easier to get fatter and impairs muscle growth.

You see, as body fat levels rise, insulin sensitivity drops, which means that cells become less responsive to insulin's signals.[6] As the body becomes more insulin resistant, its ability to burn fat decreases, and the likelihood of storing carbohydrates as fat increases.[7] Furthermore, insulin resistance suppresses intracellular signaling responsible for protein synthesis, which means less total muscle growth.[8]

Research has also shown that as we get fatter, our free testosterone levels drop and estrogen levels rise.[9] As testosterone plays a vital role in the process of muscle building, and high levels of estrogen promote fat storage, the downsides of these consequences are clear.[10]

The reality is that excessive weight gain during a "dirty" or "dreamer bulk," which involves eating obscene amounts of food every day, is incredibly counterproductive. It gets in the way of muscle growth and makes subsequent efforts to get rid of the excess body fat even harder.

This is why I always recommend that guys don't bulk if they're over 15 percent body fat and that they end their bulks once they reach 15 to 17 percent and begin cutting (as this is where the above problems start to kick in). Then, once they've reached the 10 percent body fat range, they're ready to bulk again and add more muscle to their physiques.

If you're not sure how to determine your body fat percentage, most experts agree that hydrostatic and DEXA X-ray are the most accurate methods. The downside, however, is inconvenience and cost.

Therefore, I recommend that you get a good fat caliper. The one I recommend in the bonus report at the end of this book is inexpensive and accurate to within 1 percent.

Now, let's shift gears and talk about two other types of people I commonly run into: the small, relatively lean guy who's a bit too worried about putting on some body fat while bulking properly, and the guy who wants to get *really* lean as the first order of business.

The trap the first guy is likely to fall into is simple: he chronically undereats and then usually makes strength gains in the gym but fails to add any real size. Eventually, he quits out of frustration.

Don't make this mistake. If you're gaining strength but not size, you're not eating enough. And some guys need to eat a *lot* to make steady progress on the scale. I've worked with 170-pound guys who had to eat more than 4,000 calories per day just to gain 0.5 to 1 pound per week!

And the relatively lean guy who wants to get shredded first? Well, even if he's new to lifting and can build some muscle while losing fat, it won't be enough to keep him from looking absolutely scrawny at the 7 to 8 percent body fat range.

What many guys don't realize is how much visual size you lose once you get below 10 percent. The body fat that you're stripping "pads" all your muscles, making them look larger, and unless you have considerable actual lean mass, you just look small.

This is why I recommend that you juggle your cuts and bulks to remain in the 10 to 15 to 17 percent body fat range until you reach a point where you're absolutely satisfied with your overall size at 10 percent, and *then* cut below this point. In fact, many guys (including me) find that they need to reach a point where they feel they're too big at 10 percent to have the look they want at 7 percent.

So, that's the theory of bulking, cutting, and maintaining. Let's now get into the dietary numbers and details of how to do each.

Earlier in the book, you learned how to calculate your BMR and TDEE and then later learned some basic guidelines on how you should break those calories down into daily macronutrient targets.

I also said that I was going to simplify the whole affair for you and give you easy formulas to follow. Well, this is where we get to that simplification.

Before we get to the numbers, I want to note that you shouldn't add or subtract from your total calorie intake based on the exercise you do in the program. The formulas I give below assume that you will be doing four to six hours of exercise per week, which is what the program calls for.

If you're going to be doing significantly more or less exercise than this, you can start with the formulas and adjust up or down based on how your body responds (which we'll talk more about in the sections below).

So, let's look at cutting, bulking, and maintaining separately.

CUTTING 101:
HOW TO EAT FOR MAXIMUM FAT LOSS

Cutting requires a bit more dietary precision and compliance than bulking and maintaining because if you overeat a bit on a bulk or maintenance diet, you still gain muscle and weight. Overeat on a cut, though, and you can quickly get stuck in a rut.

You're looking to lose between 0.5 and 1 pound per week when cutting, and if that sounds low to you, remember that weight loss that is too rapid is undesirable as it means you're losing a fair amount of muscle as well as fat.

If you have quite a bit of fat to lose, you may find you lose upward of 2 to 3 pounds per week for the first few weeks, and that's fine. As time goes on, though, you should see it slow down to a rate of 0.5 to 1 pound lost per week.

Calculating Your Cutting Diet

When you cut, you will first calculate a starting point and adjust as needed. Here's where you start:

- 1.2 grams of protein per pound of body weight per day,

- 1 gram of carbs per pound of body weight per day, and

- 0.2 grams of fat per pound of body weight per day.

For a 200-pound male, it would look like this:

- 240 grams of protein per day,

- 200 grams of carbs per day, and

- 40 grams of fat per day,

This would be about 2,120 calories per day, which is a good starting point for a 200-pound guy looking to lose weight.

If you're over 25 percent body fat, your formula is slightly different:

- 0.8 grams of protein per pound of body weight per day,

- 0.6 grams of carbs per pound of body weight per day, and

- 0.3 grams of fat per pound of body weight per day.

For a 250-pound guy, it would look like this:

- 200 grams of protein per day,

- 150 grams of carbs per day, and

- 80 grams of fat per day.

This also comes to about 2,120 calories per day, which is where a 250-pound man with a body fat percentage greater than 25 percent would want to start. (Remember that the more body fat you have to lose, the larger of a deficit you can safely place yourself in.)

If you're extremely obese—over 30 percent body fat—then I recommend that you work out your BMR as discussed earlier in this book and do the following:

1. Multiply it by 1.2. This will be your daily calorie intake.

2. Get 40 percent of those calories from protein, 30 percent from carbohydrates, and 30 percent from dietary fat.

    Here's how you figure this out:

    a. Multiply your total daily calorie intake by 0.4, and divide the resulting number by 4. This is how many grams of protein you will eat every day.

    b. Multiply your total daily calorie intake by 0.3, and divide the resulting number by 4. This is how many grams of carbohydrate you will eat every day.

    c. Multiply your total daily calorie intake by 0.3, and divide the resulting number by 9. This is how many grams of dietary fat you will eat every day.

    For example, if your total daily calorie intake is 2,200, here's how this looks:

    (2200 x 0.4) / 4 = 220 grams of protein per day
    (2200 x 0.3) / 4 = 165 grams of carbohydrate per day
    (2200 x 0.3) / 9 = 73 grams of dietary fat per day

General Cutting Recommendations

While overeating is the more common mistake when cutting, some people tend to undereat. If taken too far, this can be worse than overeating because it can cause significant muscle loss.

During your first week or two of cutting, you can expect to be a little hungry at times and to run into some cravings. This doesn't mean that you're losing muscle or that anything else is wrong. It just comes with the territory, but it passes after a few weeks. A proper cut is *not* supposed to be a grueling test of your will.

When I'm cutting, I try to be within 50 calories of my daily target. Some days I'm a little higher and some a little lower, but I don't have any major swings in my intake.

Stick to lean sources of protein, and you won't have trouble putting together a meal plan that works. If your protein sources contain too much fat, you're going to find it hard to keep your calories where they need to be with proper macronutrient ratios.

After seven to ten days of sticking to your cutting diet, you should assess how it's going. Weight loss isn't the only criterion to consider when deciding if your diet is right or wrong, however.

You should judge your progress based on the following criteria:

- your weight (did it go down, go up, or stay the same?),

- your clothes (do they feel looser, tighter, or the same?),

- the mirror (do you look thinner, fatter, or the same?),

- your energy levels (do you feel energized, tired, or somewhere in between?),

- your strength (is it going up, going down, or staying about the same?), and

- your sleep (are you exhausted by the end of the night, do you have trouble winding down, or has nothing changed?).

Let's talk about each point briefly.

Your Weight

Generally speaking, if your weight is going up on a cut, you're eating too much or moving too little.

The exception, however, is when someone is new to weightlifting as he not only builds muscle while losing fat, which adds weight, but his muscles also suck up quite a bit of glycogen and water, which can easily add a few pounds in the first month.

Considering that you generally lose about 1 pound of fat per week, you can see how the fat loss can be obscured on the scale.

So, if you're new to weightlifting and starting with a cut, I recommend tracking your waist measurement along with your weight for the first four to six weeks. If your waist is shrinking, you're losing fat, regardless of what the scale shows.

In time, your muscles' glycogen and water levels will stabilize. While you can continue building muscle while losing fat, you'll eventually lose more fat (in pounds) each week than you gain in muscle, resulting in net weight loss over time.

If you're a more experienced weightlifter, however, and your weight is remaining the same after several weeks of cutting, you're likely just eating too much or moving too little.

Your Clothes

Your waist measurement (at the navel) shrinking is a reliable sign that you're losing fat, so if your jeans are loosening, that's a reliable indicator of fat loss.

Your Mirror

Although it can be tough to observe changes in our bodies when we see them every day, you should definitely notice a visual difference after several weeks of cutting. You should look leaner and less puffy.

If you don't, chances are your weight hasn't changed either or has gone up, and your jeans aren't feeling looser. This is a clear sign that something is off, and it's time to reassess your food intake or exercise schedule.

Your Energy Levels

You should never feel starved and running on empty when cutting. Depending on how you ate before starting the cut, you may feel a little hungry for the first week or two, but after that, you should feel comfortable throughout the day.

We all have high- and low-energy days, but if you're having more lows than usual, then chances are you're not eating enough or are relying on too many high-glycemic carbohydrates.

Your Strength

If you're new to weight training and start with cutting, you can expect to make strength gains.

If you're an experienced weightlifter, however, it's normal to lose a few reps across the board when cutting, but you shouldn't be squatting 30 pounds less by the end of the first week. If your strength drops by a considerable amount, chances are, you're undereating and need to increase your food intake.

Your Sleep

If you're dead tired by bedtime, that's not necessarily a bad sign. It's common when people start training correctly.

What's important, however, is that you sleep long and deeply. If your heart is beating quickly at night and you're anxious, tossing and turning in bed, and if you wake up more often at night, you might be overtraining or undereating.

THE DANGER OF HIDDEN CALORIES

A huge, killer diet trap that many people fall into is eating a lot of "hidden calories" throughout the day. Then they wonder why they aren't losing weight.

Hidden calories are those that you don't realize are there and account for, such as the following:

- the 2 tablespoons of olive oil used to cook your dinner (240 calories),

- the 2 tablespoons of mayonnaise in your homemade chicken salad (200 calories),

- the 3 cubes of feta cheese on your salad (140 calories),

- the 3 tablespoons of cream in your coffee (80 calories), and

- the 2 pats of butter with your toast (70 calories).

These "little" additions add up every day and are by far the number-one reason why people fail to get results from what would otherwise be a proper dietary regimen. There just isn't a large margin for error when you're trying to maintain a moderate calorie deficit every day.

For example, let's say you're looking to maintain a 500-calorie deficit every day to lose about a pound of fat per week, but you accidentally eat 400 more calories than you should have, leaving you in a 100-calorie deficit instead. It'll now take a month or longer to lose that pound of fat. It's that simple.

It might seem paranoid to be careful about how many tablespoons of ketchup you have in a day, but if you watch your calories that closely when cutting, you're *guaranteed* to get results.

The best way to avoid hidden calories is to prepare your food yourself so you know exactly what went into it. For most people, this just means preparing a lunch to bring to the office, as they usually eat breakfast and dinner at home.

ADJUSTING YOUR NUMBERS

If your weight has remained the same for seven to ten days and you haven't gotten any leaner, and you've stuck 100 percent to your numbers, you simply need to move more or reduce your calorie intake.

My first choice is always "move more," but you can only do so much exercise. I recommend doing no more than five 60-minute weightlifting and four 30-minute cardio sessions per week. This is quite a bit, and any more will place too much stress on the body when you're in a calorie deficit.

If you're already doing that much exercise and you're not getting leaner, then you need to reduce your daily calorie intake. You do this by removing 25 grams of carbs from your daily numbers (cutting your daily intake by 100 calories) and then give this new intake seven to ten days and reassess.

It's worth noting that you don't want to reduce intake below your BMR, as this can cause too much metabolic slowdown. In case you don't remember, here's how you calculate your BMR:

$$BMR = 370 + (21.6 * LBM \text{ [lean body mass in kg]})$$

This answers the question of how long you can cut for: you can cut until your intake reaches BMR, but don't reduce your intake lower than that.

If you're doing the maximum amount of exercise recommended, you have gradually reduced your intake to your BMR, and your weight loss has stalled but you want to keep losing fat, first you will need to speed your metabolism back up. You do this by slowly increasing your food intake back up to your TDEE, at which point you can flip back to a normal deficit and continue to lose fat.

This is known as "reverse dieting," and it's something I talk more about in the sequel to this book, *Beyond Bigger Leaner Stronger*, which was written for more advanced weightlifters. Reverse dieting is more relevant to the experienced and well-developed weightlifter looking to get to the 6 to 8 percent body fat range while retaining strength and lean mass than the beginner looking to build muscle and get to the 10 percent range, but you should know about it nonetheless.

Last but not least, let's talk about how to eat on the days when you're not lifting or exercising at all. In the case of cutting, it's simple: keep your numbers the same. You don't need to adjust up or down.

BULKING 101:
HOW TO EAT FOR MAXIMUM MUSCLE GAINS

As you know, if you're in the 10 to 12 percent body fat range and looking to put on muscle as quickly as possible, you want to bulk.

Yes, you'll gain some fat along the way, but if you do it right, it won't be excessive, and it'll come off easily once you're ready to cut.

Based on my experience working with thousands of people, the average guy on a proper bulk will gain muscle and body fat at a ratio of about 1:1 (1 pound of fat gained for every pound of muscle.

In terms of weight gain while bulking, you want to see your weight going up at a rate of 0.5 to 1 pound per week. Any more than that, and you'll be gaining too much fat.

If you're new to weightlifting, however, then you'll probably gain 2 to 3 pounds per week for the first few weeks while your muscles fill up with water and glycogen. This doesn't mean you're gaining too much fat, and you should see this number settle into the 0.5 to 1-pound range within your first four to six weeks on the program.

When you have your bulk dialed in, you should be increasing reps on your major lifts every week and weight on the bar every three to four weeks.

Calculating Your Bulking Diet

As you know, a proper bulking diet requires that you eat more calories than you burn every day. While this sounds like a great idea now, don't be surprised if you get sick of eating "all of this food" at some point along the way. You won't be slamming down thousands of extra calories every week like some programs would have you doing, but even slight overfeeding over time can get a little uncomfortable.

You can also expect to hold more water than normal, as you'll be eating a substantial amount of carbohydrate every day. This makes you look kind of "puffy." Again, it's just part of the "price" you have to pay for optimizing muscle growth.

So, let's get to the actual dietary numbers for bulking. Here's where you start:

- 1 gram of protein per pound of body weight per day,

- 2 grams of carbs per pound of body weight per day, and

- 0.4 grams of fat per pound of body weight per day.

That's where you start. For a 150-pound guy, it would look like this:

- 150 grams of protein per day,

- 300 grams of carbs per day, and

- 60 grams of fat per day.

This would be about 2,340 calories per day (remember that protein and carbs contain about 4 calories per gram and fat contains about 9), which is the right place to start bulking for a 150-pound man.

Chances are these numbers are lower than other recommendations you've seen on the Internet. That's because many bulking programs out there are just overkill. They put you in a huge calorie surplus with the explanation that you have to "eat big to get big."

Well, while it's true you have to eat more than you normally would to maximize muscle growth, you don't have to eat nearly as much as some would have you believe.

GENERAL BULKING RECOMMENDATIONS

When I'm bulking, I try to be within 100 calories of my daily target, and I err on the high side (it's better to be over your target than under).

Don't think of a bulk as a license to eat whatever you want whenever you want it, as this will inevitably lead to excessive overeating and thus excessive fat storage, which will slow down your gains in the long run.

You can have a cheat meal every week, but keep it moderate. We'll talk about why soon, but a high-protein, high-carbohydrate cheat meal is preferable to a high-fat one.

I recommend eating plenty of meat while bulking because it's particularly effective for building muscle. Generally speaking, I eat two servings of meat per day (lunch and dinner) and alternate between various types such as ground turkey, chicken, lean beef, and fish.

ADJUSTING YOUR NUMBERS

The numbers given in the formula above are *starting points*, and there's a chance that you will need to eat more to effectively gain strength and muscle (especially if you have an ectomorphic body that is naturally skinny and lean). Part of the game is finding your body's "sweet spots" for bulking, cutting, and maintaining.

Fortunately, this is easy to do. Most guys will find their sweet spots to be within 10 to 15 percent of the targets they originally calculated, but some need to eat more to steadily gain weight (it's rare for a guy to gain fat too quickly on the above recommendations and have to reduce intake).

So, if, after seven to ten days, your weight hasn't gone up despite pushing yourself hard in your workouts, you're just not eating enough. Increase your daily intake by 100 calories (by adding more carbs, preferably) and reassess over the next seven to ten days. If this doesn't result in weight gain, increase again and repeat the process until you're gaining weight at a rate of about 0.5 to 1 pound per week.

If you're like most guys, here's how it's going to go: you're going to start with the above formula and gain weight for the first month or two, and then you're going to stall. You then will increase your daily intake once or twice and start gaining again. At some point, you'll probably stall again, increase again, and start gaining again. After a bit more progress, your body fat percentage will eventually reach the 15 percent range, and you'll have a month or so left to bulk before you cut to strip away the fat and repeat the process.

You can reduce your calories to a maintenance level on your rest days if you want, or you can stick to your bulking numbers. The small reduction won't make a difference in terms of overall fat storage, but some guys like to take a break from all the eating a couple of days per week.

MAINTENANCE 101:
HOW TO EAT FOR SLOW AND STEADY "LEAN GAINS"

Maintenance refers to eating more or less how much energy you burn on a daily or weekly basis and is recommended for when you want to maintain a certain level of body fat while still being able to make slow gains in the gym.

Generally speaking, guys switch to maintenance if they want to stay lean through a certain time period like summer or if they've achieved the overall body composition they want and are looking to simply maintain that look (me, for example).

If neither of those circumstances describes your current needs, don't bother with maintenance. You should be bulking and cutting until you're happy with your size and overall development and *then* you use a maintenance diet to stay lean.

Don't think of "maintaining" as "staying the same," though. I think you should always have the goal of getting at least a little stronger every month, and most guys always want to get a little bigger in certain areas of their body. For me, I'd like a little more shoulders, calves, and lats, for instance. Always set goals and be looking to improve. Don't just try to stay the same, because things tend to either get better or get worse.

Generally speaking, I like to see 0.25 to 0.5 pounds gained per month when maintaining, depending on how lean I'm trying to stay.

For example, if I maintain a very lean 6 to 7 percent body fat, I find that I can't eat enough to gain much muscle and thus may only see my weight go up about 0.25 pounds per month; in some months, it may not change at all. On the other hand, if I maintain 8 to 9 percent body fat, I'm able to eat more food every day and have seen closer to 0.5 pounds per month in gains.

As you can see, when maintaining, your weight is less of an immediate indicator of progress than when cutting or bulking. Your strength progression is, though—you should see a steady increase in reps and weight over time.

You should also notice little positive changes in the mirror and in how your clothes fit; your shirts should be getting tighter as well as the upper leg areas of your pants.

You can still cheat once per week when maintaining so long as you don't go overboard. If you do go too far in your cheating, I recommend that you reduce your intake to a cutting level for a few days to lose the little bit of fat you'll have gained.

CALCULATING YOUR MAINTENANCE DIET

Here's your starting point for maintenance:

- 1 gram of protein per pound of body weight per day,

- 1.6 grams of carbs per pound of body weight per day, and

- 0.35 grams of fat per pound of body weight per day.

For a 180-pound male, it would look like this:

- 180 grams of protein per day,

- 290 grams of carbs per day, and

- 63 grams of fat per day.

That's about 2,450 calories per day, which should work for making slow, steady muscle and strength gains with little to no body fat added along the way.

ADJUSTING YOUR NUMBERS

Dietary formulas are never one-size-fits-all. Part of proper dieting is learning what ranges work best with your body, and this applies to maintaining as much as cutting and bulking.

The good news is that this is simple. If your weight and body fat are rising too quickly, you're overeating, either daily or in your weekly cheat meal(s), or you need to add some exercise to your routine.

If overeating is the culprit, reduce your daily intake by 100 calories by reducing your daily carbohydrate intake by 25 grams. See how your body responds over the next seven to ten days. If your weight stabilizes and your training is still good, you stay there. If your weight still increases too quickly, reduce again and reassess. Chances are you won't need to do this at all, but if you do, one or two adjustments are all it should take. On the other hand, if your weight is going down and you're getting leaner, you're in a calorie deficit and need to eat more to come out of it. Remember that while getting leaner is always gratifying, your body's ability to build muscle is dramatically reduced when in a calorie deficit.

I should also warn you of a trap many people trying to maintain fall into: they severely overeat two to three days per week and then have to go into a deficit the rest of the week to undo the damage. This is fine for maintaining a certain body composition but does *not* work well if you also want to progress in the gym. This will stick you in a rut every time.

If you go slightly over your normal intake one day, you can go slightly under the next day and it balances out. Don't get too sloppy though, dramatically overeating one day and undereating the next. Maintenance is a bit more relaxed than bulking and cutting, but you still want a relatively steady, balanced intake to ensure you continue progressing in your training.

FLEXIBLE DIETING 101: MEAL PLANNING MADE EASY

You're going to love me for this section of the book.

This is where I get to tell you that you get to more or less eat whatever you want to reach your daily macronutrient targets.

As you know, I recommend that you stick to nutritious foods, but beyond that, there are no rules besides *hit your numbers every day.* Do you like starchy carbs? Great, eat them every day. How about whole grains? Awesome, me too. Dairy products? They're a staple in my diet. Red meat every day? Why not. A little bit of dessert after dinner? I *recommend* it.

Now, some people abuse this dietary freedom and try to eat as much junk food as possible while staying within their numbers. While this technically "works" for the sole purpose of building muscle and losing fat, the inevitable micronutrient deficiencies get in the way of your performance and thus your long-term gains (not to mention your health).

Just because you can eat a box of Pop Tarts every day and lose weight doesn't mean you should. Sure, our bodies can use McDonald's burger patties to build muscle (to some degree, at least), and we could use flexible dieting to eat them every day, but is it worth the potential health risks associated with regular consumption of low-quality meat?[11]

I don't think so. Being shredded doesn't matter if your hormone profile is whacked, your immune system is overwhelmed, and your body is starving for nutrients.

So, here are some good rules of thumb for your meal planning:

> *Get at least 80 percent of your daily calories from healthy (micronutrient-dense) foods that you like.*

One of the biggest problems people run into when dieting is they get to a point where they just can't stomach chicken and steamed veggies anymore, and one taste of something savory leads to an all-out binge.

Well, the best way to avoid this is to simply eat foods that you like every day.

For instance, if you would rather have a steak than chicken, work it into your meal plan (adjust for the additional fat). If you would like some whole-wheat pasta (low-GI, great source of fiber), adjust your meals for the day to allow for it. If some whole-fat Greek yogurt would hit the spot, cut out the olive oil or cheese on your lunch salad to fit it in.

Don't be afraid of little indulgences.

So long as the vast majority of your daily calories come from healthy foods full of micronutrients, feel free to include some treats if you so desire.

For instance, if you love chocolate, work some into your numbers for the day. If you've been eyeing that exquisite gelato for a couple of days now, don't be afraid to make room for 100 or so calories' worth after dinner.

Personally, I get about 90 to 95 percent of my daily calories from relatively unprocessed, nutritious foods, but I'm not afraid to work in a a bit of sugar or "junk" here and there.

MEAL PLANNING 101: HOW TO MAKE ENJOYABLE, EFFECTIVE MEAL PLANS

You now know how to work out your calorie and macronutrient targets based on your goals and so that you get to enjoy foods you actually like. The last step is learning how to turn those numbers into a meal plan that you can follow every day.

And thanks to the amount of flexibility you have in both the foods you eat and when you eat them, this is easy to do. Let's quickly recap the things to keep in mind:

- Be within 50 to 100 calories of your target number depending on what you're doing with your diet (cutting or bulking).

- Get the majority of your calories from nutrient-dense foods listed earlier in the book:
  - avocados;
  - greens (chard, collard greens, kale, mustard greens, and spinach);
  - bell peppers;
  - Brussels sprouts;
  - mushrooms;
  - baked potatoes;
  - sweet potatoes;
  - berries;
  - low-fat yogurt;
  - eggs;
  - seeds (flax, pumpkin, sesame, and sunflower);
  - beans (garbanzo, kidney, navy, and pinto);
  - lentils and peas;
  - almonds, cashews, and peanuts;
  - whole grains, such as barley, oats, quinoa, and brown rice;
  - salmon, halibut, cod, scallops, shrimp, and tuna;
  - lean beef, lamb, and venison; and
  - chicken and turkey.
- Eat foods you like.

- Don't be afraid to include a little treat every day.

- Eat as many or few meals per day as you'd like, although I recommend eating every 3 to 4 hours as you'll probably find this most enjoyable.

- Eating protein more frequently is likely superior to less frequently, and each protein feeding should contain at least 30 to 40 grams of protein.

- Eat 30 to 40 grams of protein and 40 to 50 grams of carbohydrate 30 minutes before training.

- Eat 30 to 40 grams of protein and 1 gram of carbohydrate per kilogram of body weight after your weightlifting workout.

- Consider eating 0.5 grams of carbohydrate per kilogram of body weight 2 hours after your weightlifting workout.

Those are the rules. Let's now look at the process of making a meal plan.

First, I recommend making a long list of nutritious foods that you like and that you could eat every day. You can break them up into breakfast foods, snack foods (mainly quick and easy sources of protein and carbs, like Greek yogurt, cottage cheese, nuts, fruit, and so forth), and lunch and dinner foods.

You should make these lists in a spreadsheet on your computer with separate sheets for each meal type and then columns for food, amount, protein, carbohydrate, fat, and calories, like this:

FOOD	AMOUNT	PROTEIN	CARBS	FAT	CALORIES
Oatmeal	1/2 cup	3	14	2	83

Build these lists out using www.calorieking.com or caloriecount.about.com to look up the various foods you like.

Once you're happy with your food lists, it's time to start making the actual meal plan. As you know, the primary goal is to end up within 50 calories of your target numbers.

I like to make my meal plans in a spreadsheet as well, and I lay it out like this (this was an actual cutting meal plan of mine):

MEAL	FOOD	PROTEIN	CARBS	FATS	CALS
1	1 cup rice milk	1	25	2	122
1	1 banana	1	25	0	104
1	1 scoops protein	24	3	1	117
2	2 scoops protein	48	6	2	234
2	1 banana	1	25	0	104
2	2 cups rice milk	1	56	2	246
3	4 tbs PB2	8	12	2	98

MEAL	FOOD	PROTEIN	CARBS	FATS	CALS
3	English muffin	1	25	1	113
3	Jelly	0	18	0	72
4	4.5 oz meat	30	0	4	156
4	veggies	1	10	0	44
4	dressing	0	0	8	72
5	1 scoop protein	30	5	0	140
5	4.5 oz meat	30	0	3	147
5	veggies	1	20	0	84
5	carbs	1	50	0	204
5	dessert	2	40	10	258
6	1 cup greek yogurt	23	10	5	177
supps	fish oil	0	0	8	72
TOTALS		203	330	48	2564

I use formulas to calculate the "CALS" and "TOTALS" automatically so I can easily see how things are looking as I play with the various foods and meals.

I start by entering my pre- and post-workout nutrition numbers, as these are "fixed." For me, that's meals 1 and 2 above (1 is pre-workout and 2 is post-workout).

Once you have your pre- and post-workout nutrition in place, you have free rein to "spend" your macronutrients however you please. If you like a big breakfast, put it together and see what that leaves you for the rest of the day. If you prefer a light morning and a big lunch or dinner, go that route and see how it looks.

As you can also see in my example above, I have entries for "meat," "veggies," "carbs," and "dessert" because I switch them around daily based on what I feel like eating. One day my veggies might be peas, the next green beans, the next a medley of peppers and mushrooms, and so forth. I just have simple options worked out for my allotment of "veggie carbs."

You may have also noticed that I included fish oil in my meal plan. Don't forget to account for the calories in any supplements you take.

As you play with foods and your numbers, you'll quickly see what works and what doesn't. For example, extremely fatty foods generally don't work because they eat up too much of your daily allotment of dietary fat in one go. Most people will find it more enjoyable to eat a variety of lower fat foods throughout the day than one high-fat meal that leaves them with little fat left for everything else.

On the following pages, you'll find several examples of custom meal plans my team has created for our clients.

BULKING PLAN FOR 150LBS MALE

MEAL	FOOD	CALORIES	PROTEIN	CARBS	FAT
BREAKFAST (1)	2 Sweet Potato Protein Pancakes from The Shredded Chef	358	24	59	3
	1 tablespoon syrup	52	0	13.4	0
	1 tablespoon butter	102	0	0	11.6
	multivitamin, 3g fish oil	30	0	0	3
TOTAL	MEAL 1	542	24	72.4	17.6
LUNCH (2)	2 slices whole grain bread	160	8	28	0.2
	100g extra lean 5% fat ham	107	23.2	0	1.3
	lettuce, mustard, tomato, hot sauce (if desired)	10	0	2.5	0
	1 tablespoon mayo	90	0	0	10
TOTAL	MEAL 2	367	31.2	30.5	11.5
PRE WORKOUT SNACK (3)	1 scoop whey (I recommend Legion Whey+)	100	22	2	0
	1 medium banana	105	1.3	27	0.4
	pre-workout	5	0	1	0
TOTAL	MEAL 3	210	23.3	30	0.4

WEIGHTLIFTING

MEAL	FOOD	CALORIES	PROTEIN	CARBS	FAT
POST WORKOUT SHAKE (4)	1 scoop whey	100	22	2	0
	300ml rice milk	152	1.3	31.7	2.5
	2 medium bananas	210	2.6	54	0.8
	1 tablespoon peanut butter	94	4	3.2	8.1
	5g creatine	0	0	0	0
TOTAL	MEAL 4	556	29.9	90.9	11.4
DINNER (5)	100g chicken breast, trimmed of fat	107	23.2	0	1.3
	200g (cooked) whole wheat pasta	249	10.7	53.1	1.1
	100ml tomato pasta sauce	96	1.9	16.3	1.9
	2 tablespoons Parmesan cheese	42	3.8	0.4	2.8
	30g milk chocolate	159	2.1	18	9
	3g fish oil	30	0	0	3
TOTAL	MEAL 5	683	41.7	87.8	19.1
	TOTALS	2358	150.1	311.6	60
	TARGET	2340	150	300	60

BULKING PLAN FOR 175LBS MALE

MEAL	FOOD	CALORIES	PROTEIN	CARBS	FAT
BREAKFAST	1 scoop whey (I recommend Legion Whey+)	105	22	2	0
	1 cup whole milk	150	8	12	8
	1/2 cup blueberries	42	0.6	10.5	0.3
	1/4 cup (measured dry) old fashioned oats	75	2.5	13.5	1.5
	multivitamin, 3g fish oil, fiber	30	0	0	3
TOTAL	**MEAL 1**	**402**	**33.1**	**38**	**12.8**
SNACK	2 slices whole grain bread	160	8	28	0.2
	2 tablespoons peanut butter	188	8	6.3	16.1
	1 tablespoon jam	56	0.1	13.8	0
TOTAL	**MEAL 2**	**404**	**16.1**	**48.1**	**16.3**
LUNCH	4 ounces chicken breast, trimmed of fat	120	26	0	1.5
	1/2 cup (measured dry) basmati rice	300	6	66	1
	3 ounces vegetables (cauliflower, asparagus, zucchini, string beans, onions. cucumbers, carrots)	29	2.4	5.6	0.3
	1/2 tablespoon butter	51	0	0	5.8
	lemon juice, cilantro (if desired)	10	0	2.5	0
TOTAL	**MEAL 3**	**510**	**34.4**	**74.1**	**8.6**
DINNER	4 ounces chicken breast, trimmed of fat	120	26	0	1.5
	8 ounces sweet potato	195	3.5	45.7	0.2
	3/4 cup peas	88	5.9	15.8	0.5
	1/2 tablespoon butter	51	0	0	5.8
	cinnamon for potato (if desired)	4	0	1	0
	3g fish oil, multivitamin	30	0	0	3
TOTAL	**MEAL 4**	**488**	**35.4**	**62.5**	**11**
PRE WORKOUT SHAKE	1 scoop whey	105	22	2	0
	1 cup rice milk	120	1	25	2
	pre-workout	5	0	5	0
TOTAL	**MEAL 5**	**230**	**23**	**32**	**2**

WEIGHTLIFTING

MEAL	FOOD	CALORIES	PROTEIN	CARBS	FAT
POST WORKOUT SHAKE	1 scoop whey	100	22	2	0
	1 cup rice milk	120	1	25	2
	2 large bananas	242	3	62	0.9
	2 tablespoons peanut butter	188	8	6.3	16.1
	creatine	0	0	0	0
TOTAL	**MEAL 6**	**650**	**34**	**95.3**	**19**
	TOTALS	**2684**	**176**	**350**	**69.7**
	TARGET	**2730**	**175**	**350**	**70**

MUSCLE
FOR LIFE

CUTTING PLAN FOR 200LBS MALE

MEAL		FOOD	CALORIES	PROTEIN	CARBS	FAT
1	BREAKFAST	5 egg whites	85	18	1	0.5
		2 tablespoons salsa (if desired)	10	0	2.5	0
		40g (measured dry) old fashioned oats	150	5	27	3
		cinnamon, stevia, nutmeg, vanilla extract (if desired)	10	0	1.3	0
		1 scoop whey (I recommend Legion Whey+)	100	22	2	0
		250ml almond milk (unsweetened)	30	1	1	2.5
		vitamins	0	0	0	0
	TOTAL	MEAL 1	385	46	34.8	6
2	PRE WORKOUT SHAKE	2 scoops whey protein	210	44	4	1
		250ml almond milk (unsweetened)	30	1	1	2.5
		1 medium apple	95	0	25.1	0
		2 tablespoons peanut butter	188	8	6.3	16.1
		pre-workout	5	0	5	0
	TOTAL	MEAL 2	528	53	41.4	19.6

WEIGHTLIFTING

MEAL		FOOD	CALORIES	PROTEIN	CARBS	FAT
3	LUNCH	200g shrimp	214	46.4	0	2.7
		250g (cooked) brown rice	257	5.1	54.8	1.7
		100g steamed vegetables (broccoli, cauliflower, asparagus, bell pepper, string beans, carrots, onions)	34	2.8	6.6	0.3
		creatine	0	0	0	0
	TOTAL	MEAL 3	505	54.3	61.4	4.7
4	DINNER	250g chicken breast	268	58	0	3.3
		200g white potato	155	2.8	36.3	3
		side salad (60g spinach, 1/2 carrot, 1/2 cucumber, 1 stalk celery)	47	2.4	6	0.3
		2 tablespoons balsamic vinegar	20	0	4	0
		1 teaspoon butter	34	0	0	3.9
	TOTAL	MEAL 4	524	63.2	46.3	10.5
5	SNACK	200g 0% Greek yogurt	118	21.2	8.2	0
		100g strawberries	28	0	7.2	0
	TOTAL	MEAL 5	146	21.2	15.4	0
		TOTALS	2088	237.7	199.3	40.8
		TARGET	2120	240	200	40

CUTTING PLAN FOR 220LBS MALE

MEAL	FOOD	CALORIES	PROTEIN	CARBS	FAT
PRE WORKOUT	pre-workout	5	0	1	0
	Recommended: 10g BCAAs (needed for fasted training)	0	0	0	0
	Recommended: yohimbine (for fasted training)	0	0	0	0
TOTAL	MEAL 1	5	0	1	0

WEIGHTLIFTING

MEAL	FOOD	CALORIES	PROTEIN	CARBS	FAT
BREAKFAST	2 High Protein Banana Oatcakes from The Shredded Chef	351	31	45	6
	1/4 cup blueberries	21	0	5.3	0
TOTAL	MEAL 2	372	31	50.3	6
LUNCH	6 ounces chicken breast	180	39	0	2.3
	salad (2 cups spinach, 1/2 carrot, 1/2 cucumber, 1/2 medium tomato)	54	2.9	8.4	0.5
	2 cup balsamic vinegar	20	0	4	0
TOTAL	MEAL 3	254	41.9	12.4	2.8
SNACK	1 slice whole grain bread	80	4	14	0.1
	2 tablespoons peanut butter	188	8	6.3	16.1
	1 scoop whey (I recommend Legion Whey+)	105	22	2	0.5
	1 cup almond milk (unsweetened)	30	1	1	2.5
TOTAL	MEAL 4	403	35	23.3	19.2
DINNER	6 ounces sirloin, trimmed of fat	228	38.4	0	6.6
	6 ounces potato	131	3.4	29.7	0.2
	2 tablespoons sour cream	60	1	1	5
	1 tablespoon butter	102	0	0	11.6
	3 ounces vegetables (broccoli, cauliflower, asparagus, zucchini, string beans, bell peppers, carrots, onions)	29	2.4	5.6	0.3
TOTAL	MEAL 5	550	45.2	36.3	23.7

HIIT CARDIO

MEAL	FOOD	CALORIES	PROTEIN	CARBS	FAT
SNACK	6 ounces 2% Greek yogurt	150	20	8	4
	stevia (if desired)	0	0	0	0
	15 almonds	104	3.8	3.9	9
TOTAL	MEAL 6	254	23.8	11.9	13
	TOTALS	1838	176.9	135.2	64.7
	TARGET	1826	176	132	66

If you'd like to get some help with your meal planning, you can learn more about my custom meal plan service at www.muscleforlife.com/mp.

HOW TO "CHEAT" WITHOUT RUINING YOUR DIET

Many people struggling with diets talk about "cheat days." The idea is that if you're good during the week, you can go buck wild on the weekends.

Well, unless you have a *very* fast metabolism, that's not how it works. If you follow a strict diet and exercise program, you can expect to lose 1 to 2 pounds per week. And if you get too crazy with your cheating, you can gain it right back (and more!) over a weekend. And if you're bulking, you can gain double the fat you normally would have that week.

There are much smarter ways to go about cheating.

First, I want you to think in cheat *meals*, not *days*. No sensible diet should include entire days of overeating, but a single bout of moderate overeating every week is advisable when you're dieting to lose weight.

Why?

Well, there's the psychological boost, which keeps you happy and motivated, which ultimately makes sticking to your diet easier.[12]

There's also a physiological boost, but it's not the metabolic boost that you might be thinking. Yes, studies on overfeeding (the scientific term for bingeing on food) show that doing so can boost your metabolic rate by anywhere from 3 to 10 percent, but this doesn't mean much when you consider that you would need to eat anywhere from a few hundred to a few thousand extra calories in a day to achieve this effect, thus negating the metabolic benefits.[13]

The psychological effect we're after relates to the hormone *leptin*, which regulates hunger, your metabolic rate, appetite, motivation, and libido, among many other functions.[14]

When you're in a caloric deficit and lose body fat, your leptin levels drop.[15] This, in turn, causes your metabolic rate to slow down, your appetite to increase, your motivation to wane, and your mood to sour.

When you give your leptin levels a dramatic boost, however, this can have positive effects on fat oxidation, thyroid activity, mood, and even testosterone levels.[16]

Eating carbohydrates is the most effective way to raise leptin levels, eating protein is moderately effective, eating dietary fat has little to no effect on leptin levels, and drinking alcohol lowers them.[17]

Thus, a good cheat meal is a high-protein, high-carbohydrate, low-fat, and alcohol-free meal that doesn't put you in a large calorie surplus for the day.

It's totally fine to end the day a few hundred calories over your normal intake, but you're going to have problems if you eat 1,000+ more calories than you burned for the day, especially when a large percentage of those surplus calories came from dietary fat. Add in some alcohol, which will not only blunt leptin production but will also accelerate the storage of the dietary fat as body fat, and you can undo a nice chunk of your week's progress in one meal.[18]

CONSIDER "REFEEDING" INSTEAD OF CHEATING

Another enjoyable way to get a psychological break from your diet and boost leptin levels is the "Refeed Day."

It's simple. Here's how it works:

Take your current daily calorie intake and increase it by 30 percent. This will provide enough of a surplus to confer the benefits of refeeding without adding too much body fat.

Next, break the calories into the following macronutrient profile:

- 1 gram of protein per pound of body weight,

- as little dietary fat as possible (most recommendations call for 20 grams or fewer for the day), and

- the rest from carbohydrate.

This is your macronutrient target for your Refeed Day. For example, I recently finished a cut at 187 pounds, eating about 2,200 calories per day. Here's how my Refeed Day looked:

- Calorie target: 2,900

- 190 grams of protein

- 15 to 20 grams of fat (incidental in other foods)

- 500 grams of carbohydrate

In case you're wondering how I calculated 500 grams of carbohydrate, I simply subtracted the calories from my protein and fat (760 and 135, respectively) from 2,900, giving me 2,000, and divided the sum by 4 to convert the calories into grams of carbohydrate.

And in case you're wondering how I possibly followed these numbers, I got my protein from chicken, protein powder, and 0 percent fat Greek yogurt and my carbs from fruit, potato, sweet potato, whole-wheat pasta, and pancakes.

I recommend planning your refeed on a day that's followed by a training day. Many guys plan it for the day before they train their lagging muscle group(s) because the boost in carbs results in higher energy in the gym.

The net effect of a refeed is that you feel better both physically and psychologically, you're much less likely to give in to temptations and set yourself back, and you can even experience a nice acceleration of fat loss over the following 3 to 5 days.

That said, there's a caveat: the refeed requires self-control.

If you abuse these controlled bouts of overfeeding, then you will simply gain too much fat as a result to make them effective weight-loss aids.

If you'd rather not refeed, however, and would prefer to stick to one moderate cheat meal per week, that's totally fine. Go to your favorite restaurant, eat your favorite high-carb dish, have some dessert, and enjoy knowing that it's not getting in the way of achieving your goals.

THE BOTTOM LINE

Dieting is much easier and enjoyable than most people think. While eating whatever you want whenever you want doesn't work, with a little creativity and forethought in your meal planning, you can make an infinite variety of meals that you look forward to every day.

You shouldn't feel overly stuffed or starved, deprived, or stressed out about what you should or shouldn't or can and can't eat, and it shouldn't take more than minor adjustments of intake and exercise to keep your body progressing toward your ultimate goals.

CHAPTER SUMMARY

INTRODUCTION

- *Cutting* is "fitness speak" for feeding your body less energy than it burns every day to maximize fat loss while minimizing muscle loss. Generally speaking, you can't build muscle when you're cutting.

- *Bulking* refers to feeding your body slightly more energy than it burns every day so as to maximize muscle growth. You also gain body fat while bulking.

- *Maintaining* refers to feeding your body the energy it burns every day, which enables you to make slow muscle gains without the adding any fat.

- Restricting calories hinders your body's ability to build muscle, and eating a slight surplus of calories maximizes it.

- The only people who can effectively (and naturally) build muscle and lose fat simultaneously are newbies who have a fair amount of fat to lose and people who used to be in great shape and are now getting back at it ("muscle memory" allows you to rapidly regain muscle you once had).

- I recommend that you juggle your cuts and bulks to remain in the 10 to 17 percent body fat range until you reach a point where you're absolutely satisfied with your overall size at 10 percent, and *then* cut below this point.

CUTTING

- You're looking to lose between 0.5 and 1 pound per week when cutting, and if that sounds low to you, remember that rapid weight loss is undesirable as it means you're losing a fair amount of muscle as well as fat.

- If you have quite a bit of fat to lose, you may find you lose more than 2 to 3 pounds per week for the first few weeks, and that's fine. As time goes on, though, you should see it slow down to a rate of 0.5 to 1 pound lost per week.

- During your first week or two of cutting, you can expect to be a little hungry at times and to run into some cravings. This doesn't mean that you're losing muscle or that anything else is wrong.

- When I'm cutting, I try to be within 50 calories of my daily target. Some days I'm a little higher and some a little lower, but I don't have any major swings in my intake.

- Generally speaking, if your weight is going up on a cut, you're eating too much or moving too little.

- Your waist measurement (at the navel) shrinking is a reliable sign that you're losing fat, so if your jeans feel looser, that's a good sign.

- Although it can be tough to observe changes in our bodies when we see them every day, you should definitely notice a visual difference after several weeks of cutting. You should look leaner and less puffy.

- We all have high- and low-energy days, but if you're having more lows than usual, then chances are you're not eating enough or are relying on too many high-glycemic carbohydrates.

- If your strength drops considerably, chances are you're undereating and need to increase your food intake.

- If your heart is beating quickly at night and you're anxious, tossing and turning in bed, and if you wake up more often at night, you might be overtraining, or undereating.

- The best way to avoid hidden calories is to prepare your food yourself so you know exactly what went into it.

- If your weight has remained the same for seven to ten days and you haven't gotten any leaner, and you've stuck 100 percent to your numbers, you simply need to move more or reduce your calorie intake.

- You don't want to reduce intake below your BMR as this can cause too much metabolic slowdown.

BULKING

- As you know, if you're in the 10 to 12 percent body fat range and looking to put on muscle as quickly as possible, you want to bulk.

- Based on my experience working with thousands of people, the average guy on a proper bulk will gain muscle and body fat at a ratio of about 1:1 (1 pound of fat gained for every pound of muscle).

- In terms of weight gain while bulking, you want to see your weight going up at a rate of 0.5 to 1 pound per week. Any more than that, and you'll be gaining too much fat. If you're new to weightlifting, however, then you'll probably gain 2 to 3 pounds per week for the first few weeks while your muscles fill up with water and glycogen.

- When you have your bulk dialed in, you should be increasing reps on your major lifts every week and weight on the bar every 3 to 4 weeks. You can also expect to hold more water than normal, as you will eat a substantial amount of carbohydrate every day.

- When I'm bulking, I try to be within 100 calories of my daily target, and I err on the high side (it's better to be over your target than under).

- Don't think of a bulk as a license to eat whatever you want whenever you want it. As you know, this will result in rapid fat storage, which will slow down your gains in the long run.

- You can have a cheat meal every week, but keep it moderate. Remember that a high-protein, high-carbohydrate cheat meal is preferable to a high-fat one.

- I recommend eating plenty of meat while bulking because it's particularly effective for building muscle. Generally speaking, I eat two servings of meat per day (lunch and dinner) and alternate between various types such as ground turkey, chicken, lean beef, and fish.

- You can reduce your calories to a maintenance level on your rest days if you want, or you can stick to your bulking numbers.

- If, after seven to ten days, your weight hasn't gone up despite pushing yourself hard in your workouts, you're just not eating enough. Increase your daily intake by 100 calories (by adding more carbs, preferably) and reassess over the next seven to ten days. If this doesn't result in weight gain, increase again and repeat the process until you're gaining weight at a rate of about 0.5 to 1 pound per week.

MAINTENANCE

- You should be bulking and cutting until you're happy with your size and overall development and then you can use a maintenance diet to stay lean.

- Generally speaking, I like to see 0.25 to 0.5 pounds gained per month when maintaining, depending on how lean I'm trying to stay.

- You can still cheat once per week when maintaining so long as you don't go overboard. If you do, I recommend that you reduce intake to a cutting level the next day or two to lose the little bit of fat you'll have gained.

MEAL PLANNING

- I recommend sticking to nutritious foods, but beyond that, there are no rules besides hit your numbers every day.

- Get at least 80 percent of your daily calories from healthy (micronutrient-dense) foods that you like.

- So long as the vast majority of your daily calories come from healthy foods full of micronutrients, feel free to include some treats if you so desire.

- Eat as many or few meals per day as you'd like, although I recommend eating every 3 to 4 hours as you'll probably find this most enjoyable.

- Eating protein more frequently is likely superior to less frequently, and each protein feeding should contain at least 30 to 40 grams of protein.

- Eat 30 to 40 grams of protein and about 40 to 50 grams of carbohydrate 30 minutes before training.

- Eat 30 to 40 grams of protein and 1 gram of carbohydrate per kilogram of body weight after your weightlifting workout.

- Consider eating 0.5 grams of carbohydrate per kilogram of body weight 2 hours after your weightlifting workout.

- I like to make my meal plans in a spreadsheet, and I use formulas to calculate the "CALS" and "TOTALS" automatically so I can easily see how things are looking as I play with the various foods and meals.

- Once you have your pre- and post-workout nutrition in place, you have free rein to "spend" your macronutrients however you please.

- Don't forget to account for the calories in any supplements you take.

- If you'd like to get some help with your meal planning, you can learn more about my custom meal plan service at www.muscleforlife.com/mp.

CHEATING

- If you follow a strict diet and exercise program, you can expect to lose 1 to 2 pounds per week. And if you get too crazy with your cheating, you can gain it right back (and more!) over a weekend. And if you're bulking, you can gain double the fat you normally would have that week.

- I want you to think in cheat meals, not days. No sensible diet should include entire days of overeating, but a single bout of moderate overeating every week is advisable when you're dieting to lose weight.

- A good cheat meal is a high-protein, high-carbohydrate, low-fat, and alcohol-free meal that doesn't put you in a large calorie surplus for the day.

REFEEDING

- The net effect of a refeed is that you feel better both physically and psychologically, you're much less likely to give in to temptations and set yourself back, and you can even experience a nice acceleration of fat loss over the following 3 to 5 days.

- I recommend that you plan your refeed on a day that's followed by a training day. Many guys plan it for the day before they train their lagging muscle group(s) because the boost in carbs results in higher energy in the gym.

- The refeed requires self-control. If you abuse these controlled bouts of overfeeding, then you will simply gain too much fat as a result to make them effective weight-loss aids.

15

HOW TO EAT HEALTHY FOODS ON A BUDGET

Don't measure yourself by what you have accomplished, but by what you should have accomplished with your ability.
— JOHN WOODEN

BY GETTING THE MAJORITY OF YOUR calories from nutritious foods, you'll enjoy improved energy levels, immune health, cognitive performance, and a general sense of well-being. And anecdotally speaking, the guys I know with the best physiques are "clean" eaters, getting only a small portion of their daily calories from "unhealthy" indulgences.

The benefits of eating nutritious foods aren't news to anyone, though. Willpower aside, there's another major problem people trying to eat healthily wrestle with: cost.

According to research conducted by scientists from the University of Washington, eating healthfully can cost up to *10 times* as much as living off cheap, heavily processed "junk food."[1]

Sure, a good argument can be made to eat mainly organic foods, but it costs an arm and a leg. Eating too many low-quality, highly processed meats poses serious health risks, but finding healthy, affordable alternatives can be tough.[2] Thus, it's no surprise that many people think that eating healthfully requires that you blow half your paycheck on groceries every week.

Well, fortunately, eating well doesn't have to be as expensive as you might think. With a little forethought, you can pack your meal plans full of nutritious foods without breaking the bank.

CHEAP SOURCES OF HEALTHY PROTEIN AND FAT

No matter what your goal is with your body, it's going to require eating a lot of protein. And this can add up quickly.

Here are my favorite high-quality, affordable types of protein.

EGGS

Eggs are one of the best all-around sources of protein, with about 6 grams per egg, and they are also a great source of healthy fats.

Eggs also have several health benefits, such as reducing the risk of thrombosis and raising blood concentrations of two powerful antioxidants, lutein and zeaxanthin.[3]

Oh, and if you're afraid that the cholesterol in eggs will increase your risk of heart disease, this myth has been thoroughly debunked by both epidemiological and clinical research.[4]

With an average price of about $0.20 per egg, or $2 per dozen, they're hard to beat in terms of nutrition and price.

Chicken Breast

There are several reasons why fitness-minded people eat so much chicken: it's cheap, high in protein, and low in fat.

And while it's true that poultry's omega-6 and -3 ratios are out of whack (about 10:1, whereas beef is about 2:1), we can easily handle any fatty acid imbalances by supplementing with fish or krill oil or eating fatty fish like salmon, tuna, trout, herring, sardines, or mackerel.

A pound of chicken breast has about 100 grams of protein and will cost you about $3.50.

Almonds

Almonds are by far my favorite type of nut. They're delicious and nutritious, with a handful (about 15) weighing in at 9 grams of healthy fat, 4 grams of protein, and just under 4 grams of carbs. Like eggs, they have also been associated with various health benefits, such as a reduced risk of diabetes and lower body weight.[5]

Almonds cost about $0.50 per ounce (25 to 30 nuts), making them easy to fit into any budget. They're great by themselves and go well in cold cereals like granola or muesli and hot cereals like oatmeal.

However, my favorite way to eat them is to buy freshly ground almond butter. It's delicious by itself, but it shines when you combine it with fruits like bananas or apples.

Low-Fat Cottage Cheese

You can buy a ½-cup serving of low-fat cottage cheese for less than a dollar, and you get 14 grams of protein and only 1 gram of fat.

I think it tastes great with just a dash of salt and pepper, but I also like it with fruit, such as pineapple or berries.

Protein Powder

Many people are surprised to learn that protein powder can be cost efficient.

For instance, my naturally sweetened, 100 percent whey isolate protein (which you can learn more about at the end of the book) costs about $18 per pound. That's about 400 grams of the highest-quality whey protein for $18!

Avocado

Avocadoes are a great source of dietary fat and of monounsaturated fat in particular (one avocado contains about 15 grams), which has been associated with better cholesterol levels,[6] a reduced risk of cardiovascular disease, and improved brain function.[7] On top of that, avocadoes are full of cancer-fighting phytochemicals.[8]

You can do more with them than just make guacamole, as well—they go great with eggs, soups, and salsas.

Although the prices fluctuate due to seasonal highs and lows in both demand and production, they usually range between $1 to $2 per fruit.

CHEAP SOURCES OF HEALTHY CARBS

The most popular forms of carbohydrate here in the United States are processed junk foods, which, as you know, can pose serious health risks if consumed too regularly for too long.[9] On the other hand, the regular intake of nutritious carbohydrates has been associated with a reduced risk of chronic disease.[10]

Here are my favorite sources of cheap, healthy carbs:

OATS

One cup of dry steel cut oats packs just over 50 grams of carbs, 10 grams of protein, and 6 grams of fat.

You can buy it in bulk for about $1 per pound, and it's a great source of medium-GI carbohydrate and dietary fiber. Research has also demonstrated that oats can reduce levels of LDL ("bad") cholesterol.[11]

"Oatmeal in a bowl" is a staple in many bodybuilders' diets, but you can even substitute blended oats for flour when baking or use them as breadcrumbs or breading for spicing up chicken dishes.

BLACK BEANS

Black beans are an awesome source of carbohydrates as well as protein, potassium, calcium, folic acid, and fiber.

One cup of these beans contains about 40 grams of carbs, 15 grams of protein, and 1 gram of fat, and you can buy them for about $1 per can, or in bulk (dry) for even less.

Boil them up, and they make a great side to any protein dish, but they're also perfect for making soups and dips.

BROWN RICE

Like oatmeal, brown rice is a go-to food for the fitness-minded, and for good reason.

You can pick it up dirt cheap—around $2 per pound—and one cup provides close to 45 grams of carbs, 5 grams of protein, and 2 grams of fat. Brown rice has nearly four times the fiber as white rice as well as more vitamins, minerals, and other beneficial micronutrients.

QUINOA

It might be hard to pronounce (keen-wah), but it's easy to prepare, extremely tasty, cheap (about $4 per box), and full of healthy protein and carbs.

One cup of dry kernels has a 110 grams of carbs, 24 grams of protein, and 10 grams of fat, and it can be prepared in the same ways as brown rice.

FRUIT

You can't go wrong with fruit. My favorite choices are grapes, apples, bananas, and oranges, which are full of a variety of antioxidants, vitamins, minerals, and fibers, and which range between $0.60 and $1.50 per pound.

If you're worried that the fructose in fruit might be bad for your health, though, you can rest easy. You'd have to eat an absolute ridiculous amount of fruit every day to ever have a problem.

According to a meta-analysis of clinical trials evaluating fructose intake, 25 to 40 grams of fructose per day has no negative impact on our health.[12] That's 3 to 6 bananas, 6 to 10 cups of strawberries, 10 to 15 cherries, or 2 to 3 apples per day. Or, as the old advice goes, a few servings of fruit every day.

Problems with fructose intake are only seen among those who regularly eat large amounts of refined sugars, like HFCS or sucrose.

For instance, a 20-ounce bottle of soda sweetened with HFCS contains about 35 grams of fructose. One gram of sucrose is about half glucose, half fructose, so if you eat a dessert with 50 grams of sugar, you're getting about 25 grams of fructose. Even agave nectar, which is touted as healthy by many due to its low-glycemic properties, can be as high as 90 percent fructose. Other less processed forms can be as low as 55 percent.

The bottom line is that you can avoid all the health complications associated with fructose intake by limiting your intake of foods with added sugars like agave, sucrose, honey, maple syrup, raw sugar, molasses, brown sugar, HFCS, turbinado sugar, and on and on.

Sweet Potato

Sweet potatoes can hit the spot when you want something sweet and nutritious. They're extremely tasty when prepared well (salt, cinnamon, pumpkin spice, and a little bit of butter is my jam), and they're in the middle of the glycemic index and full of vitamin A and other micronutrients.

One cup of mashed sweet potato provides you with about 60 grams of carbs, 4 grams of protein, and less than 1 gram of fat. And at a paltry cost of about $1 per pound, you can't afford to *not* include sweet potato in your meal plans.

THE BOTTOM LINE

So there you have it: it *is* possible to eat healthfully without maxing out your credit cards.

In fact, you may even *save* money if you use a few other tricks like buying frozen veggies, buying in bulk, paying attention to sales and what's in and out of season, and preparing your food in batches so you can use everything you buy.

And let's not forget that the ultimate value of eating well—longevity, vitality, and disease-free living—is hard to put a price tag on.

Now, I know this section of the book has given you a *lot* to process, but I have good news: you've learned just about everything you'll ever need to know about dieting. You'll never struggle with building muscle or losing fat again if you just follow the principles and advice I've shared. Feel free to reread this section of the book to let everything sink in.

Let's now move on to the subject of training and learn how to get the most out of our time in the gym every day.

SECTION IV:

TRAINING

16

THE BIGGER LEANER STRONGER TRAINING PHILOSOPHY

Far too many bodybuilders spend too much time exercising the smaller muscle groups such as the biceps at the expense of the larger muscle groups such as the thighs, and then they wonder why it is that they never make gains in overall size and strength.
— RORY "REG" PARK

TOO MANY OF THE TRAINING PROGRAMS touted in the magazines and infomercials are essentially the same: lots of machines, lots of isolation exercises, lots of reps with little weight, and lots of time in the gym.

These programs are better than nothing, I suppose, but that's about the only compliment I can pay them. There are just *vastly* superior ways to spend your time and energy if your goal is to build a physique, not just move your body.

Ironically, machines became a staple of gyms not because they're particularly effective or even safe, but because they're inviting. They don't look nearly as intimidating as dumbbells, bars, and plates.

Well, while a small number of machines are worth using, such as the leg press machine or cable setup, the vast majority are inferior to dumbbell and barbell exercises in terms of producing bigger, stronger muscles. This includes the Smith machine, which has been proven to be less effective for squatting and bench pressing than the free weight barbell squat and bench press.[1]

Therefore, the *Bigger Leaner Stronger* program will focus on free weights and not on machines.

We've already talked about the inferiority of isolation exercises, but you're probably wondering why they're so popular among bodybuilders, whose lives revolve around sculpting every last muscle fiber in their bodies for competitive shows. Many of those guys are freakishly huge, and if that's how they train, there must be something to it right? I mean hell, if we could just get one-third as big as them, we'd be happy.

Well, there's more to the story.

Here's what it boils down to: every professional bodybuilder going anywhere in the sport is on drugs. A *lot* of drugs. Like $50,000 to $100,000 of drugs per year. Yes, every single one, regardless of what they say.

And while there are different schools of thought as to the optimal style of training when you're on drugs, many chemically enhanced lifters have success just sitting in the gym for hours every day doing set after set after set with relatively light weights.

You see, thanks to the drugs they're on, their bodies are able to synthesize muscle proteins at alarmingly high rates, and this alone allows them do a lot of things with their training and diets that just wouldn't work if they were natural.

The big problem with focusing on isolation exercises is that the average guy needs to build a strong overall foundation of strength and muscle, not gain an extra half inch on his rear delts or extend his lats an inch lower down his torso.

There's only one way to build that base naturally: you have to do a lot of heavy, compound weightlifting. And even then, it takes a couple of years to gain the 25 to 35 pounds of muscle that takes a guy from "normal" to "ripped."

That's why the *Bigger Leaner Stronger* program is built around heavy, lower-rep weightlifting and compound exercises like the squat, deadlift, military press, bench press, and many others.

Emphasizing heavy weightlifting is the only way to continue to progressively overload your muscles, and compound exercises like those listed above give you the most bang for your buck— the most total-body strengthening and conditioning for the time and effort spent.

The *Bigger Leaner Stronger* training program follows a formula that looks like this:

$$1\text{--}2 \mid 4\text{--}6 \mid 9\text{--}12 \mid 3\text{--}4 \mid 60\text{--}65 \mid 5\text{--}7 \mid 8\text{--}10$$

No, that isn't a secret code that you have to break. Let's go through this formula one piece at a time.

1-2
TRAIN 1 TO 2 MUSCLE GROUPS PER DAY

To achieve maximum overload and muscle stimulation, you will train one or two muscle groups per workout (per day).

While upper/lower and full-body splits can work if programmed correctly, they come with several drawbacks.

The first is the fact that training multiple major muscle groups in one workout is *very hard* when you're focusing on heavy, compound weightlifting. When you do six sets of heavy chest pressing and then try to move on to heavy shoulder pressing, you simply won't lift as much as you would if you saved your shoulder work for another day.

By training only one or two muscle groups per day, you'll be able to give your workouts 100 percent focus and intensity and train hard without struggling through the systemic and muscular fatigue that comes with trying to do too much in a workout.

Training several major muscle groups in one workout also takes a lot of time. I used to do long, 1.5 to 2-hour workouts and, quite frankly, didn't look forward to many of them. I'm now in and out in no more than an hour and find that much more enjoyable, which helps me stick with the program for the long haul.

4–6
DO SETS OF 4 TO 6 REPS FOR NEARLY ALL EXERCISES

You knew I was going to have you lifting a lot of heavy weight, and here's what it comes down to: working in the 4- to 6-rep range for nearly all exercises (we'll go over the exceptions soon).

This means that you're going to be using weights that allow for at least 4 reps but no more than 6 reps (if you can't get 4 reps, it's too heavy; if you can get 6 or more, it's too light). Generally speaking, this is about 85 percent of your 1RM for each exercise.

You won't be doing burnout sets, supersets, drop sets, or anything else but controlled, heavy sets. Leave the light weight, muscle confusion routines to the amateurs, and it will only be a matter of time before they come to you, baffled as to how you're gaining so much by doing "so little."

The emphasis of heavy, compound weightlifting is a vitally important aspect of the program and is the "heart" of the whole training approach. It's also one of the more "controversial" recommendations in the book as the "optimal" rep range for muscle growth is still a subject of heated debate rather than scientific certainty.

That said, I didn't choose this rep range willy-nilly—it's based on a considerable amount of both clinical and anecdotal evidence, and before we go on, I'd like to share some of that here so you have a better understanding as to why I don't recommend the more traditional "hypertrophy" rep range of 10 to 12 reps.

A large review of weightlifting studies was published in 2007 by researchers from Goteborg University, and it contained two key findings for our purposes:

1. Training with weights between 70 percent and 85 percent of 1RM produced maximum hypertrophy in subjects, although lower and higher loads also produced marked results.

2. A moderate training volume of 30 to 60 reps per workout produced maximum hypertrophy in subjects. As the load decreased, the optimal number of reps increased (that is, the lighter the weights you're using, the more reps you want to do to maximally stimulate muscle growth).[2]

The American College of Sports Medicine published a paper in 2002 that, based on the study of hundreds of subjects, concluded that training with weights that allowed no more than 5 to 6 reps is most effective for increasing strength and that resting up to 3 minutes in between sets is optimal when training in this fashion.[3]

Researchers from Arizona State University reviewed 140 other weightlifting studies and concluded that training with weights that are 80 percent of your 1-rep max produces maximal strength gains.[4]

Yet another sign of the effectiveness of lifting heavy weights is found in a study published by scientists from Ohio University, who had 32 untrained men lift weights for eight weeks.[5] They were split into three groups: one worked in the range of 3 to 5 reps, another in the range of 9 to 11 reps, and the last in the range of 20 to 28 reps. By the end of the eight-week period, the group working in the 3- to 5-rep range made significantly more gains in both strength and muscle than the other two groups.

Now, if you're well read in the fitness world, you've undoubtedly come across studies with findings contrary to those above. For instance, there are at least two studies I know of commonly used to sell people on the belief that lifting light weights is as effective in building muscle as lifting heavy weights, so long as you train to failure.

There are major problems with these findings, however, because they don't jibe with real-world observations.

Namely, the people who have built impressive physiques using high-rep "burnout" training almost *always* were chemically enhanced at some point along the way. And on the flip side, nearly every person you'll meet who has built a strong, muscular body naturally will have done it by focusing on heavy weightlifting. They may now maintain their physique with higher-rep training, but they didn't *get there* with it.

I went through this with my own body. Nearly eight years of grueling high-rep training got me no more than 25 to 30 pounds of lean mass, with at least half of that coming in the first three years. Eventually, I sunk into a rut and made no real gains to speak of for several years.

I was able to progress again by applying what I'm teaching you in this book: lifting heavy weights and regulating and balancing my food intake. Since making these changes, my strength has exploded, and my physique has dramatically changed—I've increased my weights on every lift by 50 to 100 percent and went from about 197 pounds at 16 percent body fat to my current 187 pounds at 7 percent, which I maintain with ease.

I've also had the opportunity to work directly with thousands of people, and the results are the uniform from person to person regardless of age, genetics, or training history. Every day I e-mail with guys who were stuck in the same rut I was and who are now making gains again by focusing on heavy lifting and proper dieting.

So don't worry if people question your approach and tell you to lighten the load and increase the reps. There's no universally accepted answer just yet as to what is truly the absolute most effective way to train for both strength and hypertrophy, and there may never be one. The subject is just incredibly complicated with a staggering number of variables to consider and control for.

But know this: every well-designed, well-executed study I've seen agrees that training with 70 to 85 percent of your 1RM *works*. At this point, I can say with absolute certainty that there's just something "special" about emphasizing heavy, compound weightlifting in your training.

I'm in good company here as well. Many of the most respected people in this industry, such as Brad Schoenfeld, Mark Rippetoe, Layne Norton, Alan Aragon, Lyle McDonald, and Pavel Tsatsouline, also advocate the same style of training for maximal results in the gym.

And the best part is that you don't have to take my word on all of this. If you just follow the workout routine laid out in this book and in the bonus report, you *will* make startling strength and size gains.

9–12
DO 9 TO 12 HEAVY SETS PER WORKOUT

Regardless of which exercises you do, the workouts on this program will call for 9 to 12 heavy (or *working*) sets per workout, which are your muscle-building sets that you'll be doing after warming up.

As you'll see, the workouts in the 5- and 4-day plans will always contain 9 working sets for the major muscle group being trained, but will also provide 3 additional optional sets that you can do if you're feeling up to it. If you're brand new to weightlifting and are pretty spent after 9 sets, don't feel like you *have* to do the final 3. If you're more experienced or just have plenty of energy at the end of 9 sets, feel free to do the 3 extras.

Don't get overzealous and do more than this in each workout, though, even if you feel like you can keep going after 12 working sets. Doing more isn't going to help you build more muscle and can eventually lead to overtraining.

If you're used to spending a couple of hours in the gym every day, pounding out set after set after set, this style of training is going to feel strange to you. In fact, at first you'll probably feel like you're being lazy or barely even working out (that's how I felt at least). You're probably going to doubt that you can bigger and stronger than ever by working out less than everyone else. But don't worry—it won't require any great leap of faith. Trust in the program and it *will* deliver. Suspend your disbelief for just a few weeks, and the results will speak for themselves.

Research and anecdotal evidence has shown me that 50 to 70 heavy reps performed with each major muscle group every five to seven days is a "sweet spot" for getting the most out of natural weightlifting.

3–4
REST 3 TO 4 MINUTES IN BETWEEN SETS

When you lift weights, a staggering number of physiological activities are taking place to enable you to perform the exercise. For a muscle to contract, it requires cellular energy, oxygen, certain chemical reactions, and many other molecular processes, and as you perform each rep, you deplete your muscles' capacity to contract forcefully.

When you lift heavy weights, you push your muscles to their full contraction capacity. Sufficient recovery time in between sets is what allows you to repeat this process enough to achieve the optimum amount of muscle overload to stimulate and force new growth.

Basically, the whole point of resting between sets is to prepare your muscles to lift maximum weight in the next set. This isn't just theory, either—clinical research has correlated intraset rest times and gains in both strength and muscle size.

For instance, one study conducted by researchers at the Federal University of Parana in Brazil found that when subjects performed the bench press and squat with 2-minute rest intervals, they were able to perform significantly more repetitions per workout than when rest intervals were shortened to 15-second increments (1:45, 1:30, 1:15, and so forth).[6]

This is significant because, as you know, total workout volume is a major factor in achieving overload and stimulating muscle growth. Thus, it's not surprising that a study conducted by researchers at Kennesaw State University found that subjects gained more muscle when training to failure with 2.5-minute rest periods as opposed to 1-minute periods.[7]

Due to the amount of weight you're using in *Bigger Leaner Stronger* workouts, you should rest for 3 to 4 minutes in between your working sets. That might sound excessive, but that timing wasn't chosen randomly—it's based on clinical research.

For instance, an extensive review of weightlifting studies conducted by researchers at State University of Rio de Janeiro found the following:

"In terms of acute responses, a key finding was that when training with loads between 50 percent and 90 percent of one repetition maximum, 3-5 minutes' rest between sets allowed for greater repetitions over multiple sets.

"Furthermore, in terms of chronic adaptations, resting 3-5 minutes between sets produced greater increases in absolute strength, due to higher intensities and volumes of training. Similarly, higher levels of muscular power were demonstrated over multiple sets with 3 or 5 minutes versus 1 minute of rest between sets." [8]

These findings were echoed by another study conducted by scientists at Eastern Illinois University with resistance-trained men:

"The findings of the present study indicate that large squat strength gains can be achieved with a minimum of 2 minutes' rest between sets, and little additional gains are derived from resting 4 minutes between sets." [9]

In another paper, the same research team analyzed bench press performance with the same subjects and found the following:

"When the training goal is maximal strength development, 3 minutes of rest should be taken between sets to avoid significant declines in repetitions. The ability to sustain repetitions while keeping the intensity constant may result in a higher training volume and consequently greater gains in muscular strength." [10]

Just like the shorter workouts will feel strange at first, the longer rest times are going to feel *really* weird. You're going to feel like you're sitting around more than you're working out.

But again, let the results speak for themselves. You'll notice that you retain your strength *much* better set after set when you use proper rest periods, which is crucial for continuing to recruit maximal muscle fibers with each set.

Some days you'll feel energized and ready to lift again after 3 minutes, but other days you'll feel a bit slower and will need the full 4 minutes. The test isn't whether you *want* to do the next set, by the way; it's whether your body's heart rate has come down since the last set and you feel like you have the energy to do another.

60–65
TRAIN FOR 60 TO 65 MINUTES

If your workouts are going much longer than an hour, something is wrong. You should be able to finish every *Bigger Leaner Stronger* workout in 60 to 65 minutes.

Long workouts are not only unnecessary but are often counterproductive as well. As you know, despite their grueling nature, extremely high-volume workouts are just a recipe for stagnation.

When workout intensity is high, as it is with this program, workout volume needs to be moderate or you'll wind up overtraining. This means shorter workouts.

Time your rest periods and keep the chatting to a minimum and you'll get through your workouts efficiently, which will help you stay focused on your workouts and give them 100 percent.

5–7
TRAIN EACH MUSCLE GROUP ONE TO TWO TIMES EVERY 5 TO 7 DAYS

The amount of time you give a muscle group to rest before training it again plays a vital role in the process of muscle growth.

Quite a few training programs have you performing two to three full workouts for every major muscle group every week, often alternating between very heavy and lighter weights.

Some of these programs are based on good scientific research, but they fall short in one area: *recovery*.

Recovery, both muscular and nervous systemic, is what makes or breaks all of the work you put in to get you the body you want. If you don't allow your body to fully recover from a workout before you subject the same muscles to overload again, it doesn't matter how strictly you follow your diet or this training protocol—eventually you will struggle to make progress, and you will feel physically worse and worse over time.

If you continue training with insufficient recovery for too long, you can *lose* strength and muscle as well as all motivation for working out. You can also wind up with depressive and chronic fatigue-like symptoms, lose your appetite and sex drive, sleep poorly, and experience other negative effects.

One for one, natural weightlifters I've spoken with who have tried various two- or three-a-week programs have run into these types of recovery problems, *especially* when they're dieting for weight loss, as a calorie deficit makes it even easier to become overtrained.

Well, you're not going to run into any of these problems if you stick to the Bigger Leaner Stronger training schedule, which carefully balances training frequency, volume, and intensity and recovery.

As you'll see, each week on the program is going to involve hitting every major muscle group in the body with one primary, heavy, intense workout with some additional lighter (but not light!) upper-body work to ensure it doesn't fall behind and the option of additional lower-body work if it's needed.

8–10
DIAL IT BACK EVERY 8 TO 10 WEEKS

Heavy weightlifting can feel pretty brutal at first. It takes quite a bit of physical effort and mental concentration. Your muscles will ache. Your joints and tendons will have to adapt.

As if all that weren't enough, there's more: it puts the central nervous system under tremendous stress as well, which manifests in subtle ways. Although there are contradictory theories as to what is truly going on here physiologically, what we know for sure is repeated bouts of weightlifting cause a nonmuscular fatigue to develop in the body.[11] This, in turn, leads to reductions in speed, power, and the ability to perform technical movements or exercises.

Some research indicates that this may be more of a sensation or emotion rather than a true physical issue, but the bottom line is that it *will* affect you, so you need to know how to deal with it.[12] And the easiest way to "refresh" your entire body is to periodically reduce the intensity of your training or take a week off the weights altogether.

Thus, between each of its eight-week phases, the *Bigger Leaner Stronger* program includes a choice between what is known as a *deload week* and several days, or even an entire week, off the weights. We'll talk about how exactly the deload week works soon, but it simply involves lower-intensity training for a week.

The choice between a deload week and taking a short break from the weights is up to you. I recommend that you start with deload weeks, but if you don't feel reinvigorated by the end of them and physically and mentally ready to hit the heavy weights again, then I recommend that you try no training whatsoever for at least four to five days before getting back to it.

Many guys fear that they are going to shrink or come back weaker if they take a week or even a few days off the weights, but this simply isn't the case. Research has shown that even in the elderly, significant strength loss isn't seen until about five weeks of no exercise.[13]

In terms of how to eat on your deload week or week off the weights, if you're bulking, you can reduce your calories to a maintenance level, and if you're cutting, you don't have to change anything.

HOW TO PROGRESS ON THE PROGRAM

As you know, the most important aspect of weightlifting is achieving progressive overload by continuing to add weight to your lifts over time.

If you did everything else right—if you ate correctly, focused on heavy compound weightlifting, and trained with a proper frequency—but simply didn't add weight to the bar as you went along, you would quickly plateau. It's that important.

And that's why the *Bigger Leaner Stronger* program has a simple method of progression: once you hit 6 reps for *one* set, you add weight for your next set. The standard increase is a total of 10 pounds: 5 pounds added to either side of the barbell, or a 5-pound increase in each dumbbell.

For instance, if you get 225 for 6 reps on your first set of incline bench press, you then add 10 pounds (5 pounds to each side of the bar), rest, and work with 235 going forward.

If, after moving up like this, you only get 2 to 3 reps, you can reduce the weight by 5 pounds (leaving it at 5 pounds heavier than the weight with which you got 6 reps), or if your gym doesn't have 2.5-pound plates, simply drop back to the weight that you got 6 with and finish your remaining sets with that. Then, the next week, try to make the jump again starting fresh with your first set, and you should get 4 or even 5 reps. In most cases, however, you'll simply get 6 reps, add 10 pounds, rest, and then get 4 reps on subsequent sets.

Your primary goal with every workout should be beating the previous week's numbers, even if only by 1 rep. If you do that again the next week, you're ready to move up in weight.

You should know, however, that some weeks just won't go like that. Sometimes you'll only be able to lift exactly what you did the week prior. Sometimes you'll even be a rep weaker.

These things happen and don't necessarily mean anything is wrong. Just keep working at it and you should see a slow, steady increase in weight lifted over time.

WHERE'S MY PUMP!?

If you're used to high-rep "pump" training, you should know that lower-rep, heavy training is quite different. Don't be surprised if, for the first several weeks, your muscles feel less full than what you're used to. It's normal.

You see, heavy lifting does give a nice pump, but it's not the "my muscles are about to explode" type that many guys obsess over and think is so important. Remember, however, that while a huge pump might be great for peacocking in the gym, it has little to do with long-term muscle growth. *Overload* is what we want. A pump is just a by-product.

So long as you keep hitting the weights hard, your muscles will grow, and as your muscles grow, you'll get more and more of a pump from heavy lifting. And better yet, you'll be one of the rare guys who can look great without any pump at all because you have a true foundation of solid lean mass, not small muscles that need to fill up with blood to even be noticeable.

THE PROPER REP TEMPO FOR MAXIMUM GAINS

"Rep timing" refers to the speed at which you lower and raise the weights, and there are quite a few opinions out there as to what is best.

One of the more popular schools of thought is using very slow reps to maximize "time under tension" and thus muscle growth. "Your muscles don't know weight," many bodybuilders say, almost waxing philosophic, "they only know tension, and that's what stimulates growth."

Well, like the many "weird little tricks" of the fitness space—you know, the ones that are supposed to instantly increase your bench press or melt off belly fat—time under tension is not important enough to warrant special attention and is simply a by-product of proper training that can, more or less, be ignored.

You see, the more slowly you perform your reps with a given weight, the fewer reps you can perform with it.[14] Depending on how slowly you went, you might get half the reps or even less as a normal rep tempo.

As you reduce the number of reps you perform, you also reduce the total work performed by the muscle, and as you reduce the amount of work performed, you reduce the muscle- and strength-building potential of the exercise.[15]

The question, then, is whether the "trade-off" of time under tension for total work is worth it. Does increasing time under tension "make up for" the reduction in work performed and result in more strength progression and muscle growth?

The research says no. For example…

- A study conducted by scientists at the University of Sydney found that subjects following traditional "fast" training on the bench press gained more strength than slow training.[16]

- A study conducted by researchers at the University of Connecticut found that very slow training resulted in lower levels of peak force and power when compared with a normal, self-regulated tempo.[17]

- A study conducted by scientists at the University of Wisconsin found that even in untrained individuals, a traditional training tempo resulted in greater strength in the squat and greater peak power in the countermovement jump.[18]

- A study conducted by researchers at the University of Oklahoma found that four weeks of traditional resistance training was more effective for increasing strength than super-slow training.[19]

These findings aren't exactly surprising given the underlying mechanics of muscle growth and how reliant it is on building strength (if you want bigger muscles, you're going to have to get stronger).

To quote researchers from Ithaca College, who compared fast-tempo bench pressing to slow-tempo:

"One-way repeated measures analysis of variance showed tempos with a fast eccentric phase (1 second), and no bottom rest produced significantly greater (p ≤ 0.05) PO [power output] and repetitions than tempos involving slower eccentric velocity (4 seconds) or greater bottom rest (4 seconds).
"This combination of greater repetitions and PO resulted in a greater volume of work. Varying interrepetition rest (1 or 4 seconds) did not significantly affect PO or repetitions.
"The results of this study support the use of fast eccentric speed and no bottom rest during acute performance testing to maximize PO and number of repetitions during a set of bench press." [20]

It's also worth noting that back when I didn't know what I was doing, I used to do a lot of slow sets to maximize time under tension, and my results were in line with the research. I found it no more effective than my regular training routines, which were pretty crappy in reality.

So, the rep timing I recommend is either the "2–1–2" or "2–1–1" timing. This means the first part of the rep should take about 2 seconds, which is followed by a 1-second (or shorter) pause, which is followed by the final portion of the rep, which should take between 1 and 2 seconds to perform.

For example, if we apply this to the bench press, it means we are to lower the bar to our chest in 2 seconds, pause for 1 second or less, and raise it in 1 or 2 seconds.

INTENSITY AND FOCUS: YOUR TWO SECRET WEAPONS

If you've trained before, you know what makes a great workout: you're full of energy, the weights feel light, you're completely focused on your lifts, and you're able to push yourself further than you expected.

A big part of having this kind of workout as often as possible is consciously lifting with *intensity* and *focus*. And that doesn't mean loud grunting with death metal blaring in your headphones. While some of those types do train pretty intensely, none of the showmanship is necessary.

Instead, I recommend that we take a page from the famous Bulgarian powerlifters' books and imitate their counterintuitive type of training for hitting one-rep lifts. They didn't stomp around like a madman or spend 15 minutes amping themselves up to screaming guitars and vocals. Instead, they just walked up to the bar and hit the lift as calmly and solidly as they could. If they couldn't get it without overstimulating their nervous systems, they considered it to be too much weight.

You see, intensity is simply the level of physical and mental exertion you give to your workout. It's how intent you are on pushing yourself outside of your comfort zone and making progress. It's your desire to not just make it through your set but to accomplish something with it.

A high-intensity workout is one where you feel like you didn't leave anything in the tank. You didn't settle for a lighter weight when you felt you could've gone up. Your mind wasn't wandering elsewhere while you were lifting. You weren't just robotically going through the motions. You were consciously, but calmly, pounding out every rep and every set with determination.

By *focus*, I mean mental concentration: having your mind on your lifts and not on the TV show you watched last night, the party later that night, the argument with your girlfriend, or whatever else.

While there's nothing wrong with talking while resting, don't get carried away in conversation because it'll inevitably be distracting. Your rest times will drag on too long. You'll have your mind on other things when you sit down to do your set. It's just counterproductive. Save the fraternizing for after the gym.

I don't want to get too "woo-woo" on you and say you need to hypnotically visualize every lift before you perform it, but there's definitely something to be said for having 100 percent of your attention on moving the weight in front of you. It's "mind over matter," as they say.

The *Bigger Leaner Stronger* training routines are built to help you maintain a high level of intensity and focus. It's much easier to do 4 to 6 reps at maximum intensity and focus than 10 to 12. It's much easier to remain revved up and determined for 45 minutes than 90.

But the routine itself doesn't supply the intensity and focus. You have to.

DOES ANYTHING CHANGE WHEN CUTTING?

One of many terrible pieces of training advice I hear among the "bros" is to train with light weights and high reps when cutting to "bring out the cuts."

This is 100 percent wrong.

Focusing exclusively on high-rep training doesn't help burn more fat than heavier weights. It doesn't "shred you up," nor does it make you vascular.

Ironically, training heavy is *especially* important when you're cutting because the name of the game is muscle preservation, and you need to keep overloading the muscles to accomplish this.

So train hard when you're cutting and keep trying to go up in strength. Most guys experience an initial drop in strength when they switch from a bulk to a cut, but I've always managed to build my strength back up and end more or less where I began with little to no muscle loss (if I do lose any muscle when I cut, I can't see it in the mirror).

HOW TO USE CARDIO TO BUILD MUSCLE

Many guys fear cardio as if every minute spent performing it means a muscle and strength loss. Some bodybuilder types bash it simply because they don't like doing it.

While it's clearly evident that excessive cardio causes muscle loss (just look at any marathon runner), moderate amounts of regular cardio can *help* you build more muscle over time.

Let's look at how this works.

CARDIO AND MUSCLE RECOVERY

As you know, intense exercise causes damage to muscle fibers, which must then be repaired. This damage is the likely primary cause of the soreness that you feel the day or two following a workout, known as delayed onset muscle soreness, or DOMS.

Repairing the damage is a complex process that is partly regulated by two simple factors: the quantity of "raw materials" needed for repair that are brought to the damaged muscle over time and the speed at which waste products are removed.

Well, cardio can help your body repair muscle damage more quickly because it increases blood flow to various areas of the body. This type of "active recovery" delivers more "raw materials" to the muscles for use and removes the waste products, which results in an all-around quicker recovery period.[21]

It's worth noting, however, that these benefits are primarily seen in the legs because most forms of cardio don't involve the upper body. If you want to boost whole-body recovery, then you would need to do something that gets your upper body working, like a rowing machine, or using your arms to pump on the elliptical machine.

Cardio and Your Metabolism

In our collective dietary fantasy, all nutrients eaten would be sucked into the muscles and either absorbed or burned off and none would result in fat storage, and when we restricted our calories for fat loss, all of our energy needs would be met by burning only fat, not muscle.

The reality, however, is that our bodies do these things to varying degrees. Some people's bodies store less fat when they overeat than others', and some can get away with larger calorie deficits without losing muscle.

Genetics and anabolic hormone levels are the major players here, which means there just isn't much we can do about how our bodies innately respond to calorie surpluses or deficits.

All is not lost if you're not a part of the genetic elite, however, because an important factor in what your body does with the food you eat is insulin sensitivity, and this is something we can positively affect.

As discussed earlier in the book, retaining insulin sensitivity is highly beneficial when you're eating a surplus of calories to build muscle, whereas insulin resistance inhibits muscle growth and promotes fat storage.

This is where cardio comes in because it improves insulin sensitivity and does so in a dose-dependent manner (meaning the more you do, the more benefits you get).[22]

In this way, doing cardio can help your muscles better absorb the nutrients you eat, which can mean more muscle growth and less fat storage over time.

Cardio and Conditioning

A common issue in the bodybuilding world is the dramatic reduction in cardiovascular fitness when focusing only on bulking and heavy weightlifting for months on end.

Building one's cardio conditioning back up is not only uncomfortable, but going from doing absolutely no cardio to doing several sessions per week in addition to putting yourself in a calorie deficit places a lot of stress on the body. This added stress makes weight loss physically and psychologically tougher, and it can even accelerate muscle loss.[23]

By keeping regular cardio in year-round, however, you can maintain your metabolic conditioning and prevent the systemic "shell shock" that many people experience during the beginning of a cut.

It's also common for people who have bulked for months without cardio to experience an initial lag in weight loss. I've yet to find a satisfactory explanation for why this occurs, but it could be related to the fact that exercise improves the body's ability to metabolize fat, and thus regular cardio may optimize and preserve this mechanism.[24]

The Bottom Line

The bottom line is that moderate amounts of cardio most definitely don't impair muscle growth and may even accelerate it, and cardio confers other health benefits as well. I recommend that you make cardio a regular part of your routine, whether you're cutting, bulking, or maintaining.

The muscle-related benefits of cardio are especially true if the exercise closely imitates the motions used in exercises performed to build muscle, like cycling or rowing.

These benefits were demonstrated in a particularly interesting study conducted by researchers at Stephen F. Austin State University.[25] What they found is that the type of cardio done had a profound effect on the subjects' ability to gain strength and size in their weightlifting. The subjects who did running and walking for their cardio gained significantly less strength and size than those who cycled.

A similar effect was also seen in a study conducted by researchers at the University of Wisconsin.[26] They separated 30 untrained men into two groups and had one follow a weight training program three days per week and the other do the same plus 50 minutes of cycling. After 10 weeks, they found that the men who cycled in addition to training with weights gained more thigh muscle than the weights-only group.

Personally, I've been recumbent cycling two to four times per week for more than a year now, and I've enjoyed tremendous improvements in my cardiovascular endurance and resting heart rate. While I can't conclusively say that I've built more leg muscle from it, I did notice an initial increase in leg strength as they had to adapt to the new stimulus.

THE BEST TYPE OF CARDIO FOR LOSING FAT, NOT MUSCLE

Cardio machines often show pretty graphs indicating where your heart rate should be for "fat burning" versus "cardiovascular training."

You calculate this magical heart rate by subtracting your age from 200 and multiplying this number by 0.6. If you keep your heart rate at this number, you're often told, you'll be in the "fat burning zone."

Well, there's only a slight kernel of truth here.

You do burn both fat and carbohydrates when you exercise, and the proportion varies with the intensity of exercise. A very low-intensity activity like walking taps mainly into fat stores, whereas high-intensity sprints pull much more heavily from carbohydrate stores. At about 60 percent of maximum exertion, your body gets about half of its energy from carbohydrate stores and half from fat stores (which is why many "experts" claim that you should work in the range of 60 to 70 percent of maximum exertion).

Based on the above, you might think that I'm arguing for steady-state cardio (cardio that involves steadily keeping your effort and heartbeat in a certain range), but there's more to consider.

The first issue is total calories burned while exercising. If you walk off 100 calories, 85 of which come from fat stores, that isn't as effective as spending that time in a moderate run that burns off 200 calories with 100 coming from fat. And that, in turn, isn't as effective as spending that time doing sprint intervals that burn off 500 calories with 150 coming from fat.

Sprinting's benefits extend beyond the calories burned while exercising, though. A study conducted by scientists at the University of Western Ontario gives us insight into just how much more effective high-intensity cardio is.[27] Researchers had 10 men and 10 women train three times per week, with one group doing between four and six 30-second treadmill sprints (with four minutes of rest in between each), and the other group doing 30 to 60 minutes of steady-state cardio (running on the treadmill at the "magical fat-loss zone" of 65 percent VO_2 max).

The results: after six weeks of training, the subjects doing the intervals had lost significantly more body fat. Yes, four to six 30-second sprints burn more fat than 60 minutes of incline treadmill walking.

These findings are supported by several other studies, such as those conducted by researchers at Laval University, East Tennessee State University, Baylor College of Medicine, and the University of New South Wales, which have all shown that shorter, high-intensity cardio sessions result in greater fat loss over time than longer, low-intensity sessions.[28]

Although the exact mechanisms of how high-intensity cardio trumps steady-state cardio for fat-loss purposes aren't fully understood yet, scientists have isolated quite a few of the factors, which include the following:

- increased resting metabolic rate for more than 24 hours after exercise,

- improved insulin sensitivity in the muscles,

- higher levels of fat oxidation in the muscles,

- significant spikes in growth hormone levels (which aid in fat loss) and catecholamine levels (chemicals your body produces to directly induce fat mobilization), and

- post-exercise appetite suppression.[29]

High-intensity interval training not only burns more fat in less time than steady-state cardio, but it also preserves muscular size and improves performance as well.

Research has shown that the longer your cardio sessions are, the more they impair strength and hypertrophy.[30] Thus, keeping your cardio sessions *short* is important when we're talking about maximizing your gains in the weight room and preserving your muscle. Only high-intensity interval training allows you to do this *and* burn enough fat to make it worthwhile.

I like the recumbent bike for my cardio, and here's how I do it:

1. I start my workout with 2 to 3 minutes of low-intensity warm-up on the lowest resistance.

2. I then bump the resistance up several notches to give me something to pedal against but not so much that my quads get fried in just one bout, and I pedal as fast as possible for 60 seconds. If you're new to HIIT, you may need to start with 30- to 45-second sprints.

3. I then reduce the resistance to its slowest setting and pedal at a moderate pace for the same amount of time as my high-intensity interval (60 seconds). If you're new to HIIT, you may need to extend this rest period to 1.5 to 2 times your high-intensity intervals (if you sprint for 30 seconds, you may need 45 to 60 seconds of recovery).

4. I then repeat this cycle of all-out and recovery intervals for 25 to 30 minutes.

5. I finish with a 2- to 3-minute cool-down at a low intensity.

That's it. I'll bring my iPad and read or watch something and the time flies by.

If you'd like to do a different form of HIIT cardio, such as rowing, sprinting, swimming, jump roping, or anything else that permits it, go for it. You can apply the same simple principles: relatively short bursts of maximum effort that spike your heart rate followed by low-intensity recovery periods that bring it down to normal levels.

If you want to include some steady-state cardio in your routine, that's fine as well. Just know that it's not as effective for fat loss purposes and that if you do too much of it, you can impair muscle growth. Personally, I wouldn't do more than 45 to 60 minutes of steady-state cardio in one session, and in terms of weekly frequency, we'll talk about that in a minute.

THE BEST TIME TO DO CARDIO

When you do your cardio in relation to your weightlifting matters.

Researchers from RMIT University worked with well-trained athletes in 2009 and found that "combining resistance exercise and cardio in the same session may disrupt genes for anabolism."[31] In laymen's terms, they found that combining endurance and resistance training sends "mixed signals" to the muscles. Cardio before the resistance training suppressed anabolic hormones such as IGF-1 and MGF, and cardio after resistance training increased muscle tissue breakdown.

Several other studies, such as those conducted by researchers from the Children's National Medical Center, the Waikato Institute of Technology, and the University of Jyvaskyla in Finland, came to the same conclusions: training for both endurance and strength simultaneously impairs your gains on both fronts.[32] Training purely for strength or purely for endurance in a workout is far superior.

Cardio before weightlifting also saps your energy and makes it much harder to train heavy, which in turn inhibits your muscle growth.

Therefore, I recommend that you separate your weightlifting and cardio sessions by at least a few hours if at all possible. Personally, I lift early in the morning and do my cardio after work, before dinner.

If there's no way that you can split up your cardio and weightlifting, do your weight training first, as cardio first will drain energy that you'll want for your lifting. While this arrangement isn't *ideal*, it's not a huge problem. You can still do well on the program.

If you can, I recommend having a protein shake after your weightlifting and before your cardio as this will help mitigate the muscle breakdown.

HOW OFTEN YOU SHOULD DO CARDIO

In terms of frequency, here's how I do it:

- When I'm bulking, I do two 25-minute HIIT sessions per week.

- When I'm cutting, I do three to five 25-minute HIIT sessions per week.

- When I'm maintaining, I do two to three 25-minute HIIT sessions per week.

- I never do more than five cardio sessions per week, as I've found my strength begins to drop off in the gym if I do.

Many people are shocked to learn that I do no more than 1.5 to 2 hours of cardio per week while cutting but am able to get to the 6 to 7 percent body fat range with ease. Well, the idea that you have to do a ton of cardio to get shredded is a complete myth. It's not only unnecessary but unhealthy as well.

You don't have to do cardio to lose fat, but if you want to get down to the 10 percent range or below, I can pretty much guarantee you'll have to do at least two to three sessions per week.

If you'd like to stick with steady-state cardio or include it in your routine, stick with the frequency recommendations given above. You can mix and match modalities (HIIT vs low-intensity steady-state, or LISS) but I still wouldn't do more than five sessions per week.

THE BOTTOM LINE

Congratulations! You've just learned the core principles of the *Bigger Leaner Stronger* training program. Chances are that this is a new approach to training for you, and if that's the case, you should be excited.

Soon you're going to be enjoying explosive muscle growth and rapid fat loss by doing relatively short, stimulating workouts that you look forward to every day and that get the kind of results other guys can only dream about.

You're never going to burn yourself out with hours and hours of grueling cardio either. In fact, if you're like me, you'll come to enjoy your cardio sessions because they'll noticeably improve your performance and overall health without eating up large chunks of your free time.

Next on the agenda is the discussion of the individual weightlifting exercises you're going to be performing on the program. Carry on to find out!

CHAPTER SUMMARY

WEIGHTLIFTING

- While a small number of machines are worth using, such as the leg press machine or cable setup, the vast majority are inferior to dumbbell and barbell exercises in terms of producing bigger, stronger muscles.

- The average guy needs to build a strong overall foundation of strength and muscle, and there's only one way to do that naturally: you have to do a lot of heavy, compound weightlifting.

- To achieve maximum overload and muscle stimulation, you will train one or two muscle groups per workout (per day).

- You're going to be working in the 4- to 6-rep range for nearly all exercises.

- The workouts on this program will call for 9 to 12 heavy (or *working*) sets per workout.

- Due to the amount of weight you're using in *Bigger Leaner Stronger* workouts, you should rest for 3 to 4 minutes in between your working sets.

- You should be able to finish every *Bigger Leaner Stronger* workout in 60 to 65 minutes.

- Between each of its eight-week phases, the *Bigger Leaner Stronger* program includes a choice between what is known as a *deload week* and several days, or even an entire week, off the weights.

- I recommend that you start with deload weeks, but if you don't feel reinvigorated by the end of them and physically and mentally ready to hit the heavy weights again, then I recommend that you try no training whatsoever for at least 4 to 5 days before getting back to it.

- The *Bigger Leaner Stronger* program has a simple method of progression: once you hit 6 reps for *one* set, you add weight for your next set. The standard increase is a total of 10 pounds: 5 pounds added to either side of the barbell or a 5-pound increase in each dumbbell.

- So long as you keep hitting the weights hard, your muscles will grow, and as your muscles grow, you'll get more and more of a pump from heavy lifting.

- The rep timing I recommend is either the "2–1–2" or "2–1–1" timing. This means the first part of the rep should take about 2 seconds, which is followed by a 1-second (or shorter) pause, which is followed by the final portion of the rep, which should take between 1 and 2 seconds.

- Training heavy is *especially* important when you're cutting because the name of the game is muscle preservation, and you need to keep overloading the muscles to accomplish this.

- A high-intensity workout is one where you feel like you didn't leave anything in the tank. You didn't settle for a lighter weight when you felt you could've gone up. Your mind wasn't wandering elsewhere while you were lifting. You weren't just robotically going through the motions—you were consciously, but calmly, pounding out every rep and every set with determination.

- By *focus*, I mean mental concentration: having your mind on your lifts and not on the TV show you watched last night, the party later that night, the argument with your girlfriend, or whatever else.

CARDIO

- Cardio can help your body repair muscle damage more quickly because it increases blood flow to various areas of the body.

- Cardio improves insulin sensitivity and in this way can help your muscles better absorb the nutrients you eat, which can mean more muscle growth and less fat storage over time.

- By keeping regular cardio in year-round, you can maintain your metabolic conditioning and prevent the systemic "shell shock" that many people experience during the beginning of a cut.

- The muscle-related benefits of cardio are especially true if the exercise closely imitates the motions used in exercises performed to build muscle, like cycling or rowing.

- HIIT not only burns more fat in less time than steady-state cardio, but it preserves muscular size and performance better as well.

- If you'd like to do a different form of HIIT cardio, such as rowing, sprinting, swimming, jump roping, or anything else that permits it, go for it.

- If you want to include some steady-state cardio in your routine, that's fine as well. Just know that it's not as effective for fat loss purposes and that if you do too much of it, you can impair muscle growth.

- I recommend that you separate your weightlifting and cardio sessions by at least a few hours if at all possible. If there's no way that you can split up your cardio and weightlifting, do your weight training first as cardio first will drain energy that you'll want for your lifting.

- When I'm bulking, I do two 25-minute HIIT sessions per week. When I'm cutting, I do three to five 25-minute HIIT sessions per week. When I'm maintaining, I do three 25-minute HIIT sessions per week.

- I never do more than five cardio sessions per week, as I've found my strength begins to drop off in the gym if I do.

- You don't *have* to do cardio to lose fat, but if you want to get down to the 10 percent range or below, I can pretty much guarantee you'll have to do at least two or three sessions per week.

17

THE BIGGER LEANER STRONGER TRAINING PROGRAM

There is no reason to be alive if you can't do the deadlift!
— JON PALL SIGMARSSON

NOW THAT YOU UNDERSTAND THE BASIC principles and premises of the *Bigger Leaner Stronger* training methodologies, let's look at the exercises you'll be performing and how to train each major muscle group properly.

MEET YOUR MAKERS: THE FOUR LIFTS THAT BUILD STRONG, MUSCULAR BODIES

Out of the hundreds and hundreds of exercises you could possibly do, four reign supreme. If you neglect them like I did when I started lifting, you're guaranteed to never reach your genetic potential in terms of size, strength, and performance.

These exercises are the squat, deadlift, bench press, and military press, and their timeless power has been proven beyond the shadow of a doubt by over a century of bodybuilders, strongmen, and athletes.

There are popular training programs out there that have you do nothing but these four exercises, such as Starting Strength and 5 x 5, and one of your primary goals with your *Bigger Leaner Stronger* training is to improve your performance of these key lifts. If you can do that, you're going to be able to build the body you want—it's that simple.

Unfortunately, however, many guys neglect these exercises (with the exception of the bench press, of course) or do them incorrectly, thus robbing themselves of potential gains.

Most guys stop their bench press six inches or more above their chests and their military press above their chins because it's "better for the shoulders." They load up a bunch of plates and squat down a foot or two and stand back up because they "don't want to hurt their knees." They round their backs when deadlifting so they can "really go heavy."

Well, not only does improper form dramatically reduce the effectiveness of exercises, but it also opens the door to injury. Heavy half-reps, whether on the bench press, military press, or squat, put large amounts of strain on your joints, tendons, and ligaments—much more than if you were moving less weight through a proper, full range of motion, gradually strengthening the muscles and supporting tissues. When deadlifting, hunching your back to get the weight up and then severely arching your lower back during the lockout is just all wrong—a nasty injury waiting to happen.

On the flip side, if you lift with strict attention to form and a full range of motion, you'll enjoy full development of your muscles, steady strength gains, and no unnecessary injuries or pains.

Ignorance is certainly one of the primary reasons why so many guys lift with poor form—they just never learned how to train correctly, and there is a bit of technical skill to it—but laziness is another main reason. These four exercises are *hard* when performed correctly. A full, butt-below-parallel squat is brutal when compared to a wussy little half rep. If everyone had to touch the bar to their chest when bench pressing, you'd see a lot less weight on the bars and a lot of sour faces.

There's also the problem of determining what proper form is. There are quite a few authoritative opinions as to what a proper squat, deadlift, bench press, and military press look like. One well-respected coach might say your toes should never go past your knees when you squat, while another says it's natural and recommended. One might say rounding the upper part of the spine when you deadlift is okay, while another says it's dangerous.

Who's right? How can we know? And why should you listen to me?

Well, in this case I'm going to pass the buck to the man whose work taught me—and hundreds of thousands of others—how to squat, bench press, deadlift, and military press heavy and pain-free: Mark Rippetoe.

"Rip," as he's known, has been in this game for nearly four decades and is a renowned and highly respected strength coach. He's the author of several books, including the iconic *Starting Strength*, and his weightlifting methods are used by professional athletes of all kinds and laymen alike.

I'm going to teach you Rip's methods of pushing, pulling, and squatting because they've withstood the tests of time and large numbers. They're safe and effective, and they don't require anything special in terms of physical prowess.

I'm going to give you everything you need to perform the exercises properly and safely, but I definitely recommend that you read *Starting Strength* if you want to dive into the biomechanics of each movement.

So, let's start our discussion of the exercises you'll be performing on the program with the most important lifts and learn exactly how to do them correctly.

THE SQUAT

Many guys think leg training consists of loading up the leg press with every plate in the gym and using tourniquet-tight knee wraps and a weight belt cinched to its tightest notch, only to wiggle into the sled, grind out a few excruciating quarter reps, and celebrate with an ear-splitting yell and high-fives with his buddies.

Good news: that's not going to be you. You're going to be the guy in the corner with the squat rack—you know, the loneliest place in the gym—quietly going about your business with deep, heavy squats. No wraps, no belts, no swagger—just a bar bending across your back, loaded with a "measly" few hundred pounds (yes, you'll get there) and a puddle of sweat on the ground.

Who's going to be the winner in the end? Who's going to consistently get bigger and stronger, and who's the least likely to get hurt? You, of course.

While many guys will do *anything* for leg training before putting the barbell on their backs, they're missing out on what many of the top strength coaches in the world consider the absolute toughest and most rewarding exercise we can do.

To nobody's surprise, squatting strengthens every muscle in your legs, which doesn't just increase the amount of weight you can lift—it also helps you run faster and jump higher, and it improves flexibility, mobility, and agility.[1] And as if those aren't reasons enough to squat regularly, it's also an incredibly effective core workout.[2]

Laziness aside, why do so many people avoid squatting? Well, more often than not, they've fallen victim to the myths that the squat is bad for your back and knees—a lie that has been perpetuated for about five decades now.

It all started with work done in the 1960s, when research concluded that a deep squat stretched the knee ligaments too far, increasing the risk of injury. These findings spread like wildfire through the fitness world, and some U.S. military services even cut squatting movements out of their training programs.

It was noted at the time that the studies had serious flaws, including the choice of subjects and researcher bias, but that wasn't enough to stop the uprising against the squat. For instance, one of the studies was done with parachute jumpers, whose knees had been repeatedly pounded with violent impacts and twisted all over the place in parachute lines.

Well, much more research has been done since then, and a much different picture has emerged.

A rigorous study conducted by scientists at Duke University involved the analysis of more than two decades of published literature to determine, in great detail, the biomechanics of the squat exercise and the stresses it places on the ankles, knees, hip joint, and spine.[3]

Highlights from the paper, and many studies reviewed within, set the record straight on how the squat affects our bodies and teach us a lot about proper squat form:

- The hamstrings counteract the pull on the shinbone, which neutralizes the shearing force placed on the knee and alleviates stress on the ACL.

- Even in extreme cases, such as powerlifters lifting 2.5 times their body weight, the compressive forces placed on the knee and its tendons are well within its ranges of ultimate strength.[4]

- Stress placed on the ACL is negligible considering its ultimate strength (in one study, the highest ACL force recorded when squatting was a mere 6 percent of its ultimate strength).[5] The highest recorded PCL forces were well within natural strength limits.[6]

- If you maintain a neutral spine position while squatting (instead of a rigidly flexed position), you greatly reduce the shearing force placed on your vertebrae (your spine is better at dealing with compressive force than shearing).[7]

- Maintaining a posture as close to upright as possible further reduces this force, as does increasing intra-abdominal pressure, which you can create by holding your breath while you squat and gazing straight ahead instead of down.[8]

In closing, researchers from Duke University concluded that the squat "does not compromise knee stability, and can enhance stability if performed correctly."[9] Furthermore, any risks of spinal injury can be avoided by simply minimizing the shearing force placed on the spine.

After their own extensive review of the literature, the National Strength and Conditioning Association came to the same conclusion:

"Squats, when performed correctly and with appropriate supervision, are not only safe, but may be a significant deterrent to knee injuries." [10]

So rest easy: as long as you use proper squat form, the squat does *not* put your back or knees at risk of injury.

The real problem with the squat is that few people do it correctly. The most common error is, of course, doing partial reps by not lowering the body until the hips drop lower than the knees. There are other common mistakes, though: too narrow of a stance, too wide of a stance, bowing the knees, the early "butt wink," and more.

Well, let's make sure you don't make any of the same mistakes by breaking the lift down into its different parts and analyzing how it works.

The Squat Setup

I recommend that you always squat in a power rack or squat rack with the safety bars/pins set six inches or so below the height of the bar at the bottom of the rep (which you'll learn about in a minute). Do this even if you have a spotter.

Position the bar on the rack so it cuts across the upper half of your chest. This might feel a bit low, but it's better to have it on the low side than trying to tippy-toe heavy weight off the rack.

Face the bar so you can walk it out backward. Don't ever walk the bar out forward, as trying to rerack it by walking backward is dangerous.

Get under the bar and place your heels at about shoulder-width apart, with the toes rotated out by about 20 to 25 degrees (your right foot should be at about 1 o'clock and your left at about 11 o'clock).

When you're ready to unrack the bar, bring your shoulder blades together, tighten your entire upper back, raise your chest up, and straighten your lower back. Put the bar below the bone at the top of your shoulder blades, solidly across your upper back muscles and rear deltoids. Do *not* put the bar on your neck.

Use a narrow grip because this helps you maintain upper-back tightness. Place your thumbs on top of the bar.

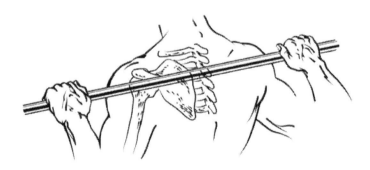

Notice how all of the weight is resting on his back, with none on his hands. This is important. The wide grip that many people use slackens the back muscles, which provide crucial support for the weight and transfers the load to the spine. Don't follow their lead.

This tight, hands-in position will probably feel a bit awkward at first, and you might need to improve your shoulder flexibility to get there. If you're not flexible enough yet, that's okay—get as close to the proper position as you can, ensuring that your shoulder blades are pinched and that the weight is solidly on your back (you're not holding the load in your hands). As you continue to train and stretch, you'll be able to get your hands in close.

The Squat Movement

Once you've unracked the weight, take one or two steps back and assume the proper squatting position as outlined above (heels shoulder-width apart, toes pointed out).

Pick a spot on the floor about six feet away, and stare at it for the entirety of the set. Don't look up at the ceiling, as this makes it hard to reach the proper bottom position, can throw off proper hip movement and chest positioning, and can even cause a neck injury.

You're now ready to start the downward motion, which is accomplished by shifting the hips back and sitting the butt straight down while keeping the chest up and the entire back straight and tight.

Many people have the tendency to want to transfer the load to the quads as they descend and accomplish this by sliding the knees too far forward. Well, if your knees push too far past your toes as you descend, they're put in a compromising position that can lead to all kinds of pains and problems, particularly with the patellar tendon under the kneecap.

A good rule of thumb is that the forward motion of the knees should occur in the first third or half of the descent, and they should go no further than just in front of the toes. Once the knees are out of the way and in place, the movement becomes a simple drop of the hips straight down followed by a rise straight up.

The bottom of the squat is the point where your hips are back and slightly lower than your kneecaps (which causes your femurs to be a little lower than parallel with the ground). Your knees are just a little forward of the toes and the back is straight, but not necessarily *arched*, and at an angle that places the bar over the middle of the foot.

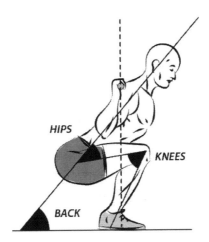

I recommend that you practice this movement with no bar to get a feel for it. If you want to score bonus points, put yourself on camera so you can ensure that what you *think* you're doing is actually what you're doing.

Once you've reached the bottom of the squat, you drive your butt straight up—not forward—and raise your shoulders at the same pace. To do this, you must maintain a back angle that keeps the weight over the middle of your foot. If your hips rise faster than your shoulders, you'll start tipping forward, which puts heavy strain on the neck and back.

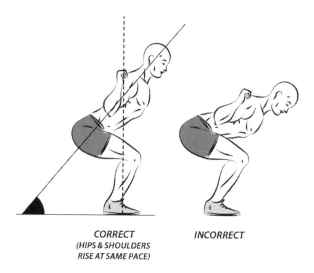

CORRECT
(HIPS & SHOULDERS
RISE AT SAME PACE)   INCORRECT

Don't think about anything but driving your hips straight up while keeping your chest up and maintaining the proper spine angle, and you'll ascend correctly.

Squat Tips

If you're having trouble getting your knees to remain in line with your feet as you descend and ascend, you can do a simple mobility exercise that works like this: squat with no weight and, at the bottom, place your elbows against your knees and the palms of your hands together, and nudge your knees out. Work your knees in and out for a good 20 to 30 seconds, rest, and repeat this a few times. If you do this several times per week, you'll quickly notice a difference in your ability to maintain the proper position when you start adding weight.

If you need to place the bar a bit higher on your back due to shoulder stiffness, the angles change slightly. Here's another diagram to help:

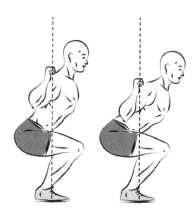

The figure on the left is in what's called a "high-bar squat" position, and the right is the "low-bar squat" position, which I prefer. While the low-bar squatting position produces less torque on the knees than the high-bar position, the magnitude of both forces are well within tolerable ranges, making neither position "better" than the other in this regard.[11] Use whichever squatting position is most comfortable for you.

Squatting too rapidly increases the shearing and compressive forces placed on your knees.[12] Make sure your descent is controlled—don't simply drop your hips as quickly as you can.

Take a deep breath at the top of the first rep—when you're standing tall—and hold it, tightening your entire torso. You can hold your breath as you perform the rep or exhale slightly (maybe 10 percent of the air you're holding) on the way up, and then fill up with air again at the top.

Don't squat on a Smith machine unless you have no other choice. It forces an unnatural range of motion that can be quite uncomfortable, and research has shown it's less effective than the barbell squat performed with free weight.[13]

If your back tends to round as you descend, causing what's known as the "butt wink," it's because your hamstrings are too tight. Stretch them every day (but not before lifting, as studies have shown that this saps strength and does nothing to prevent the risk of injury), and as they loosen, you'll find that you can keep your lower back in a neutral position until you hit the very bottom, when your pelvis naturally rotates down a little.[14]

Don't point your feet straight forward, as this can increase stress on the knees. As the stance widens, the body naturally wants the feet to be parallel with the thighs. By twisting them in and squatting, you force an unnatural torque on the knees that can lead to bowing them in as you ascend, which increases the risk of injury.

You can start your ascension by creating a little "bounce" at the bottom of the squat as your hamstrings, glutes, and groin muscles stretch to the limit of their natural ranges of motion.

Don't use a powerlifter's super-wide squatting stance unless you're actually powerlifting. This type of stance does allow for more weight to be lifted, but it reduces the role of the quads in the lift.

If you feel the need to squat with blocks or plates under your heels, it's because you need more hamstring and/or ankle flexibility. Check out Dr. Kelly Starrett's work on improving hamstring and ankle mobility so you can squat as described in this chapter.

Believe it or not, the wrong shoes can make squatting significantly harder. Bad shoes are those with a soft or unstable sole or raised heel, as this promotes instability during the lift, and those with too high of a heel, which shifts your body weight and thus your knees too far forward as you descend and ascend.

By using shoes with flat soles or proper weightlifting shoes with a slight, rigid heel elevation, you'll find it much easier to sit back onto your heels and engage your hamstrings and glutes more effectively. (You'll find my shoe recommendations in the bonus report at the end of the book.)

Squat Variations

There are quite a few variations of the squat, but the majority are inferior to the basic movement and thus not recommended.

That said, there is one variation that is fantastic and included in the *Bigger Leaner Stronger* program: the front squat.

Front Squat

The front squat emphasizes the quadriceps and core and creates less compression of the spine and less torque in the knees, which makes it particularly useful for those with back or knee injuries or limitations.[15] It also makes it easier to achieve proper depth.

Like the back squat, you set up for a front squat with your feet about shoulder-width apart and your toes slightly pointed out.

There are different ways to grip the bar, but I recommend the position used for the Olympic lift known as the *clean*, which looks like this:

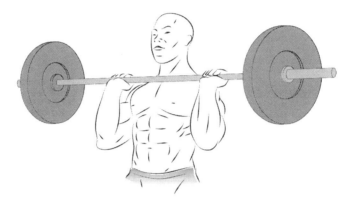

If this places too much stress on your wrists, you can alleviate this by removing a finger or two from under the bar, such as the thumb and pinky.

In this position, the barbell sits on the front of your shoulders, which requires that your upper-back muscles work harder, that your torso stays upright, and that your chest and elbows remain up and forward. Don't try to hold the bar above your shoulders with your hands or your wrists will start hurting. It's uncomfortable at first, but you want your shoulders to carry the load.

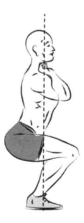

Maintain this tight, vertical position for the entire lift.

To begin the descent, take a deep breath and stabilize your core. Push your hips out and squat straight down, keeping your knees in line with the toes, until your thighs are just below parallel to the ground. You'll notice that this pushes your knees a bit more forward than the back squat, which is normal.

Drive through your heels to begin the ascent and keep your chest up, back tight, and elbows high.

The Bench Press

If you're new to weightlifting, get ready for every guy you know to start asking how much you bench. Although it's one of the easier exercises to perform (squatting and deadlifting are *much* harder), bench pressing a lot of weight is just synonymous with being manly and strong I guess.

Thus, guys rarely miss chest day, and the strong desire to bench a few plates or more often leads to many mistakes: failing to bring the weight all the way down, overarching the back, raising the butt off the bench, shrugging or rolling the shoulders at the top, flaring the elbows, and more.

Well, while you can cheat on something like dumbbell curls without risking much in the way of injury, the bench press is different. If you don't know what you're doing and try to press large amounts of weight with poor form, it's easy to hurt your shoulders, which can then take what feels like *forever* to heal and rehab.

Bench press properly, however, and you'll keep your shoulders safe and your chest growing bigger and stronger. Let's talk about how this works.

Bench Press Setup

A strong bench press starts with a strong base, and here's how it works:

Lie down on the bench and "screw" your shoulder blades in by retracting them in toward each other and down toward your waist. Create an arch in your lower back that's big enough to fit a fist between it and the bench. Your chest should be raised as if you're going to show it to someone, and you'll want to keep it "up" like this for the entire lift.

Your grip should be a few inches wider than shoulder-width (about 22 to 28 inches, depending on your build). If you get too narrow, you'll be relying too much on the triceps (incidentally, the close-grip bench press is a fantastic triceps exercise, but we'll talk about that later), and if you get too wide, you'll reduce the range of motion and overall effectiveness of the exercise.

Don't use a "thumbless" or "suicide" grip (as its aptly called), which has your thumbs next to your index fingers as opposed to wrapped around the bar. While people give various reasons for liking the thumbless grip, its disadvantage is obvious: when you're going heavy, it's surprisingly easy for the barbell to slip out of your hands and crash down on your chest, or worse, your neck (just Google "thumbless grip bench press accident" if you don't believe me!).

Put the bar in the palm of your hand, not in your fingers, because this leads to wrist pains.

Grip the bar *hard.* Try to crush it like spaghetti, as this will give you a little boost in strength.

Create a stable lower body base by placing your feet directly beneath your knees, which should be angled outward, tightening your quads and activating your glutes. The upper part of your leg should be parallel to the floor, and the lower part should be perpendicular (forming a 90-degree angle), which allows you to push through your heels as you ascend, creating the "leg drive" that you've probably heard of (the powerlifting style of bench press, with the heels elevated, is fine too if you prefer it).

Once you've done all the above, you've put yourself in the position that you want to maintain throughout the entire lift.

Bench Press Movement

Unrack the bar by locking your elbows out to move the bar off the hooks, and move the bar into position with your elbows still locked. Don't try to bring the weight straight from the hooks to your chest, and don't drop your chest and loosen your shoulder blades when unracking, because it will make you shrug the bar off with your shoulders.

Research has shown that keeping your arms at about a 45-degree angle relative to your torso and using a medium grip are the best ways to protect your shoulders while performing the bench press.[16] However, 45 degrees on the nose isn't necessarily right for everyone—you'll want to find the position between 30 and 60 degrees that is most comfortable for you.

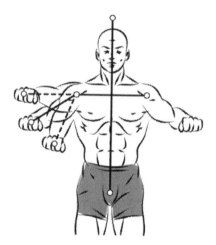

The lowest position above is about 20 degrees and commonly seen in powerlifting. The middle position is about 45 degrees and is what I find most comfortable. The top position is 90 degrees, which places the shoulders in a compromising position.

The proper bench press movement is a controlled lowering of the bar all the way down to the bottom of your chest (over your nipples), followed by an explosive drive upward. The bar should move in a straight line up and down, not toward your face or belly button.

There's a never-ending debate over whether you should bring the bar to your chest. Many fitness "experts" claim that you should lower the weight no further than the point where your upper arms are parallel to the floor, as going any deeper places too much stress on the shoulders. This is nonsense.

Reducing the range of motion only reduces the effectiveness of the exercise, and the shoulders are only at risk of injury when with improper technique. By using a full range of motion with proper form, you'll maximize muscle growth while preventing injury.

Don't watch the bar as it moves, as this will likely cause you to vary its angles of descent and ascent. Instead, pick a spot on the ceiling to look at during the exercise and see the bar going down and up in relation to it. The goal is to bring it up to the same spot for each rep.

Keep your elbows "tucked" in the starting position the entire time, paying special attention during the ascension (as this is when people usually flare them out to gain leverage). Increasing the angle relative to your torso makes it easier to get the weight up but puts undue stress on the shoulders.

Bench Press Tips

Don't allow your chest to go flat while doing the press, and don't allow your shoulders to shrug or roll forward at the top of a rep. Keep your chest up, elbows tucked, and shoulder blades pinched and retracted.

Use your legs to drive against the floor. This transfers force up through the hips and back, which helps maintain proper form and can increase the pushing force you can generate.

Keep your butt on the bench at all times. If your butt is lifting, the weight is probably too heavy. The three points of contact that you should always maintain are the upper back (stays down on the bench), the butt (ditto), and the feet (stay planted on the floor).

Don't bounce the bar off your chest. Lower it in a controlled manner, keeping everything tight. Then let it touch your chest and drive it up.

Don't smash the back of your head into the bench, as this can strain your neck. Your neck will naturally tighten while doing the exercise, but don't forcefully push it down.

When you're lowering the weight, think about the coming drive up. Visualize the explosive second half of the exercise the entire time, and you'll find it easier to control the descent of the weight, prevent bouncing, and even prepare your muscles for the imminent stress of raising the bar. (This technique is good for all exercises, by the way.)

Make sure to finish your last rep before trying to rack the weight. Many guys make the mistake of moving the bar toward their faces on the way up during their last rep. What if they miss the rep and it starts coming down or misses the hooks? It's not pretty.

Instead, press the weight straight up as a usual, lock your elbows out, move the bar back to the rack until it hits the uprights, and then lower it to the hooks.

Bench Press Variations

As a part of the *Bigger Leaner Stronger* program, you're going to do two variations of the basic bench press: the incline bench press and close-grip bench press.

<u>Incline Bench Press</u>

The "upper chest" debate is one of the many "controversial" subjects in the world of weightlifting.

Do you need to do chest exercises specifically for the upper chest? Or do all chest exercises stimulate all available muscle fibers? And even more to the point, is there even such a thing as the "upper chest?"

Well, I'll keep this short and sweet.

There is a portion of the "chest muscle" that forms what we call the "upper chest." It's known as the *clavicular pectoralis*, and here's what it looks like:

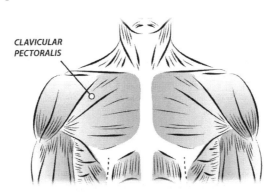

While this muscle is a part of the big chest muscle, the pectoralis major, the angle of the muscle fibers is quite different. Thus, certain movements can emphasize the main head of the pectoralis and others can emphasize the clavicular head.

Notice that I say *emphasize*, not *isolate*. That's because all movements that emphasize one of the two do, to some degree, involve the other. Nevertheless, proper chest development requires a *lot* of emphasis on the clavicular pectoralis for two simple reasons:

1. It's a small, stubborn muscle that takes its sweet time to grow.

2. The movements that are best for developing it also happen to be great for growing the pectoralis major.

The best way to ensure your upper chest doesn't fall behind your pec major in size is to do a lot of incline pressing, Hence, my inclusion of the incline bench press in the program, which emphasizes the clavicular pectoralis more than flat or decline pressing.[17]

When doing this exercise, the angle of incline in the bench should be 30 to 45 degrees. I prefer 30 degrees, but some people prefer an incline closer to 45. I recommend that you try various settings ranging between 30 and 45 degrees and see which you like most.

The basic setup and movement of the incline bench press is just as you learned for the regular bench press, with a small exception: the bar should pass by the chin and touch just below the collarbones to allow for a vertical bar path.

Close-Grip Bench Press

As I mentioned earlier, as you narrow your grip on the bar, the triceps have to do more of the work. This is undesirable when you're focusing on training your chest, but it's one of my favorite ways to train the triceps.

When doing a close-grip bench press, your grip should be slightly narrower than shoulder-width and no closer. You'll see many guys place their hands just a few inches apart, and this is a bad idea—it puts the shoulders and wrists in a weakened, compromised position.

The rest of the setup and movement are the same as the regular bench press: the shoulder blades are "screwed" into the bench, there's a slight arch in the lower back, the feet are flat on the floor, and the bar moves straight down, touches the bottom of your chest, and moves straight up.

If your shoulders or wrists feel uncomfortable at the bottom of the lift, simply widen your grip by about the width of a finger and try again. If this doesn't handle it, widen your grip by another finger width and repeat until it's comfortable (but not so wide that you're turning it into a standard bench press!).

The Deadlift

The deadlift is the ultimate full-body workout, training just about every muscle group in the body: leg muscles, glutes, the entire back, core, and arm muscles. Basically, any muscle that's involved in producing whole-body power is involved in the deadlift, and that's why it's an integral part of every serious strength training program.

While few people argue its effectiveness for building muscle and strength, some claim it's also one of the "dangerous" exercises that we should avoid unless we want to have serious back problems one day.

At first glance, this fear would seem to make sense: lifting hundreds of pounds off the ground—putting all that pressure on your back, particularly your low-back and erector spinae muscles—would be a recipe for thoracic and lumbar disaster, right?

Well, let's start by reviewing a study conducted by researchers at the University of Valencia that set out to determine the most effective way to train the paraspinal muscles, which run down both sides of your spine and play a major role in the prevention of back injuries.[18]

Researchers had 25 people with no low-back pain perform two types of exercise for their backs: (1) bodyweight exercises like lumbar extensions, forward flexions, single-leg deadlifts, and bridges and (2) two weighted exercises, deadlifts and lunges, using 70 percent of their 1RM weight. Muscle activity was measured using electromyography, a technique of measuring and analyzing muscle contractions via electrical activity that occurs in the muscles.

The result: deadlifts most activated the paraspinal muscles. And it wasn't even close. The deadlift's average electromyographic muscle activity was 88 percent and peaked at 113 percent, whereas the back extension produced an average activity of 58 percent and a peak of 55 percent, and the lunge produced an average of 46 percent and a peak of 61 percent. The rest of the exercises' average activities ranged between 29 and 42 percent muscle activity, with the supine bridge on a BOSU ball being the least effective.

Thus, researchers concluded, the deadlift is an incredibly effective way to strengthen the paraspinal muscles.

Another study conducted by researchers at the University of Waterloo was done to determine how much low-back flexion deadlifting caused and thus how much strain it put on the vertebrae and lumbar ligament.[19] Did the exercise put the back, and low-back in particular, under excessive strain that could lead to injury?

Researchers used real-time X-ray imaging (called *fluoroscopy*) to watch the spines of elite powerlifters while they fully flexed their spines with no weights and while they deadlifted more than 400 pounds. With the exception of one trial of one subject, all men completed their deadlifts within the normal range of motion they displayed during full flexion. Ligament lengths were unaffected, indicating that they don't help support the load but instead limit the range of motion.

So, as we can see, a proper deadlift effectively strengthens your entire back, including your erector spinae muscles, and doesn't force anything unnatural in terms of range of motion.

As with the squat and bench press, poor form is what gives the deadlift a bad name. There are many mistakes you can make, but the major "no-no" is rounding your lower back during the lift, as this shifts much of the stress away from the erector spinae muscles to the vertebrae and ligaments.

So, with that out of the way, let's now learn how to deadlift properly.

Deadlift Setup

Always start with the bar on the floor—not on the safety pins or on the rack.

Your stance should be a bit narrower than shoulder width, and your toes should be pointed slightly out. You should stand with the bar above the middle of your feet (the top of your instep).

Stand up tall with your chest out, and take a deep breath of air into your diaphragm (not your lungs), bracing your abs as if you were about to get punched in the stomach.

Bend through your knees until your shins touch the bar and your knees are slightly past it, and then lift your chest until your back is in a neutral position and tight. Don't overarch your lower back, and don't squeeze your shoulder blades together like with the squat. Just push your chest up and your shoulders and back down.

Don't make the newbie mistake of bringing your hips too low with the intention of "squatting" the weight up. The lower your hips are below optimal, the more they will have to rise before you're able to lift the weight off the floor, which is just wasted movement.

Instead, you should feel tightness in your hamstrings and hips as you wedge yourself into what's essentially a "half-squat" position.

Your arms should be completely straight and locked and just outside your legs, leaving enough room for your thumbs to clear your thighs.

Grip the bar by placing it into the middle of your palms, not in your fingers. Both palms should be facing in to build grip strength. The other grip option is the "mixed grip," where one palm faces in (usually the nondominant hand) and the other faces out, which can allow you to lift heavier weight.

Here's what the starting position looks like:

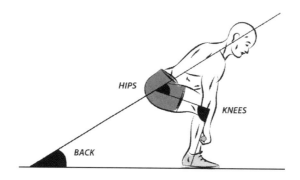

You're now ready to pull.

Deadlift Movement

Drive your body upward and slightly back *as quickly as you can* by pushing through your heels. Keep your elbows locked in place and your lower back slightly arched (no rounding!).

Ensure that your hips and shoulders move up simultaneously: don't shoot your hips up without also raising your shoulders.

You'll feel your hamstrings and hips working hard as you continue to rise. Keep your back neutral and tight the whole way up, and try to keep the bar on as vertically straight of a path as possible (there should be little lateral movement of the bar as you lift it up).

The bar should move up your shins and roll over your knees and thighs, at which point your glutes contract forcefully to bring you into a standing position. At the top, your chest should be out and your shoulders down. Don't lean back, shrug the weight, or roll your shoulders up and back.

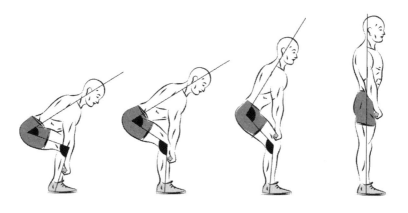

The next half of the movement is lowering the weight back down to the floor in a controlled manner (yes, it must go all the way back to the floor!). This is basically a mirror image of what you did to come up.

You begin lowering the bar by pushing your *hips* back first, letting the bar descend in a straight line, sliding down your thighs, until it reaches your knees. You then bend your knees and lower it down your shins. The back stays locked in its tight, neutral position the entire time.

Don't try to deliberately slow down the lowering of the weight, especially as you get the bar to your knees. The entire second half of the lift should take about 1 to 2 seconds.

There are two ways of transitioning into your next rep: the tap-and-go and stop-and-go methods. The tap-and-go method has you tap the floor with the plates and move directly into your next rep, whereas the stop-and-go method has you fully release the plates on the floor for a second before starting your next rep.

The latter is harder than the former but not necessarily *better*. It's more a matter of finding what feels best for you. I prefer the tap-and-go method, but sometimes I use the stop-and-go method if I'm going particularly heavy.

Deadlift Tips

Wear long pants and long socks on the day that you'll be deadlifting to prevent shin scraping. This can be caused by poor form but can also be unavoidable depending on the relationship between your limbs and torso and lower body.

As with squatting, deadlifting in shoes that have air cushions or gel fillings or overly elevated heels is a bad idea. They compromise stability, cause power loss, and interfere with proper form. Get shoes with flat, hard soles or weightlifting shoes for your deadlifting and squatting and you'll be better for it.

If you start it with bent elbows, you'll end up putting unnecessary strain on your biceps. Keep your elbows straight for the entire lift.

Stick with the overhand grip if possible as it's great for strengthening your grip. As you get stronger, however, you may find that the bar starts falling out of your hands during your sets. If this happens, you can switch to the alternating grip and, if you like, include some grip-specific training in your routine, which you can find here: http://bit.ly/grip-training.

Too wide of a stance or grip will make the exercise awkward. The deadlift stance is narrower than the squat stance, and it requires that the hands be just outside the legs.

Try to crush the bar with your grip. If your knuckles aren't white, you're not squeezing hard enough.

If you start the ascension with your hips too high, you'll turn the deadlift into a stiff-legged deadlift, which is more stressful on the lower back and hamstrings. Make sure that you get your hips low enough in the starting position.

A common mistake guys make is starting the ascension slowly, which makes it *much* easier to get stuck. Explode the bar up from the floor as fast as you can by applying as much force through your heels as possible.

When you're lowering the weight, if you break your knees too early, you'll hit them with the bar. To avoid this, begin your descent by pushing your hips back first and don't bend your knees until the bar reaches them.

Don't strain to look up while deadlifting. Keep your head in a neutral position and in line with your spine.

Deadlift Variations

Sumo Deadlift

The sumo deadlift uses a wide stance (1.5 to 2 times the width of your shoulders) to shorten the range of motion and limit the shearing force on the lower back.[20] It also can feel more comfortable in the hips than a conventional deadlift, depending on your biomechanics (if you walk with your toes pointed out, the sumo may be better for you).

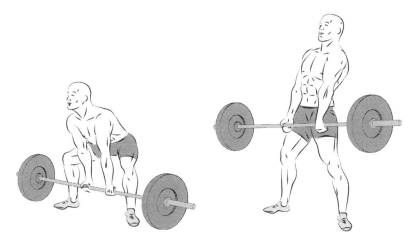

The downside of the sumo deadlift is the reduced range of motion, which results in less work done, which means less overall muscle development.[21] Nevertheless, give this variation a try if you lack the flexibility to do a conventional deadlift, if it just feels uncomfortable (certain people's bodies are better suited to the sumo deadlift), or if it's causing low-back pain.

Hex Bar Deadlift

The hex bar—or trap bar—deadlift is a great way to learn to deadlift, because it doesn't require as much hip and ankle mobility to get to the bar and puts less shearing stress on the spine.[22] It also allows you to lift more weight than the conventional deadlift, which may make it a more effective exercise for developing overall lower body power.[23]

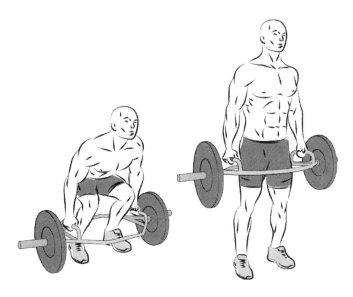

The conventional deadlift is more effective in strengthening the erector spinae and hip muscles, however, because the hex bar deadlift is more like a squat due to the increased load it places on the quadriceps.

Romanian Deadlift

The "RDL," as it's often called, was started by a Romanian powerlifter named Nicu Vlad, who would perform outrageous feats of strength like front squatting 700 pounds while only weighing 220 pounds.

The RDL is a variation of the deadlift that targets the glutes and hamstrings and minimizes the involvement of the quads and hip muscles.

The RDL starts with the weight on safety pins or the lower portion of the rack. You use the same stance and grip as with the regular deadlift, and you walk the weight back a step or two. In the start position, your knees are locked, your chest is up, your back is straight and tight, and your eyes should focus on a point on the floor about 10 feet away.

When you begin the movement, you unlock your knees just enough to put some tension on the quads, and your back should be slightly arched. Start the bar down the thigh in a straight line by pushing the hips back, and your torso should lean forward to keep your shoulders directly over the bar.

The bar passes over your knees and travels down the shins, and you go as low as you can without breaking the extension of your back. Because of the increasing angle of the torso, you probably won't be able to go much further than a few inches past your knees, and that's okay. In fact, if the weight is touching the floor, you're doing it wrong (you're bending your knees).

Resist the temptation to relax the tension in the knees at the bottom by flexing them, as this transfers the load from the hamstrings to the quads.

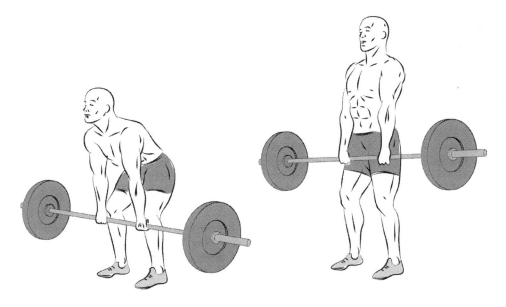

Once you've achieved a good stretch in your hamstrings and your back is ready to unlock, start back up. On the way up, keep your chest and back tight and locked into position, and move the bar straight up your legs.

Hold your back rigid for the entire lift. Don't let the chest sag or the lower back loosen.

The Military Press

The military press is the best all-around shoulder exercise you can perform. It's a simple, easy to learn movement that allows for the safe lifting of heavy weights.

There are two variations of the military press: standing and seated. The standing variation requires tremendous core and lower back strength to maintain balance, which in turn limits the weight you can lift. While there's nothing inherently wrong with this, I find that heavy deadlifting and squatting every week builds more than enough core and lower back strength, and I prefer to use this lift to maximize the overload on my shoulders.

Thus, I go with the seated press and recommend that you do the same. That said, the seated press requires a proper military press station, which looks like this:

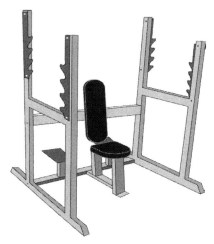

If your gym doesn't have this piece of equipment or if you can't rig something like it using a power rack and utility bench, then you can opt for the standing variation, which you can perform in a squat rack.

Let's now talk form, starting with the seated press.

The Seated Military Press Setup

Place your feet flat on the ground about shoulder-width apart with your toes and knees slightly turned out. Press your heels into the ground to keep your upper back and butt rooted in place against the back of the bench.

Grip the bar slightly wider than you would to bench press (slightly wider than shoulder-width) and place the bar over your wrists, not in your fingers. Your back should be in a neutral position and stay there throughout the lift.

The Seated Military Press Movement

To begin the descent, take a deep breath, tighten your abs and glutes, and press your chest up. Bring the bar straight down toward your clavicle, and keep your elbows tucked like you would during the bench press (don't force them to stay right at your sides and don't let them slide too far behind you).

Tilt your head back to allow the bar to pass your nose and chin and look forward, not straight up. (This is why a full bench doesn't work for the military press: you can't tilt your head back to get it out of the way and are forced to lower the weight lower down your chest, which is incorrect.) There should be a slight arch in your lower back at the bottom of the lift, but don't overdo this as it can cause injury when you start loading more and more weight. If you're arching too much, the weight is probably too heavy.

Once the bar has reached your clavicle, raise it straight up along the path of descent, and once it passes your forehead, shift your torso a little forward and squeeze your glutes. Keep raising the bar until your elbows are locked: your shoulders, traps, and back should be tight and squeezed.

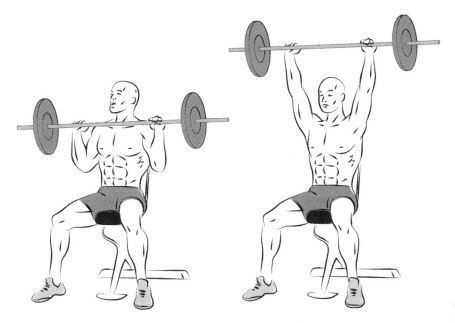

The Standing Military Press Setup & Movement

The standing press is performed in exactly the same way—you're just standing.

The bar rests on the squat rack at the same height as if you were squatting, and once you've unracked it, the movement is as described above. To recap: place the feet and grip shoulder-width apart, grip the bar like the bench press, keep the back neutral, descend straight to the clavicles, tilt the head back while looking forward, raise the bar along the same path, shift the torso forward slightly, squeeze the glutes, and lock out.

HOW TO TRAIN THE BIGGER LEANER STRONGER WAY

While the theory of "muscle confusion" is silly and scientifically bankrupt, it's true that your body can respond favorably to doing new exercises after doing the same routine for a bit. Changing things up can also help keep you excited for and interested in your workouts, which improves overall results.

Thus, the *Bigger Leaner Stronger* program calls for changing your routine every eight weeks. We'll get more into the actual programming in the next chapter, but first I want to give you the list of "approved" exercises so you can build your own workouts as well as some general tips on training each muscle group.

The exercises I recommend are the ones I've found most effective for building a big, strong body. They are listed in order of seniority (the first exercise is what I feel is most important for developing the muscle group, the second is second-most important, and so forth). As you'll see in the bonus report, the program I've developed has you performing all of them over the course of your first year.

You might be surprised at how few choices there are for each muscle group, and that's because while there are an overwhelming number of exercises we *could* do to train the various muscle groups in our body, a small minority actually deliver the goods (Pareto's 80/20 principle at work).

In terms of how to do the exercises, instead of filling another 30 pages with images and descriptions, I'd rather share videos with you instead. You can find links to videos on proper form for all exercises in the bonus report.

Chest

Your goal shouldn't be to just have a "big chest" because just adding size willy-nilly won't necessarily give you the look you want. The goal is to have a big, *proportionate* chest that has fully developed upper and lower portions.

The exercises that best accomplish this are few, and they maximally recruit muscle fibers and allow for heavy, progressive overload without dramatically increasing the risk of injury.

Here they are:

Incline Barbell Bench Press
Incline Dumbbell Bench Press
Flat Barbell Bench Press
Flat Dumbbell Bench Press
Dip (Chest Variation)

These are the exercises you *must* master if you want to build an impressive chest. Period. Forget cable work, dumbbell flys, push-up variations, machines, and every other type of chest exercise out there for now. They just aren't nearly as effective as the above core, foundation-building lifts and are only for advanced weightlifters who have already paid their dues with the heavy pressing to build big, strong pecs.

Another common exercise I've left off the list is any type of decline press. This wasn't a mistake.

The reason I'm shunning this popular exercise is that decline pressing is simply less effective than incline and flat pressing for training the pecs. Due to its reduced range of motion, it causes less stimulation of both the pectoralis major and clavicular pectoralis.[24]

A common argument for doing decline presses is to work the lowest portion of the pectoralis major, but dips are a far superior exercise for accomplishing this while also training more muscles overall and building upper body balance and coordination.

As you know, a major part of building a great chest is focusing on your incline pressing more than anything else. If you don't, your upper chest *will* fall behind in development, which will look stranger and stranger as your pectoralis major gets larger and larger.

As most people's upper chests are already behind, this usually means starting each chest workout with 3 to 6 sets of incline pressing for four to six months straight. Flat pressing is done as well, but always after the incline pressing.

I usually rotate between dumbbell-centric and barbell-centric routines. For example, I'll do a routine of incline dumbbell presses, flat dumbbell press, and weighted dips for eight weeks and then switch to a routine of flat bench press, incline bench press, and flat dumbbell press for the next eight.

BACK

There are a handful of muscles that make up the bulk of the back, and they need to be well developed, including the *trapezius, rhomboids, latissimus dorsi, erector spinae, teres major* and *minor,* and *infraspinatus.* Here's how they look:

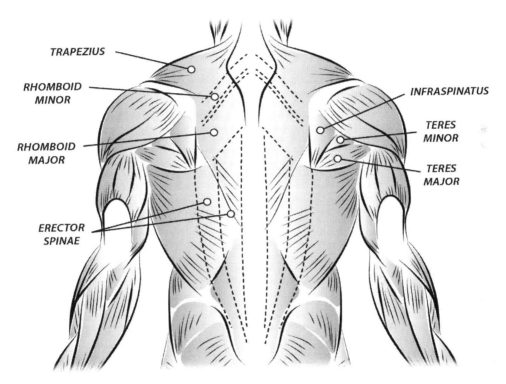

Here's the goal in terms of overall back development:

- large, but not overdeveloped, traps that establish the upper back,

- wide lats that extend low down the torso, creating that pleasing V-taper,

- bulky rhomboids that create "valleys" when flexed,

- clear development and separation in the teres muscles and infraspinatus, and

- a thick, "Christmas tree" structure in the lower back.

And here are the exercises that get the job done:

Barbell Deadlift
Barbell Row
One-Arm Dumbbell Row
Pull-Up

Lat Pulldown (Front and Close-Grip)
T-Bar Row Seated Cable Row (Wide- and Close-Grip)
Chin-Up
Barbell Shrug

The deadlift is, by far, the most effective back exercise you can do. You just can't beat it for all-around development and strength, and that's why you'll be doing it every week. Every back workout will start with it. You're going to need all the energy you can muster to pull heavy weight.

The barbell row, one-arm dumbbell row, and pull-up (especially the wide-grip pull-up) are almost tied in my book as each is a fantastic all-around back builder. The shrugs are listed last because they only train the traps and are only included in workouts if trap development is lagging.

In terms of programming your own workouts, I highly recommend that you always start with the deadlift. From there, move to a wide-gripped pulling movement like the barbell or T-bar row or front lat pulldown or wide-grip pull-up (weighted, if you can), followed by a more narrow-gripped pulling movement like the one-arm dumbbell row, close-grip lat pulldown, close-grip seated row, or chin-up.

SHOULDERS

Your shoulders consist of three major muscles known as *deltoids,* and here's how they look:

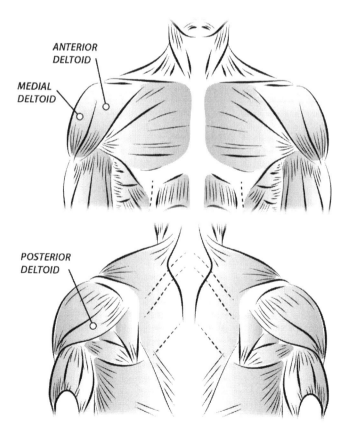

It's important to develop all three heads of this muscle group, because if one is lagging, it will be painfully obvious.

In most cases, the medial and posterior deltoids need the most work because the anterior deltoids get worked pretty intensely with proper chest training. The other two heads don't, however.

Here are the exercises I recommend focusing on in your shoulder training:

Seated Barbell Military Press or Standing Barbell Military Press
Seated Dumbbell Press or Arnold Dumbbell Press
Dumbbell Side Lateral Raise or One-Arm Dumbbell Side Lateral Raise
Rear Delt Raise (Bent-Over or Seated)
Face Pull
Barbell Rear Delt Row
Dumbbell Front Raise

As you can see, I'm a fan of pressing. As with the chest, you just can't beat heavy pressing for developing your shoulders. And as a natural weightlifter, you're going to need as much help as you can get in this department.

If all you do is press, however, you'll find that your middle and rear heads of your deltoids fall behind in development. This is why a good shoulder workout trains all three heads of the muscle by having you press as well as do side raises and something for the rear delts. Just like any other muscle group, the shoulders can benefit from higher-rep work, but you have to emphasize the heavy weightlifting if you want them to grow.

As a side note, the dumbbell front raise is a good exercise, but don't do this in place of a barbell or dumbbell press as it simply doesn't build mass like they do. If you're particularly weak on your presses, the front raise can be helpful in strengthening many of the small, supporting muscles required for the tougher lifts, but I recommend that you do it after your pressing, not instead of it.

LEGS

I understand the temptation to skip legs day. I used to do it all the time and am paying the price now. My legs have come a long way but are still behind my upper body in overall development, and my calves are still too small (I'm working on it!).

Before we get to the training, I'd like to quickly review the major muscles of the leg so we know what we're looking to develop.

The quadriceps is a group of four muscles that compose the bulk of the muscle on the front of the thigh. The four "heads" of the quadriceps are the *rectus femoris, vastus lateralis, vastus medialis,* and *vastus intermedius.* Here's how they look:

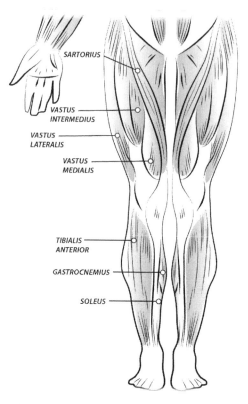

The back of the leg is dominated by three muscles that contract the hamstring tendon, which are the *semitendinosus*, *semimembranosus*, and *biceps femoris*. Here's how they look:

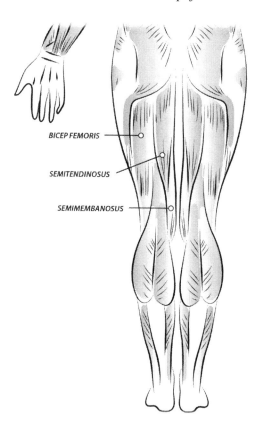

And last but not least is the calf muscle, which consists of two muscles: the *gastrocnemius* and *soleus*. And here's how they look:

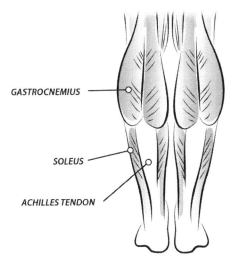

The gastrocnemius is the most externally visible muscle, and the soleus is a deep muscle that lies underneath the gastrocnemius. These two muscles work together to manipulate the foot and ankle joint as well as flex the leg at the knee joint.

When it comes to just looks, we're most concerned with the gastrocnemius, but a properly developed soleus "props up" the gastrocnemius, making it look more impressive.

So, those are the major muscle groups that we're concerned with in terms of visual development. There are quite a few smaller muscles that will greatly affect our ability to properly train the larger muscles, but we don't need to review each of them. By following the advice in this chapter, they will develop along with the larger groups.

My list of favorite leg exercises is pretty short and simple. They are compound movements, they allow for heavy weights, and they are safe.

These are the exercises I've used to dramatically improve my own legs, and they will do the same for you:

Barbell Squat
Front Squat
Hack Squat (sled, not barbell)
Leg Press
Barbell Lunge (Walking or In Place)
Dumbbell Lunge
Romanian Deadlift
Leg Curl (Lying or Seated)
Calf Raise (Donkey, Standing or Seated)
Calf Press on the Leg Press

Working legs is very simple. Rule #1: Always do squats. Rule #2: Always do squats. Rule #3: You get the point.

The bottom line is that every leg workout should begin with either the back or front squat, with the former focusing on the hamstrings and the latter on the quadriceps. Next, I like to focus on the other major muscle group of the pair, with the back squat my exercise of choice for hamstring emphasis and the front squat, hack squat, leg press, or a lunge movement for the quadriceps. I then usually finish with some hamstring-centric work like the Romanian deadlift or even the leg curl.

That leaves the calves—the most stubborn muscle group you can probably find on your body and the embarrassment of weightlifters everywhere.

Why is this? Why are great calves so rare, and why do many of the guys who have them almost never train them?

Well, many cases of "baby calves" are caused by simple neglect. As with their abs, many people forget to train their calves or think it's unnecessary.

That's not the whole story, though; there are genetic barriers to work through as well, which explains why some people tend to have small calves that basically refuse to grow no matter what they do, whereas others develop bulging calves despite hardly trying.

The answer to this "mystery" lies in the composition of the calf muscle fibers themselves. You see, there are two primary groups of muscle types: Type 1, also known as "slow twitch" fibers, and Type 2, also known as "fast twitch" fibers.

Type I muscle fibers have the lowest potential for growth and force output.[25] However, they are dense with capillaries (small blood vessels) and rich in mitochondria (which produce energy for cells) and myoglobin (which provides extra oxygen to the muscles), which makes them resistant to fatigue. Type II fibers, on the other hand, have a much higher potential for growth and force output than Type I fibers, but they fatigue quickly.[26]

Research has shown that the muscle fibers of the gastrocnemius—the calf muscle we see and are primarily concerned with developing for aesthetic purposes—can vary in composition from person to person.[27] One guy's gastrocnemius might be composed of as much as 60 percent Type 2 fibers, whereas another's is as little as 15 percent. And thus, the former will find it easy to add mass to his calves, but the latter (me) will find it a slow, frustrating grind.

Furthermore, research has also shown that the ratio of Type 1 to Type 2 fibers in various muscles is determined by how we primarily use the muscles.[28] As the calf is mainly used in low-intensity, endurance activities like walking, jogging, biking, and so forth, there's a greater need for Type 1 than Type 2 fibers, further predisposing us to having pretty little "dress legs."

Fortunately, our genetics don't ultimately decide whether we are stuck with tiny calves. With proper training, anyone can build muscular calves, but you should just know that it may or may not come quickly depending on your DNA.

Now, speaking of calf training, some people say it's like ab training: you don't need to bother with it if you're doing a lot of squats and deadlifts. Well, I disagree (on both counts, actually, but we'll talk abs soon).

Unless you're bringing better-than-usual calf genetics to the game, you're going to have to work these little suckers quite a bit to maintain proportions with your thighs and arms. And if you're like me and your body somehow decided it didn't need any calves whatsoever (before I started training my calves regularly and correctly, I had *nothing* no matter how much I squatted and deadlifted), you're going to have to work them even more.

I've tried a lot of calf routines, and I've learned a couple of things:

Like the abs, the calves seem to recover from workouts more quickly than other muscle groups and thus can be trained more intensively.

I've yet to find concrete scientific evidence of this, but the anecdotal evidence goes back decades. Arnold even noticed that his calves recovered faster than other muscle groups.

The calves seem to respond particularly well to periodized training that includes high-rep work.

Periodized training has you work a muscle group with various rep ranges, and the calves seem to particularly benefit from the inclusion of higher-rep ranges. (And in case you're wondering, a periodized approach works well on other muscle groups as well, but it's best suited to advanced weightlifters and is discussed in the sequel to this book, *Beyond Bigger Leaner Stronger*.)

There are various theories as to why this is but no definitive answers that I know of. Nevertheless, success leaves clues, and this is one you'll often come across in talking with guys who have built impressive calves and had to actually work for it.

Based on these two points, the calf routine I'm going to recommend works as follows:

- Do 2 calf workouts per week with at least one day in between each.

- Do 6 sets per workout.

- For the first set, point your toes forward. For the second, point them slightly out (about 20 degrees). For the third set, point them slightly inward. Repeat for the next 3 sets.

- Use a 2-1-2 rep tempo: 2 seconds to full contraction, a slight pause while contracted, and 2 seconds to release.

- Once you hit the top of your rep range with a given weight, add 10 pounds.

Here are the workouts:

Calf Workout A

Standing Calf Raise – 3 sets of 4 to 6 reps
Seated Calf Raise – 3 sets of 4 to 6 reps
Rest 2 to 3 minutes in between these sets

Calf Workout B

Leg Press Calf Raise – 3 sets of 8 to 10 reps
Donkey Calf Raise (or Leg Press Calf Raise) – 3 sets of 8 to 10 reps
Rest 1 to 2 minutes in between these sets

Simple enough. Personally, I do Workout A on Tuesdays and B on Thursdays.

As with all exercises, form is extremely important in calf training. If you shortchange yourself by reducing the range of motion, you'll find the workouts far less effective.

The proper form with these calf exercises is simple: at the bottom of a rep, your heels are as low as they'll go and you feel a deep stretch in your calves, and at the top of a rep, you're up on your tippy-toes like a ballerina. Many people simply use too much weight and can't make it anywhere near as high as they should at the top of their reps and then wonder why their calves never get bigger or stronger. Don't make the same mistake.

ARMS

While I think the arms get a bit *too* much attention in the overall scheme of things, I definitely agree that a physique isn't complete without big, developed arms.

As you probably know, the largest arm muscles are the biceps and triceps, but let's look at them in a little more detail, as well as the forearms, so we know exactly what we're training.

The biceps (or, formally, *biceps brachii*) is a two-headed muscle that looks like this:

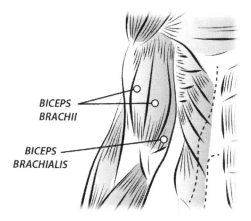

You can also see the *biceps brachialis*, which lies beneath the biceps brachii. While this muscle isn't nearly as prominent as the biceps brachii when developed, it plays an important role in the overall look of your arms.

It looks like a mere "bump" in between the biceps brachii and triceps, but its level of development affects the amount of "peak" your biceps appear to have (ultimately, peak is mostly determined by genetics, but increasing the size of the brachialis can give the *appearance* of a better peak).

The next muscle group to talk about is the triceps, or *triceps brachii*, which has three heads:

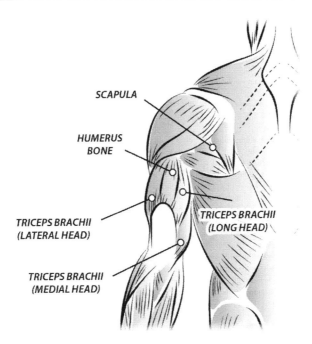

As you can see, the three heads combine to form the distinctive "horseshoe" that can become quite pronounced when properly developed.

While the biceps are usually the focus of arms workouts, many people don't realize that the triceps account for quite a bit of your arm's size. Small triceps mean small, disproportionate arms, regardless of the size of the biceps.

Last but not least are the forearms, which consist of several smaller muscles:

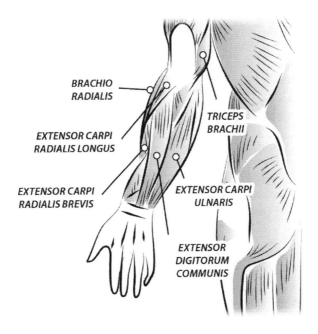

Forearms are like the calves of the arms. They aren't the immediate focus, but if they're underdeveloped, it's sorely obvious.

Now let's get to the exercises, starting with the biceps:

Barbell Curl

E-Z Bar Curl

Dumbbell Curl

Hammer Curl

Chin-up

By now, you're probably not surprised that the list is short and sweet. These exercises plus your heavy back training are all you need to build big, thick, strong biceps.

In terms of programming, you have quite a bit of flexibility. What I like to do is at least one barbell and one dumbbell exercise per workout for the biceps. Most of the time it's the barbell curl followed by the hammer curl.

Let's move on to the triceps:

Close-Grip Bench Press

Seated Triceps Press

Dip (Triceps Variation)

Lying Triceps Extension ("Skullcrusher")

Triceps Pushdown

I like to start my triceps training with something I can push some weight on, like the close-grip bench press or seated triceps press. There's no real rule of thumb for what comes next—I simply rotate through the other exercises on the eight-week schedule that you'll be following.

It's worth noting that you may run into some pretty intense forearm soreness with the arm workouts in this program and with the biceps training in particular. It can almost feel like your *bones* are aching. If you experience this, simply reduce your working set weight to the 6- to 8-rep range (enough weight to allow for 6 reps but no more than 8) and build your strength here for the first couple of months. You should then be able to return to the 4 to 6 rep work and be pain-free.

CORE

Everyone wants it…the elusive six pack. The hallmark of the fitness elite, the proof that you know the inside "secrets" of getting ripped.

Unfortunately, the amount of bad advice out there on how to get them is just staggering. Some trainers say you just have to do special types of ab exercises…and they're wrong. Others say you just have to get lean and you'll have an awesome core…and they're wrong. Others still say you just have to do a lot of squatting and deadlifting…and they're wrong too. And let's not forget the quacks who say the real secret is avoiding certain types of foods and taking weird pills and powders—they're *really* wrong.

Like most things fitness, the real way to get six-pack abs—for both guys and gals—is pretty straightforward.

When people talk about "abs," what they're referring to is the pair of muscles that make up the *rectus abdominis:*

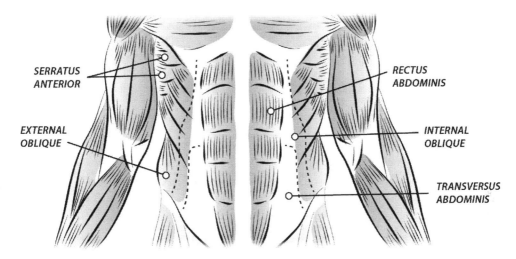

SERRATUS
ANTERIOR

EXTERNAL
OBLIQUE

RECTUS
ABDOMINIS

INTERNAL
OBLIQUE

TRANSVERSUS
ABDOMINIS

As you can see, however, these muscles aren't the whole story of the full six-pack look that people want, however. There are other "core" muscles that must be properly developed as well such as the obliques (external mainly), the *transversus abdominis* (or "TVA" as it's commonly referred to), and the *serratus anterior.*

How do you get these muscles to pop, you're wondering? Well…

No number of ab exercises alone will give you a great six pack.

No matter how simple or fancy the exercises, they are not the "shortcut to six-pack abs."

Yes, ab exercises are necessary for developing a solid core, but it takes more than weekly ab challenges to get the look you desire.

Just deadlifting and squatting isn't enough.

I don't know how many times I've heard the following: "I don't train abs; I squat and deadlift." And these guys and girls usually have unimpressive cores.

The reality is these two exercises, even when performed with heavy weight (80+ percent of 1RM), just don't involve the "show" muscles of the rectus abdominis, the tranversus abdominis, and the external obliques as much as people think.[29]

Now, don't get me wrong: heavy squatting and deadlifting do help build an all-around great core, but they aren't enough on their own.

Just being lean isn't enough, either.

It's true that you need to have low levels of body fat for your abs to fully show. For us guys, they start becoming visible as you get under 10 percent body fat (20 percent body fat for girls).

But you can get very lean and still not have the six-pack look you want because most people's cores aren't naturally developed enough to have the deep cuts and pronounced lines that make for a truly outstanding six pack.

What does it take to get a killer core, then?

The full six-pack look requires both low body fat levels *and* well-developed core muscles, and that means doing two things:

Reducing your body fat percentage.

Our rectus abdominis doesn't start showing until we reach the 10 percent range, and the rest of the core muscles don't pop until we reach the 8 percent range.

Just know that no matter how great your core muscles are developed, you will not achieve the look you want if your body fat percentage is too high.

Regularly performing the right ab and core exercises.

Building a great six-pack requires that you do both ab exercises that train your rectus abdominis and exercises that train the other core muscles that complete the look we want.

What are the right exercises, then? Let's find out…

Cable Crunch
Hanging Leg Raise
Captain's Chair Leg Raise
Ab Roller
Air Bicycles
Flat Bench Lying Leg Raise
Decline Crunch

I didn't just choose these at random. Research led by Peter Francis, PhD at the Biomechanics Lab at San Diego State University showed them to be the most effective for training the rectus abdominis and obliques.

One of the biggest ab training mistakes most people make is that they don't perform any weighted ab exercises. The result is the ability to do a bazillion crunches or leg raises…but with abs that look small and underdeveloped.

The abs are like any other muscle: they require progressive overload to grow, and that can only be accomplished by adding resistance to exercises. You don't have to add weight to all of your ab training, but you must do some if you want abs that pop.

I've found that abs seem to respond best to a combination of weighted and unweighted work. Here's how I like to do it:

• Do a set of a weighted exercise like the cable crunch, captain's chair leg raise, or hanging leg raise for 10 to 12 reps (you can add weight to the latter two by snatching a dumbbell in between your feet).

• Go directly into 1 set of an unweighted exercise, to failure.

• Go directly into 1 set of an unweighted exercise, to failure.

• Rest 2 to 3 minutes.

For example:

- Do a set of cable crunches in the 10- to 12-rep range.

- Go directly into 1 set of captain's chair leg raises, to failure.

- Go directly into 1 set of air bicycles, to failure.

- Rest 2 to 3 minutes.

Do 3 of these circuits two or three times per week, and your abs and obliques *will* develop.

In terms of developing the rest of your core muscles, heavy compound weightlifting exercises like the deadlift, squat, and military press get the job done better than special "core exercises,"[30] particularly when performed with heavy weight.[31] Nothing else is needed here.

All right then, that's it for the exercises you'll be doing on the *Bigger Leaner Stronger* program. In the next chapter, you're going to learn how to build workouts with them!

BOTTOM LINE

Building muscle and strength doesn't require that you constantly "challenge" your muscles with new, exotic exercises. It only requires that you make progress with a relatively small number of exercises that maximally challenge each muscle group and enable you to safely overload them over time.

This not only simplifies your goals, but it also makes working out more enjoyable. You go into every workout knowing exactly what you're doing and why, and you're able to easily track your progress over time.

CHAPTER SUMMARY

INTRODUCTION

- Out of the hundreds and hundreds of exercises you could possibly do, four reign supreme: the squat, deadlift, bench press, and military press.

- Heavy half-reps, whether on the bench press, military press, or squat, put large amounts of strain on your joints, tendons, and ligaments—much more than if you were moving less weight through a proper, full range of motion, gradually strengthening the muscles and supporting tissues.

THE SQUAT

- As long as you use proper form, the squat does *not* put your back or knees at risk of injury.

- If you can avoid it, don't squat on a Smith machine.

- Don't use a powerlifter's wide squatting stance unless you're actually powerlifting.

- If you feel the need to squat with blocks or plates under your heels, it's because you need more hamstring and/or ankle flexibility. Check out Dr. Kelly Starrett's work on improving hamstring and ankle mobility so you can do the squat as described in this chapter.

- By squatting in shoes with flat soles or proper weightlifting shoes with a slight, rigid heel elevation, you'll find it much easier to sit back onto your heels and engage your hamstrings and glutes more effectively.

- The front squat emphasizes the quadriceps and core and creates less compression of the spine and less torque in the knees, which makes it particularly useful for those with back or knee injuries or limitations.

THE BENCH PRESS

- If you don't know what you're doing and try to bench press large amounts of weight with poor form, it's very easy to hurt your shoulders. Bench press properly, however, and you'll keep your shoulders safe and your chest growing bigger and stronger.

- Don't bounce the bar off your chest. Lower it in a controlled manner, keeping everything tight. Then let it touch your chest and drive it up.

- When you're lowering the weight, think about the coming drive up.

- Make sure to finish your last rep before trying to rack the weight.

- The best way to ensure your "upper chest" doesn't fall behind your pec major is to do a lot of incline pressing.

- As you narrow your grip on the bar, the triceps have to do more of the work.

THE DEADLIFT

- The deadlift is the ultimate full-body workout, training just about every muscle group in the body.

- The sumo deadlift uses a wide stance (1.5 to 2 times the width of your shoulders) to shorten the range of motion and shearing force on the lower back. It also can feel more comfortable in the hips than a conventional deadlift, depending on your biomechanics (if you walk with your toes pointed out, the sumo may be better for you).

- The hex bar—or trap bar—deadlift is a great way to learn to deadlift, because it doesn't require as much hip and ankle mobility to get to the bar, and it puts less shearing stress on the spine.

- The RDL is a variation of the deadlift that targets the glutes and hamstrings and minimizes the involvement of the quads and hip muscles.

THE MILITARY PRESS

- The military press is the best all-around shoulder exercise you can perform. It's a simple, easy to learn movement that allows for the safe lifting of heavy weights.

- The standing variation requires tremendous core and lower back strength to maintain balance, which in turn limits the amount of weight you can lift.

- I find that heavy deadlifting and squatting every week builds more than enough core and lower back strength and thus prefer the seated variation.

CHEST TRAINING

- Forget cable work, dumbbell flys, push-up variations, machines, and every other type of chest exercise out there for now. They just aren't nearly as effective as the core, foundation-building lifts and are only for advanced weightlifters who have already paid their dues with the heavy pressing to build big, strong pecs.

- Due to its reduced range of motion, decline pressing causes less stimulation of both the pectoralis major and clavicular pectoralis.

- A major part of building a great chest is focusing on your incline pressing more than anything else.

- I usually rotate between dumbbell-centric and barbell-centric routines.

BACK TRAINING

- In terms of programming your own back workouts, I highly recommend that you always start with the deadlift.

- From there, move to a wide-gripped pulling movement like the barbell or T-bar row, front lat pulldown, or wide-grip pull-up (weighted, if you can), followed by a more narrow-gripped pulling movement like the one-arm dumbbell row, close-grip lat pulldown, close-grip seated row, or chin-up.

SHOULDER TRAINING

- In most cases, the medial and posterior deltoids need the most work because the anterior deltoids get worked pretty intensely with proper chest training. The other two heads don't, however.

- As with the chest, you just can't beat heavy pressing for developing your shoulders. And as a natural weightlifter, you're going to need as much help as you can get in this department.

- If all you do is press, however, you'll find that your middle and rear heads of your deltoids fall behind in development. This is why a good shoulder workout trains all three heads of the muscle by having you press as well as do side raises and something for the rear delts.

LEG TRAINING

- The bottom line is that every leg workout should begin with either the Back or Front squat.

- Next, I like to focus on the other major muscle group of the pair with the back squat—my exercise of choice for hamstring emphasis—and the front squat, hack squat, leg press, or a lunge movement for the quadriceps.

- I usually finish with some hamstring-centric work like the Romanian deadlift or even the leg curl.

- Unless you're blessed with great calf genetics, you're going to have to work your calves quite a bit to maintain proportions with your thighs and arms.

- Research has shown that the muscle fibers of the gastrocnemius—the calf muscle we see and are primarily concerned with developing for aesthetic purposes—can vary in composition from person to person.

- Like the abs, the calves seem to recover from workouts more quickly than other muscle groups and thus can be trained more intensively.

- The calves seem to respond particularly well to periodized training that includes high-rep work.

- Proper form with calf exercises is simple: At the bottom of a rep, your heels are as low as they'll go and you feel a deep stretch in your calves, and at the top of a rep, you're up on your tippy-toes like a ballerina.

ARM TRAINING

- In terms of programming, you have quite a bit of flexibility. What I like to do is at least one barbell and one dumbbell exercise per workout for the biceps. Most of the time it's the barbell curl followed by the hammer curl.

- I like to start my triceps training with something I can push some weight on like the close-grip bench press or seated triceps press.

- You may run into some pretty intense forearm soreness with the arm workouts in this program and with the biceps training in particular. If you experience this, simply reduce your working set weight to the 6- to 8-rep range (enough weight to allow for 6 reps but no more than 8) and build your strength here for the first couple of months.

CORE TRAINING

- The full six-pack look requires both low body fat levels and well-developed core muscles.

- The squat and deadlift, even when performed with heavy weight (80+ percent of 1RM), just don't involve the "show" muscles of the rectus abdominis, the transversus abdominis, and the external obliques as much as people think.

- The abs are like any other muscle: they require progressive overload to grow, and that can only be accomplished by adding resistance to exercises. You don't have to add weight to all of your ab training, but you must do some if you want abs that pop.

18

THE BIGGER LEANER STRONGER WORKOUT ROUTINE

No matter what you do or how satisfying it is in that beautiful moment in time, immediately you want more. You have to, if you want to find out how good you can be.
— GLENN PENDLAY

NOW THAT YOU KNOW WHICH EXERCISES you should be doing and how to train each muscle group properly, let's take a look at how to build actual workout routines using everything you've learned.

Just as all *Bigger Leaner Stronger* workouts should be built using the exercises given in the previous chapter, they should also follow certain guidelines:

Don't forget the formula discussed in chapter 16, as this is the "engine" that makes the program work.

How you train is just as important as the exercises you do. If you do all the right exercises but fail to follow the formula by doing things like lifting too little weight, resting too little, doing too few or too many sets per workout, and so forth, you'll make less-than-optimal gains.

Lift weights three to five times per week, with four being better than three, and five being better than four.

You can certainly make gains lifting 3 or 4 times per week, and I'm going to show you exactly how to do this, but you will do best if you can somehow work in five sessions every week.

If you're going to train five days per week, use the following training template:

<u>Day 1:</u>

Chest and Abs

<u>Day 2:</u>

Back and Calves

Day 3:

Shoulders and Abs

Day 4:

Legs

Day 5:

Upper Body and Abs

Your "Upper Body" day consists of 3 sets for the chest performed in the 8- to 10-rep range with 1 to 2 minutes of rest in between each set followed by arms training (biceps and triceps) in the 4- to 6-rep range.

In terms of the amount of weight to use for your 8- to 10-rep sets, it should be about 10% less than your heavy, 4- to 6-rep weight (about 75% of your 1RM). And the goal is to progress here like everywhere—once you hit ten reps, add weight.

In terms of your choice of exercises for this additional chest training, I recommend that you stick to incline pressing and dips.

For example, here's a 5-day week on the program (and remember that "working sets" are your heavy, 4- to 6-rep sets and "optional" sets are for when you feel like you have a bit more juice left but aren't mandatory):

DAY 1

CHEST & ABS

Incline Barbell Bench Press – Warm-up sets and then 3 working sets
Incline Dumbbell Bench Press – 3 working sets
Flat Barbell Bench Press – 3 working sets
Face Pull – 3 working sets of 8 to 10 reps per set with 1 to 2 minutes of rest in between these lighter sets
3 ab circuits

The face pull isn't an exercise you see many people doing but it's one of my favorites for strengthening the rotator cuff muscles, which are heavily involved in pressing.

DAY 2

BACK & CALVES

Barbell Deadlift – Warm-up sets and then 3 working sets
Barbell Row – 3 working sets
Wide-Grip Pull-Up or Chin-Up – 3 working sets (weighted if possible)
Optional: Close-Grip Lat Pulldown – 3 working sets
Optional: Barbell Shrugs – 2 working sets
Calf Workout A

If you have lower-back issues, remember that you can swap the deadlift for a more lower-back-friendly variation like the sumo or hex deadlift, or you can drop it altogether and choose another "approved" exercise like the T-bar row.

DAY 3

SHOULDERS & ABS

Seated or Standing Barbell Military Press – Warm-up sets and then 3 working sets
Side Lateral Raise – 3 working sets
Bent-Over Rear Delt Raise – 3 working sets
3 ab circuits

DAY 4

LEGS

Barbell Squat – Warm-up sets and then 3 working sets
Leg Press – 3 working sets
Romanian Deadlift – 3 working sets
Calf Workout B

DAY 5

UPPER BODY & ABS

Incline Barbell Bench Press – Warm-up sets and then 3 sets of 8 to 10 reps per set
with 1 to 2 minutes of rest in between these lighter sets
Barbell Curl – Warm-up sets and then 3 working sets
Close-Grip Bench Press – 3 working sets (no need to warm up after the chest pressing)
Alternating Dumbbell Curl – 3 working sets
Seated Triceps Press – 3 working sets
3 ab circuits

If you're going to lift 5 days per week, I recommend that you start with this routine for your first eight to ten weeks. It's the first phase of the workouts you'll find in the bonus report.

In terms of which days to train on, most people like to lift Monday through Friday and take the weekends off, maybe doing some cardio on one or both of these days. This works well. Feel free to work your rest days however you want, though. Some people prefer to lift on the weekends and take off two days during the week.

Work your cardio in as needed. You can lift and do cardio on the same days without an issue.

If you're going to train 4 days per week, use the following template:

<u>Day 1:</u>

Chest & Triceps & Calves

<u>Day 2:</u>

Back & Biceps & Abs

<u>Day 3:</u>

Upper Body & Calves

<u>Day 4:</u>

Legs & Abs

In this template, your "Upper Body" day consists of 3 sets for the chest performed in the 8- to 10-rep range followed by shoulders training.

Here's an example of a 4-day week on the program:

DAY 1

CHEST & TRICEPS & CALVES

Incline Barbell Bench Press – Warm-up sets and then 3 working sets
Flat Barbell Bench Press – 3 working sets
Dip (Chest Variation, weighted if possible) – 3 working sets
Seated Triceps Press – 3 working sets
Calf Workout A

DAY 2

BACK & BICEPS & ABS

Barbell Deadlift – Warm-up sets and then 3 working sets
Barbell Row – 3 working sets
Wide-Grip Pull-Up or Chin-Up – 3 working sets (weighted if possible)
Barbell Curl – 3 working sets
3 ab circuits

DAY 3

UPPER BODY & CALVES

Incline Barbell Bench Press – Warm-up sets and then 3 sets of 8 to 10 reps per set
with 1 to 2 minutes of rest in between these lighter sets
Seated or Standing Barbell Military Press – Warm-up sets and then 3 working sets
Side Lateral Raise – 3 working sets
Bent-Over Rear Delt Raise – 3 working sets
Calf Workout B

DAY 4

LEGS & ABS

Barbell Squat – Warm-up sets and then 3 working sets
Leg Press – 3 working sets
Romanian Deadlift – 3 working sets
3 ab circuits

Again, if you're going to lift 4 days per week, start here.

In terms of which days to train on, you have the same flexibility as with the 5-day layout. Work your cardio in as needed.

If you're going to train three days per week, you have two templates to choose from:

OPTION A:

Day 1:

Back & Biceps & Abs

Day 2:

Chest & Triceps & Calves

Day 3:

Legs & Shoulders

OPTION B:

Day 1:

Pull & Abs

Day 2:

Push & Calves

Day 3:

Legs & Abs

Neither of these templates is necessarily better than the other. It comes down to personal preference.

In Option A, your first and second days consist of 9 working sets for your major muscle groups (chest and back, respectively) and 6 for your minor groups (triceps and biceps). Your final day consists of 9 sets for legs and 6 to 9 sets for shoulders (yes, this is hard).

In Option B, your "Push" day consists of training your chest, shoulders, triceps, and calves, in that order. In terms of number of sets, this should involve 6 to 9 sets for both chest and shoulders and 3 sets for triceps.

Work your cardio in as needed.

Here's an example of an "Option A" three-day week:

DAY 1

BACK & BICEPS & ABS
Barbell Deadlift – Warm-up sets and then 3 working sets
Barbell Row – 3 working sets
Wide-Grip Pull-Up or Chin-Up – 3 working sets (4 to 6 reps per set, weighted if possible)
Barbell Curl – 3 working sets
3 ab circuits

DAY 2

CHEST & TRICEPS & CALVES
Incline Barbell Bench Press – Warm-up sets and then 3 working sets
Flat Barbell Bench Press – 3 working sets
Dip (Chest Variation, weighted if possible) – 3 working sets
Seated Triceps Press – 3 working sets
Calf Workout A

DAY 3

LEGS & SHOULDERS
Barbell Squat – Warm-up sets and then 2 working sets
Leg Press – 2 working sets
Romanian Deadlift – 2 working sets
Seated or Standing Barbell Military Press – Warm-up sets and then 2 working sets
Side Lateral Raise – 2 working sets
Optional: Bent-Over Rear Delt Raise – 2 working sets

As you can see, not much changes here except day 3, which is a real ball-breaker. Some people like to do a set of legs, rest 60 to 90 seconds, then do a set of shoulders, rest 60 to 90 seconds, and alternate like this. This is tough, but it also is a workable way to save time.

And here's an example of an "Option B" 3-day week:

DAY 1

PULL & ABS

Barbell Deadlift – Warm-up sets and then 3 working sets
Barbell Row – 3 working sets
Wide-Grip Pull-Up or Chin-Up – 3 working sets (weighted if possible)
Barbell Curl – 3 working sets
3 ab circuits

DAY 2

PUSH & CALVES

Incline Barbell Bench Press – Warm-up sets and then 3 working sets
Seated or Standing Barbell Military Press – Warm-up sets and then 3 working sets
Flat Barbell Bench Press – 3 working sets
Side Lateral Raise – 3 working sets
Optional: Close-Grip Bench Press – 3 working sets
Calf Workout A

DAY 3

LEGS & ABS

Barbell Squat – Warm-up sets and then 3 working sets
Leg Press – 3 working sets
Romanian Deadlift – 3 working sets
3 ab circuits

This setup is quite different than the other workouts, but it follows simple guidelines:

- Your push day should include 6 sets for both your chest and shoulders and 3 optional sets for your triceps. Dips are great for including in this type of workout because they train the chest, shoulders, and triceps.

- Your pull day should include 9 sets for your back and 3 for your biceps.

- Your legs day is identical to the other routines.

HOW TO DO YOUR WORKOUTS

You want to do the exercises one at a time, in the order given.

So you start with the first exercise and do your warm-up sets, followed by your 3 heavy sets (with the proper rest in between each, of course), and then move on to the next exercise on the list, and so forth, like this:

Exercise 1: Set 1

Rest

Exercise 1: Set 2

Rest

Exercise 1: Set 3

Rest

Exercise 2: Set 1

Rest

And so on.

THE "SECRET" TO A PROPER WARM-UP ROUTINE

What if I told you that with one simple technique you could immediately increase your strength on every lift while also reducing the risk of injury?

Well, you can, and the "secret" lies in how you warm up each muscle group before hitting the heavy weights.

Warm up incorrectly, and you can reduce your strength and set yourself up for muscle strains or worse. Here's an example of an ineffective warm-up routine:

Put 135 pounds on the bar and do about 10 to 15 reps. Rest a few minutes and then go to 185 pounds for 12 reps. After another short rest, go up to 205 pounds for 8 reps, which is done to failure. A few minutes later, it's 4 to 6 reps with 225 pounds, followed by a longer rest and finally a monumental struggle with 275 pounds for 2 reps.

What's the problem here? Well, by the time you get to the heavy, muscle-building sets, you're so fatigued from what you've already done that you can't handle the heavy stuff nearly as well you should be able to. This leads to subpar workouts that fail to overload the muscles adequately and thus produce lackluster results over time.

Another common warm-up mistake is doing too little. Many guys are anxious to start loading the plates and thus only do one light warm-up set before hitting the heavy stuff. This can lead to muscle strains, joint impingements, or worse.

Warm up correctly, however, and you will find that you can tap into your maximum strength without increasing the risk of injury. This helps you maximally overload your muscles without having to worry about getting hurt, which in turn safely stimulates the maximum amount of muscle growth.

A proper warm-up routine has two simple goals: to introduce blood into the muscles to be trained and to progressively acclimate them to heavy weight *without* causing fatigue. You want your muscles fresh and ready for the heavy sets—the muscle-building sets—and not burned out from too much warm-up work.

Here's how you do it:

First Set:

In your first warm-up set, you want to do 12 reps with about 50 percent of your heavy, 4- to 6-rep set weight and then rest for 1 minute. This set should feel very light and easy.

For instance, if you did 3 sets of 5 reps with 225 pounds on the bench last week, you would start your warm-up with about 110 pounds and do 12 reps, followed by 1 minute of rest.

Second Set:

In your second warm-up set, you use the same weight as the first and do 10 reps, this time at a little faster pace. Then rest for 1 minute.

Third Set:

Your third warm-up set is 4 reps with about 70 percent of your heavy weight, and it should be done at a moderate pace.

This set and the following one are done to acclimate your muscles to the heavy weights that are about to come. Once again, you follow this set with a 1-minute rest.

With a working set weight of 225, this would be about 155 to 160 pounds.

Fourth Set:

The fourth warm-up set is the final one, and it's simple: 1 rep with about 90 percent of your heavy weight. Rest 2 to 3 minutes after this final warm-up set.

This would be about 200 pounds if your heavy weight were 225.

Fifth, Sixth, and Seventh Sets:

These are your working sets performed in the 4- to 6-rep range with about 85 percent of your 1RM.

Moving on to the Next Exercise:

Generally speaking, you don't need to perform more warm-up sets in a workout beyond the four laid out above. For instance, if you start your workout with the flat bench press and then move to the incline press, you don't have to do a new round of warm-up sets.

That said, I do like to do a 10- to 12-rep warm-up when moving on to an exercise that targets muscles that aren't sufficiently warmed up. For example, when I'm moving from shoulder presses to side or rear raises, I like to do a 10- to 12-rep warm-up set on the raise as I find the medial and posterior delts aren't always ready for heavy weight after pressing.

WARMING UP ON ARMS DAY

When warming up for an Arms Day, I like to do a warm-up set for biceps immediately followed by a warm-up set for triceps, followed by a 60-second rest.

I don't superset my *heavy* sets like this, but as we're not trying to lift as much weight as possible while warming up, we don't lose anything by doing it here.

THE BOTTOM LINE

The bottom line is that warming up correctly is an important part of training with heavy weight and building muscle. Trust me—it's worth spending your first 10 minutes warming up instead of just rushing into the heavy lifting.

YOUR FIRST FEW WEEKS ON THE PROGRAM

If you're new to weightlifting, you're going to find everything a bit awkward at first. You'll be working out your weights, you'll have trouble maintaining proper form on some of the exercises, and you'll probably get pretty sore from your workouts.

All of this is normal and just part of the game. However, it shouldn't take long before you're comfortable with each exercise and your weight for each, and you'll get less and less sore as time goes on.

Feel free to use your warm-up sets to get acquainted with the exercises, and feel free to work in the 6- to 8-rep or even the 8- to 10-rep range for these first few weeks to get a good feel for everything. Then, once you're comfortable, move into the 4- to 6-rep range.

Aches and soreness are to be expected, but sharp pains while lifting mean that something is wrong. Don't try to muscle through a sharp pain. Instead, drop the weight and check your form. If your form is fine, stop the exercise and do another.

Stay away from the exercise that was giving you pain for a couple of weeks and strengthen the area with an exercise that doesn't hurt. Then try the original exercise again and see whether it still bothers you. If it still does, don't do it.

If you're having any serious pains while or after training, see a doctor, as it might be an indicator of something else.

FINDING YOUR STARTING WEIGHTS

Finding your starting weights on the various exercises is more or less a matter of trial and error. As a general rule, for every 10 pounds you add to the bar, you'll lose about 2 reps. The same goes for each 5-pound increase on the dumbbells.

You can err on the side of starting too light and then just dial everything in as you familiarize yourself with the weights and exercises.

WE DON'T NEED NO STINKIN' SPOTTER...BUT SOMETIMES IT HELPS

A spotter isn't necessary because you should always use weights that you can perform clean, unassisted reps with.

That said, if you do have someone to spot you on certain exercises like the bench press and military press, it has a couple of advantages.

First, it allows you to go for that extra rep that you might not want to try otherwise.

Second, there's a strange strength benefit to having someone standing there to assist you, even if he does nothing more than put his hands under or even fingers under the bar. I know it sounds like broscience, but you'll experience it—you'll be struggling on your last rep, your buddy will just put his fingers under the bar, and suddenly you'll push it up and ask why he helped.

So, if you don't have someone to work out with, I recommend that you ask someone in the gym to give you a spot at least on those two exercises. I also recommend that you let the person know what you'd like him to do, which brings me to the proper way to spot:

1. If needed, help with the lift off.

2. Let the person do as many reps as possible without any assistance from you.

3. If he gets bogged down on a rep, place your hands under the bar, but don't take any weight off yet. Chances are this is all he'll need to finish his rep.

4. If he's still stuck, take about 10 percent of the load off.

5. If he's still stuck, take another 10 to 15 percent of the load off.

6. If he's still stuck, he's toast—take as much of the load off as you can so he can finish the rep.

I don't want to make this sound overly complicated, but a good spotter is there for safety reasons only. The rule is that if the person you're spotting is moving the weight up, even if slowly, you don't touch it. Don't accept poor spotting, as this can seriously put a damper on your gains, leading you to believe you're hitting certain strength milestones when you're not.

While the technique of spotting is self-explanatory in most cases, I'd like to mention here the proper way to spot someone who's squatting: spot the bar, not the person. Don't hook your arms under the armpits, as you're looking to reduce the load and spotting via the body isn't the safest way to do this.

Now, if there is no way to get a spot, you can still make good progress on your pushing. My first recommendation is that you do your bench and military pressing and squatting in a power cage, as it allows you to set safety bars and thus do your sets without having to worry about getting stuck with the weight on top of you.

If that's not possible, then you need to get used to ending your bench press, military press, and squat sets at the point where you have, at best, one rep left in the tank. That is, you end them at the point where you struggle to finish a rep and aren't quite sure whether you can get another. You'll become more aware of this point as you continue lifting.

THE DELOAD WEEK

As you know, I recommend that you make rest and recovery a priority every eight weeks by either taking a week off the weights or doing a deload week.

Here's how I like to program my deload weeks:

DAY 1

Deadlift – 3 sets of 8 to 10 reps with 50% of your normal (heavy) weight
Barbell Row – 3 sets of 8 to 10 reps with 50% of your normal (heavy) weight
One-Arm Dumbbell Row – 3 sets of 8 to 10 reps with 50% of your normal (heavy) weight
Pullups – 3 sets of bodyweight to failure

DAY 2

Military Press – 3 sets of 8 to 10 reps with 50% of your normal (heavy) weight
Incline Bench Press – 3 sets of 8 to 10 reps with 50% of your normal (heavy) weight
Close-Grip Bench Press – 3 sets of 8 to 10 reps with 50% of your normal (heavy) weight
Dips – 3 sets of bodyweight to failure

DAY 3

Barbell Squat – 3 sets of 8 to 10 reps with 50% of your normal (heavy) weight
Front Squat – 3 sets of 8 to 10 reps with 50% of your normal (heavy) weight
Romanian Deadlift – 3 sets of 8 to 10 reps with 50% of your normal (heavy) weight

That's it.

As you can see, the big difference is a dramatic reduction in the intensity of your workouts.

In terms of which days you should train on, I recommend that you rest one day in between each workout. Most people like to train on Mondays, Wednesdays, and Fridays.

CHANGING YOUR ROUTINE

Unless your muscles are made of brain matter, they have no cognitive abilities. They're not trying to guess what workout you're going to do today and can't be "confused" by regularly changing your workout routine. Muscle tissue is purely mechanical in nature and can contract and relax, and nothing more.

That said, there's validity to the basic premise that for your muscles to keep growing in both size and strength, they must be continually challenged. Where "muscle confusion theory" misses the boat, however, is what type of "challenge" drives muscle growth.

You see, you can change up your routine every week—hell, every *day*—and easily fall into a rut of no gains simply because "change" isn't a primary driver of muscle growth. You already know what is, however: progressive overload.

The key to building muscle and strength isn't merely *changing* the types of stimuli (new exercises) but *increasing* them. And the most effective way to do this is to force your muscles to overreach and perform more than the last time.

If you just do this with the core, muscle-building exercises you'll do in this program (squat, deadlift, bench press, and military press), you'll be miles ahead of the average gymgoer trying to continually "confuse" his muscles.

With *Bigger Leaner* Stronger, however, you're taking this approach a bit further by including other exercises that work the various muscle groups in slightly different ways and help you achieve a balanced, well-proportioned physique that can both "show" and "go."

For instance, if you only military press for your shoulders and never do any isolation work for your lateral and posterior deltoids, your shoulders are never going to "pop" like you want. If you only back squat for your legs, chances are your quadriceps aren't going to develop and separate as well as they would if you also included some exercises that emphasize them such as the front squat, leg press, or hack squat.

There's a method to proper exercise rotation, though. Namely, there are two types of exercises:

The "nonnegotiables," which are exercises you should do every week, without fail.

These are the big compound lifts vital for building a strong, muscular physique: the squat, deadlift, bench press, and military press.

The "negotiables," which can be seen as "accessory" work done in addition to the above.

These are mostly compound exercises like the dumbbell press, barbell row, and dip, but they also include isolation exercises like the side lateral raise, face pull, and dumbbell curl.

An easy, effective way to program a workout is to do 3 to 6 sets of your "nonnegotiable" exercises followed by 3 to 6 sets of your "negotiable" exercises and to change the "negotiables" every eight to ten weeks, after your rest or deload weeks.

The key to it all, however, is ensuring that you're making progress on these exercises. That is, you're increasing the number of reps you can do with given weights over time and using this to increase the amount of weight you can lift.

STRENGTH WEEK

As you know, one of your primary goals as a natural weightlifter is to get stronger, and particularly on the big compound movements.

That's why the core of the *Bigger Leaner Stronger* program, as laid out earlier, is a hybrid between traditional strength training and traditional "bodybuilding" workouts.

The program combines the compound lifting found in strength programs that builds a foundation of strength and size and the isolation work found in bodybuilding workouts that helps develop smaller muscles that contribute to overall proportions and aesthetics.

Out of these two elements, however, the former (heavy compound lifting) is far more important than the latter (doing isolation work) for reaching your goals. The bottom line is the majority of your progress with your physique is going to come from your progress in your squatting, deadlifting, and bench and overhead pressing.

That's why I recommend that you make every fourth training week on the program a "Strength Week." That is, for every three weeks of "normal" workouts, you do one Strength Week.

In this week, you will follow a more traditional strength training layout, which has you perform the same exercises several times in the week but has you do fewer sets each workout.

The purpose of the Strength Week is to give you more practice doing the key exercises (the more you do them, the better you get) and help you get stronger faster.

There are two layouts for this week that you will alternate between:

STRENGTH WEEK A

DAY 1

Barbell Squat – Warm-up sets and then 3 working sets
Seated or Standing Barbell Military Press – Warm-up sets and then 3 working sets
Barbell Deadlift – Warm-up sets and then 1 working set

DAY 2

Barbell Squat – Warm-up sets and then 3 working sets
Flat Barbell Bench Press – Warm-up sets and then 3 working sets
Barbell Deadlift – Warm-up sets and then 1 working set

DAY 3

Barbell Squat – Warm-up sets and then 3 working sets
Seated or Standing Barbell Military Press – Warm-up sets and then 3 working sets
Barbell Deadlift – Warm-up sets and then 1 working set

STRENGTH WEEK B

DAY 1

Barbell Squat – Warm-up sets and then 3 working sets
Flat Barbell Bench Press – Warm-up sets and then 3 working sets
Barbell Deadlift – Warm-up sets and then 1 working set

DAY 2

Barbell Squat – Warm-up sets and then 3 working sets
Seated or Standing Barbell Military Press – Warm-up sets and then 3 working sets
Barbell Deadlift – Warm-up sets and then 1 working set

DAY 3

Barbell Squat – Warm-up sets and then 3 working sets
Flat Barbell Bench Press – Warm-up sets and then 3 working sets
Barbell Deadlift – Warm-up sets and then 1 working set

Those familiar with strength training will immediately recognize these as basic routines from the popular program *Starting Strength.*

Some points on how to do your Strength Weeks properly:

- As you can see, Workout A emphasizes military pressing whereas Workout B emphasizes bench pressing. Alternate between these workouts for your Strength Weeks (A, B, A, B, etc.).

- As mentioned earlier, make every fourth training week a Strength Week. I say fourth *training week* because this doesn't include rest or deload weeks. Here's how most people like to do it:

3 weeks of normal workouts
1 Strength Week (A)
3 weeks of normal workouts
1 Strength Week (B)
1 Rest/Deload week
Repeat

As you can see, this setup has you train for eight weeks, take a week to rest and recover, train for eight weeks, rest and recover, and so forth.

- If you normally rest/deload every eight weeks but, for whatever reason, need to do it early— let's say after six weeks of training—just start your next training cycle anew, like this:

3 weeks of normal workouts
1 Strength Week (A)
2 weeks of normal workouts
1 Rest/Deload week
3 weeks of normal workouts
1 Strength Week (B)

3 weeks of normal workouts
1 Strength Week (A)
1 Rest/Deload week
And so on.

- If you find that you generally need to rest/deload more frequently than every eight weeks, just follow the pattern of three normal weeks followed by one Strength Week.

For example, if you need to rest/deload every six weeks, here's how it would look:

3 weeks of normal workouts
1 Strength Week (A)
2 weeks of normal workouts
1 Rest/Deload week
1 week of normal workouts
1 Strength Week (B)
3 weeks of normal workouts
1 Strength Week (A)
1 Rest/Deload week
3 weeks of normal workouts
1 Strength Week (B)
2 weeks of normal workouts
1 Rest/Deload week
And so on.

- If you're able to go longer than eight weeks before needing a rest/deload week, follow the 3:1 ratio between normal and Strength weeks until you need to take a break. Then start anew. Like this:

3 weeks of normal workouts
1 Strength Week (A)
3 weeks of normal workouts
1 Strength Week (B)
3 weeks of normal workouts
1 Strength Week (A)
1 Rest/Deload week
3 weeks of normal workouts
1 Strength Week (B)
And so forth.

(Remember that regardless of your rest/deload schedule, you never do the same Strength Week twice in a row—you always alternate between A and B.)

- I recommend that you rest at least one day in between your Strength Week workouts. Many people like to train on Mondays, Wednesdays, and Fridays.

- Your Strength Week working sets should be done with the same weight as your working sets in your normal workouts. For example, if, in your last back workout, you deadlifted

225 pounds for sets of 5, 4, and 4 reps, you use 225 pounds for your deadlifts on your Strength Week.

- You progress in your strength workouts in the same way as your normal workouts—once you get six reps, add five to ten pounds to the bar and continue working with that weight.

- Rest the normal three to four minutes in between sets.

- You can continue doing cardio (or not) as usual.

That's it for the Strength Week.

WANT A YEAR'S WORTH OF WORKOUT ROUTINES BUILT BY ME?

Feel free to take what you've learned in the book and formulate your own workout routines, but if you'd like a little help with coming up with what to do, you can find a full year's worth of training routines in the free bonus report at the end of the book.

THE BOTTOM LINE

You now know the core principles of the *Bigger Leaner Stronger* program. You also know how the program works and how to ensure you get the most out of it. If you're feeling a bit overwhelmed by all the details, I totally understand. Take a few minutes to go back over this chapter and let it all sink in.

Once you've started applying what you've learned in this chapter, you'll see how simple it is. Making great gains in the gym requires nothing more than doing a bunch of "little" things right in both your diet and training. There isn't one great "secret" to building a strong, muscular, and lean physique; you just assemble the pieces of the puzzle efficiently and correctly and it all comes together.

CHAPTER SUMMARY

WORKOUT SCHEDULE

- Lift weights 3 to 5 times per week, with 4 being better than 3 and 5 being better than 4.

- In terms of which days to train on, most people like to lift Monday through Friday and take the weekends off, maybe doing some cardio on one or both of these days. This works well. Feel free to work your rest days however you want, though. Some people prefer to lift on the weekends and take off two days during the week.

- Work your cardio in as needed. You can lift and do cardio on the same days without an issue.

- You want to do the exercises one at a time, in the order given. So you start with the first exercise and do your warm-up sets, followed by your 3 heavy sets (with the proper rest in between each, of course), and then move on to the next exercise on the list, and so forth.

PROPER WARM-UP ROUTINE

- Warm up incorrectly, and you can reduce your strength and set yourself up for muscle strains or worse.

- A proper warm-up routine has two simple goals: to introduce blood into the muscles to be trained and to progressively acclimate them to heavy weight *without* causing fatigue.

- In your first warm-up set, you want to do 12 reps with about 50 percent of your heavy, 4- to 6-rep set weight and then rest for 1 minute.

- In your second warm-up set, you use the same weight as the first and do 10 reps this time at a little faster pace. Then rest for 1 minute.

- Your third warm-up set is 4 reps with about 70 percent of your heavy weight, and it should be done at a moderate pace. Once again, you follow this set with a 1-minute rest.

- The fourth warm-up set is the final one and it's simple: 1 rep with about 90 percent of your heavy weight. Rest 2 to 3 minutes after this final warm-up set.

- Generally speaking, you don't need to perform any more warm-up sets beyond the four laid out above. That said, I do like to do a 10- to 12-rep warm-up when moving on to an exercise that targets muscles that aren't sufficiently warmed up.

- When warming up for an Arms Day, I like to do a warm-up set for biceps immediately followed by a warm-up set for triceps, followed by a 60-second rest.

YOUR FIRST FEW WEEKS ON THE PROGRAM

- Feel free to use your warm-up sets to get acquainted with the exercises and feel free to work in the 6- to 8- or even the 8- to 10-rep range for these first few weeks to get a good feel for everything. Then, once you're comfortable, move into the 4 to 6 range.

- Aches and soreness are to be expected, but sharp pains while lifting mean that something is wrong. Don't try to muscle through a sharp pain.

FINDING YOUR STARTING WEIGHTS

- Finding your starting weights on the various exercises is more or less a matter of trial and error.

- As a general rule, for every 10 pounds you add to the bar, you'll lose about two reps. The same goes for each 5-pound increase on the dumbbells.

SPOTTING

- A spotter isn't necessary because you should always use weights that you can perform clean, unassisted reps with. That said, if you do have someone to spot you on certain exercises like the bench press and military press, it has a couple of advantages.

- Don't accept poor spotting, as this can seriously put a damper on your gains. The worst mistake most people make when spotting is take weight off the bar when it's unnecessary.

- If no spot is available, I recommend that you do your bench and military pressing and squatting in a power cage, as it allows you to set safety bars and thus do your sets without having to worry about getting stuck with the weight on top of you.

CHANGING YOUR ROUTINE

- The key to building muscle and strength isn't merely *changing* the types of stimuli (new exercises) but *increasing* them. And the most effective way to do this is to force your muscles to overreach and perform more than the last time.

- An easy, effective way to program a workout is to do 3 to 6 sets of your "nonnegotiable" exercises followed by 3 to 6 sets of your "negotiable" exercises and to change the "negotiables" every eight to ten weeks, after your rest or deload weeks.

- If you find that you generally need to rest/deload more frequently than every eight weeks, just follow the pattern of three normal weeks followed by one Strength Week.

STRENGTH WEEK

- The purpose of the Strength Week is to give you more practice doing the key exercises (the more you do them, the better you get) and help you get stronger faster.

- Make every fourth training week on the program a "Strength Week." That is, for every three weeks of "normal" workouts, you do one Strength Week.

- If you normally rest/deload every eight weeks but, for whatever reason, need to do it early—let's say after six weeks of training—just start your next training cycle anew.

- If you're able to go longer than eight weeks before needing a rest/deload week, follow the 3:1 ratio between normal and Strength weeks until you need to take a break.

- Your Strength Week working sets should be done with the same weight as your working sets in your normal workouts.

- You progress in your strength workouts in the same way as your normal workouts—once you get six reps, add five to ten pounds to the bar and continue working with that weight.

- Rest the normal three to four minutes in between sets.

- You can continue doing cardio (or not) as usual.

19

TRACKING YOUR PROGRESS
IF YOU CAN'T MEASURE IT, YOU DON'T KNOW IT

Courage doesn't always roar. Sometimes courage is the quiet voice at the end of the day saying, 'I will try again tomorrow.'
— MARY ANNE RADMACHER

I USED TO BE THAT GUY who showed up to the gym every day, only to lift more or less the same weights for more or less the same reps for months on end. I saw no real difference in the mirror—no noticeable muscle growth and no reduction in body fat percentage.

What did I do in response to the seemingly never-ending problem of "no gains?" I changed things, of course. You know, I tried new exercises and routines, new diet "tricks," or new supplements.

This "shotgun" approach never worked—my strength and body composition didn't change much as time went on—but I dutifully kept searching for the "workout of the week" or dietary "insight" that would finally show me the way…only to continue to be disappointed.

While much of the blame for this long, frustrating cycle of letdowns and setbacks lay with the workout programs and diets themselves—they were so flawed that no natural weightlifter could do well with them—there was another major mistake I was making that dramatically exacerbated the problem.

Sir William Thomson, also known as Lord Kelvin, was an ingenious physicist and engineer, and he said that when you can measure something and express it in numbers, you know something about it, but when you can't, your knowledge is lacking.

This insight is applicable to training and dieting. If you can measure your progress (or lack thereof) and express it in real numbers, then you know whether you're going in the right direction. If you don't have any consistent, objective way to measure progress, then you're going at it blind, hoping for the best.

I was doing the latter, never *really* knowing whether I was increasing my strength over time or whether I was eating properly for my goals.

You see, one of the most effective ways to prevent getting stuck in a rut of no gains is simply *to track your numbers*. That is, you should keep a training journal that includes what you do in each workout, and you should either track or plan your daily food intake (and stick to the plan!).

To some, this may seem a bit obsessive, but I think you already know why it's absolutely vital to continued success in this game.

Building your ideal body takes time. As the old adage goes, it's a marathon, not a sprint. Yes, you can radically transform your body and life and enjoy the ride, but no matter how you look at it, it takes a real investment of time and effort.

The tricky thing about building muscle and strength is that it comes slowly, bit by bit. If you're just starting out, you're going to see huge jumps in strength for the first several months, but eventually, your progress will slow down. From that point on, you will have to consciously work for every rep of improvement in your lifts and every pound of muscle added to your frame.

This is where things get hazy for people who don't keep journals. Unless you have superhuman memory, you won't know exactly what you did the previous week for the various exercises in your workout. Sure, you might make a mental note of the "ego" lifts like bench press and dumbbell curls, but what about everything else? You need to approach *all* lifts with the same attention to detail.

When you don't know what you did the previous week, you don't know what you're shooting for this week. As your goal with every workout is to do just a little more than the last time you performed it—even if it's just one more rep with the same weights—you can see the problem here.

When you step up to the bar, you don't want to be trying to remember what you did last week. You want to know exactly what you're going for. Hell, some people like to even visualize themselves performing the set successfully and say it helps.

If you bench pressed 245 for 4 reps last week, all you care about when you get under that bar is pressing it for 5 reps. Go ahead and even see yourself doing it in your mind's eye. Then the next week, your goal is 6 reps on the first set, at which point you'll add weight and go for 4 reps on the second set. This is how you build strength: one rep at a time.

A successful workout is one where you made *progress*—where you got one more rep than last week or moved up in weight. If this doesn't happen, don't despair, but you need to push harder the next week. If you're stuck for several weeks or even moving backward, you need to check your nutrition and rest, because something is off.

The bottom line is that if you don't keep a training journal, it gets real sloppy real quick. Lifting random amounts of weight for random numbers of reps every week doesn't work nearly as well as an accurate, linear model of progression driven by real data.

HOW TO KEEP A TRAINING JOURNAL

You have a few options for keeping a training journal:

1. You can use an app such as the…ahem…completely awesome one I'm developing called *Stacked* (www.getstackedapp.com).

2. You can try other apps on the market but expect to be disappointed. You'll probably find it easier to just use a note-taking app on your phone or even a plain old notebook that you write in each week.

3. You can pick up the premade printed journal called *The Year One Challenge for Men*, which has an entire year's worth of *Bigger Leaner Stronger* workouts that you can fill out as you progress on the program.

If you're creating your own journal, list the exercises you're going to do for the day and look at the previous week's numbers. Assess whether your goal is to go up in reps or weight this week and start your workout, recording what you do in each set (the weight lifted, reps done, and any relevant notes).

Here's an example of how I kept my written journal before switching to an app:

Week 4

Monday

8/14/14

192 lbs.

Chest

Bench Press – 275 x 4, x 4, x 4 (feel strong)

Incline Dumbbell Press – 110 x 5, x 5, x 4

Flat Dumbbell Press – 110 x 5, x 5, x5

Simple enough. I often make notes if I feel particularly strong or weak on an exercise, if some kind of ache or pain bothers me, if I didn't sleep well the night before, etc.

The next week I would review these numbers and plan on doing something like 5 x 5 x 4 or even 5 x 4 x 4 with 275 on my bench press. If I did that and the rest of the workout was exactly the same as the previous week, that's a successful workout.

You will also want to keep track of your body weight, and you have two options here:

1. Weigh yourself once per seven days, on the same day each week, in the morning in the nude, after going to the bathroom, and on an empty stomach.

2. Weigh yourself every day under the same conditions as above and calculate the average weight once every seven days. Here's how this looks:

Day 1: 192.1

Day 2: 192

Day 3: 191

Day 4: 191.8

Day 5: 193

Day 6: 191.3

Day 7: 190.7

7-Day Average: 191.7

I prefer the averaging method because it makes sure you don't get thrown off by a bad weigh-in, which can be caused by something as simple as holding more water that day or having more food still in you that day.

THE BOTTOM LINE

No matter how good of a workout program you follow, if you don't keep a training journal and either plan or track food intake, you're almost guaranteed to run into problems.

Keeping your journal like this allows you to always have your eye on improvement and to never fall backward or get stuck for long periods. When you see your numbers plateauing, you can jump on it right away and not let months go by before you realize that nothing is changing.

And nine times out of ten, getting back on track is easy, as getting stuck is usually caused by not pushing yourself hard enough in your workouts, not eating right, or not resting enough, or a combination of the three.

CHAPTER SUMMARY

- One of the most effective ways to prevent getting stuck in a rut of no gains is simply *to track your numbers.*

- When you step up to the bar, you don't want to be trying to remember what you did last week. You want to know exactly what you're going for. Hell, some people like to even visualize themselves performing the set successfully and say it helps.

- A successful workout is one where you made *progress*—where you got one more rep than last week or moved up in weight. If this doesn't happen, don't despair, but you need to push harder the next week. If you're stuck for several weeks or even moving backward, you need to check your nutrition and rest, because something is off.

- The bottom line is that if you don't keep a training journal, it gets real sloppy real quick. Lifting random amounts of weight for random numbers of reps every week doesn't work nearly as well as an accurate, linear model of progression driven by real data.

20

THE CODE OF A GOOD TRAINING PARTNER

The question isn't who is going to let me; it's who is going to stop me.
— AYN RAND

WORKING OUT WITH A BAD PARTNER sucks. It drains your energy and motivation and can even cause you to lose enthusiasm for working out altogether.

On the other hand, working out with a good partner can go far in keeping you on track and making progress. He helps keep you accountable and wanting to show up every day, and having a spot on certain exercises helps push you for another rep and encourages you to move up in weight as you should.

These things can make a big difference as time goes on. Those workouts, additional reps, and progressions in weight that wouldn't have happened if you were solo add up to real gains.

So, I recommend that you find someone to work out with before you start, and the two of you should agree to the following code.

1. I will show up on time for every workout, and if I can't avoid missing one, I'll let my partner know as soon as I know.

2. I won't let my partner get out of a workout easily. I will reject any excuses that are short of an actual emergency or commitment that can't be rescheduled, and I will insist that he comes and trains.

3. In the case where there's a valid excuse, if at all possible, I'll offer to train at a different time so we can get our workout in.

4. I will come to the gym to *train*—not to chat. When we're in the gym, we focus on our workouts, we're always ready to spot each other, and we get our work done efficiently.

5. I will train hard to set a good example for my partner.

6. I will push my partner to do more than he thinks he can. It's my job to motivate him to do more weight and more reps than he believes possible.

7.   I will be supportive of my partner and will compliment him on his gains.

Such a code might seem cheesy, but if you and your partner agree to these six points, you'll be doing each other a huge favor and will be helping each other more than you might realize.

If your partner can't follow these points—if he is inconsistent in showing up, is more interested in chatting than lifting, trains lethargically, fails to push you to do more, etc.— he's a liability and is doing more harm than good. You're better off training alone.

21

HOW TO PREVENT WORKOUT INJURIES

Strength does not come from winning. Your struggles develop your strengths. When you go through hardships and decide not to surrender, that is strength.
— ARNOLD SCHWARZENEGGER

AT FIRST GLANCE, IT WOULD SEEM to make sense that weightlifting would, over time, lead to injuries or at least joint problems.

I mean how good can it possibly be for our bodies to squat, push, and pull hundreds of pounds over and over? Wouldn't it speed up the "wear and tear" on the joints, tendons, and ligaments and thus the onset of osteoarthritis (the degradation of the joints)?

Interestingly enough, research doesn't support these assumptions.

For example, one study conducted by researchers at the Glasgow Royal Infirmary analyzed the bodies of 25 competitive weightlifters—people who spend a lot more time training and lift a lot more weight than you or I do—and found that on the whole, their joints were as healthy, or healthier, than other people their age.[1] Furthermore, about half of the subjects admitted they were using anabolic steroids regularly, which means their joints were under even more strain than usual from the excessive weights lifted.

Researchers also found that previously injured joints were more susceptible to joint degeneration than healthy joints. Thus, those with injured joints may need to dial back the intensity of their weightlifting to preserve their joint health.

You see, the reality is that weightlifting just isn't a dangerous activity.[2] You're far more likely to get injured playing just about any sport than you are lifting weights.[3]

Nevertheless, this doesn't answer the questions as to why so many weightlifters seem to have shoulder, knees, and lower back problems. If weightlifting isn't inherently bad for your joints, what's going on here?

Well, it's true that weightlifting injuries are on the rise, and this is most likely because the number of people doing it is also on the rise. Mass movements like CrossFit don't help either, as a bad instructor is all it takes for a large group of people to dramatically increase the risk of injury.[4]

That said, as with any physical activity, the occasional ache or strain is inevitable, but if you do certain things wrong, you can get hurt, and it will probably involve a joint like the shoulder, knee, or lower back.

INJURY RISK MISTAKE #1
LIFTING MORE WEIGHT THAN YOU CAN HANDLE

According to research conducted by scientists on behalf of the Center for Injury Research and Policy, the most common way people injure themselves while weightlifting is dropping weights on themselves.[5]

And how do people increase the risk of dropping weights on themselves?

They ego-lift. They stack the plates and just hope for the best.

I cringe when I see skinny guys load three or four plates on either side of the bar, only to perform shaky quarter reps with a spot. All it will take is a slightly too fast descent or a momentary tweak of the back or knee, and Humpty Dumpty *will* have a great fall.

Trying to lift too much weight also puts excessive strain on your joints, tendons, and ligaments. By working with weights that you can properly handle, however, and by doing full, controlled reps, you not only avoid that problem, but you also make better gains[6] and improve flexibility.[7]

Here's the bottom line: if you can't get full reps, you're using too much weight, and you're increasing your risk of injury. Simply lighten the load, do full reps, improve your strength, and only move up in weight when you can keep it fully under control.

INJURY RISK MISTAKE #2
USING BAD FORM

This is similar to the first mistake, but not the same.

Form mistakes go far beyond the heavy half-repping that gives a bad name to the big compound lifts like the squat, deadlift, bench press, and military press. You can work with proper amounts of weight and use a full range of motion and still put yourself at a considerable risk of injury.

For instance, even if you're working with weights you can handle properly…

- If you round your back during a deadlift or hyperextend it too far at the top, you're asking for a lower back injury.

- If you flatten your back and round your shoulders at the top of a bench press or flare your elbows out too much, you will probably have shoulder problems at some point.

- If you let your knees bow in when you squat or extend too far past your toes, you can hurt them when going heavy.

- If you do your overhead/military presses behind your neck and your body is built like most people's, you're increasing your risk of injury. (Strangely enough, some people's bodies just mechanically can handle this type of movement, but most don't do well with it.)

Pushing yourself in the gym is good, so long as you always maintain proper form as well.

INJURY RISK MISTAKE #3
FAILING TO WARM UP PROPERLY

Many people's warm-up routines consist of a few minutes of static stretching, and this is a bad way of going about it.

Static stretching before exercise has been shown to impair speed and strength.[8] Not only can it fail to prevent injury, but it can also *increase* the risk of injury due to the cellular damage it causes to muscle and its analgesic effect.[9]

A proper warm-up routine should bring blood to the muscles that are about to be trained, increase suppleness, raise body temperature, and enhance free, coordinated movement, which is why I prescribe the warm-up routine shared earlier in the book.[10] The process of moving the muscles repeatedly through the expected ranges of motion has been shown to reduce the risk of injury.[11]

INJURY RISK MISTAKE #4:
"NO PAIN NO GAIN, BROOOOO!!!!!"

This might be obvious, but many people don't quite get it: if you experience pain, stop your set. If an exercise always bothers you, do something else.

Realize that pain is a warning that something is wrong, and if you don't heed it, serious injury can follow.

Case in point: probably the worst injury I've witnessed was a guy in his sixties at a bench press competition. He had just barely struggled out one rep with about 350 pounds, and then he started rubbing his elbow. He then told the guys to load more weight so he could go for a PR. Everyone was rooting him on.

He got under the bar, unracked it, and got it halfway down. Then we heard a *POP* above the noise of the crowd. Fortunately, the spotters were on the ball and saved him from what looked like a near decapitation. His elbow had completely blown out, and I overheard an idiot telling him to just ice it and he'd be fine. In reality, he should have been on his way to the emergency room.

The point is this: *don't be stupid.*

Aches and stiffness and such are common enough and usually go away once you warm up, but ignore and try to "alpha" your way through *pain*, and you're asking to get hurt.

The key to dealing with pain is treating it like an injury until it's better. Avoid exercises that aggravate it and let it heal. If that means no deadlifting or squatting for a few weeks, so be it. Find alternative exercises that you can do. Annoying, yes, but an injury that sets you back several *months* is much more frustrating.

HOW TO RECOVER FROM WORKOUT INJURIES

If you don't make the above mistakes, your chances for injury are quite low. But stuff can happen, so let's talk about how to recover should you get hurt.

First, if the injury is serious, you should see a doctor right away. Don't "go home and put some ice on it" and figure you'll be all right. That said, the most common injuries are minor muscle strains, which are fairly easy to recover from if you take the following actions.

Rest

The most important part of recovery is rest, and it's simple: don't put any stress on the affected body part(s) until they're fully healed. People who violate this simple principle can wind up with chronic dysfunction that can become quite a problem.

Once the injured area feels healed (no more pain through a full range of motion), start to slowly train it again. Work with lighter weights and see how you feel the next day, and gradually work back into your normal routine.

Ice

Ice helps you recover by reducing inflammation, swelling, and internal bleeding from injured capillaries and blood vessels.[12] As long as there is pain and inflammation, ice will help.

You should begin treatment with ice, not heat, and I recommend keeping a damp cloth between the ice pack and your skin to avoid discomfort.

Don't apply ice for more than 15 to 20 minutes at a time, but you can rotate on and off all day.

Compression

Like ice, compression helps you heal by reducing swelling and inflammation.[13] Use an elastic bandage or a compression sleeve, and wrap the injured part tightly, but not so tight as to impair blood flow.

You can combine compression with ice by wrapping over the ice pack or by getting a product specifically designed to combine both ice and compression, like those offered by Hyperice.

Elevation

By raising the affected part above your heart, you speed the blood's journey back to your heart, which reduces swelling and aids in removing waste products from the area.[14]

THE BOTTOM LINE

Don't think that injuries are inevitable in this game. By following the advice in this chapter, I've never had to deal with more than a strained muscle (knock on wood!), and I wish the same for you!

CHAPTER SUMMARY

- Weightlifting isn't a dangerous activity. You're far more likely to get injured playing just about any sport than you are lifting weights.

- Those with injured joints may need to dial back the intensity of their weightlifting to preserve their joint health.

- If you can't get full reps, you're using too much weight, and you're increasing your risk of injury. Simply lighten the load, do full reps, improve your strength, and only move up in weight when you can keep it fully under control.

- Pushing yourself in the gym is good, so long as you always maintain proper form as well.

- Static stretching before exercise has been shown to impair speed and strength. Not only can it fail to prevent injury, but it may *increase* the risk of injury due to the cellular damage it causes to muscle and its analgesic effect.

- If you experience pain, stop your set. If an exercise always bothers you, do something else. The key to dealing with pain is treating it like an injury until it's better. Avoid exercises that aggravate it and let it heal.

SECTION V:

SUPPLEMENTATION

22

THE NO-BS GUIDE TO SUPPLEMENTS WHAT WORKS, WHAT DOESN'T, AND WHAT TO WATCH OUT FOR

Biceps are like ornaments on a Christmas tree.
— ED COAN

THE SHELVES OF YOUR LOCAL SUPPLEMENT store are packed with all kinds of bogus junk claiming to deliver results that only steroids can achieve. You know the claims…

Advanced time-release formula guaranteed to feed your lean mass for up to 8 hours!
Kick your testosterone production into overdrive and maximize your gains!
Assault estrogen receptors in your body and completely block muscle-killing hormones!

The products include pre-, intra-, and post-workout supplements, testosterone, human growth hormone, nitric oxide boosters, anti-estrogens, aromatase inhibitors, and the list goes on and on.

If you believe half of the hype you read in supplement advertisements or on their labels, well, it would probably take a while before you realize the simple truth of the matter, which is…

Most everything you see in the world of workout supplements is utterly worthless.

Yup…a complete waste of money. Not all. But most.

How can I say that so confidently? Well, I've not only tried every type of supplement you can imagine, but I've also studied the science and am interested only in what has been objectively proven—not "gymlore" and fancy marketing pitches.

You see, the supplement companies are cashing in big on a "little" trick that your mind can play on you known as the *placebo effect*. This is the scientifically proven fact that your simple belief in the effectiveness of a medicine or supplement can make it work. People have alleviated and in many cases even cured a whole host of serious illnesses, both mental and physical, by taking medically inert (useless) substances that they *believed* had therapeutic value.

Thus, just because some guys *believe* that the shiny new bottle of "muscle-maximizing" pills will work and then "feel them working" doesn't mean they have any actual value. Unfortunately, however, the placebo effect doesn't seem to be strong enough to help us build more muscle with pixie dust, despite what we think might be happening.

And the sad reality is many (most, really) supplements hawked in gyms, magazines, and websites are nothing more than that: pixie dust. That is, the majority of ingredients in these products have never been scientifically proven to do anything like what is claimed, or better yet, they have been proven to be flat-out worthless.

If you're wondering how companies can even get away with such an egregious scam, it's simple: the supplement industry is completely unregulated. You don't have to submit products to the FDA to start selling—you just whip something together, say whatever you want in your advertising, and voilà, you're now in the supplement business. Watch the documentary *Bigger Stronger Faster* if you want to see how hilariously easy this is.

The degenerates running certain supplement companies set the standard for unethical practices by doing things like spiking pre-workouts with methamphetamine-like substances (yes, several large supplement companies were caught doing this) or adding a dangerous chemical extracted from dynamite to fat-loss pills (one of the same companies did this as well), and, well, they may get caught…one day. And fined. Or not.

I've had the displeasure of meeting several of these unsavory types, and I wasn't surprised to hear jokes about their latest "pills in a bottle" for customers to snap up; about how easy it is to just tell people what they want to hear and sell them anything; about how large the drug bills are of bodybuilders they sponsor (yeah, some supplement companies pay for their athletes' steroids, but you're led to believe the magic pixie dust is the key to their physiques); about dishonest ways to fudge ingredient dosages and nutrition facts such as "amino spiking" protein powders, which entails filling them up with scoops of cheap amino acids that can be technically displayed as grams of protein; and more.

That said, there *are* honest people and companies out there, and there *are* a handful of supplements worth buying and using. Most aren't the sexy muscle-building crap pushed by 'roid monsters in the magazines, but they are scientifically proven to help you in your journey to build muscle, get lean, and stay healthy.

So, let's go through the common types of supplements and look at what you should and shouldn't spend your hard-earned cash on. And in the bonus report offered at the end of this book, you'll find my exact product recommendations (brands and products themselves).

VITAMIN D

Just a few years ago, vitamin D was simply known as the "bone vitamin," and even today, many physicians still believe it is essential only for bone health.

Research shows otherwise, however: insufficient vitamin D levels increase the risk of many types of disease, including osteoporosis, heart disease, stroke, some cancers, type 1 diabetes, multiple sclerosis, tuberculosis, and even the flu, but we're going to focus on the positive.[1]

Thanks to the hard work of many scientists, including the notable Dr. Michael Holick, we now know that nearly every type of tissue and cell in the body has vitamin D receptors, which means it's an essential hormone that plays a vital role in a large number of physiological processes.[2]

When we ingest vitamin D or produce it in the skin (as a result of sun exposure), it gets converted into its active form, *1,25-dihydroxyvitamin D*, or vitamin D3.[3] This substance then interacts with and supports virtually every tissue type in your body, including your heart, brain, and even fat cells. It also regulates genes that control immune function, metabolism, and cell growth and development.[4]

As you can see, this vitamin deserves a *lot* more attention than it has been given over the last couple of decades. Fortunately, however, vitamin D's vital importance and amazing benefits are becoming more and more widely known and accepted.

Now, as you may already know, our body can't produce vitamin D without sun exposure, and according to research published by the Center for Disease Control in 2011, 8 percent of Americans are vitamin D deficient, and 25 percent are considered "at risk" of a deficiency.[5] According to other research, however, deficiency may be as high as 42 percent.[6]

There are two ways to ensure you get enough vitamin D:

1. Spend 15 to 20 minutes in the sun every day with at least 25 percent of your skin exposed.[7]

2. Take supplements.

As most of us aren't able to take midday tanning breaks, supplementation is the answer.

How to Take Vitamin D

According to the Institute of Medicine, 600 IU per day is adequate for ages 1 to 70 (and 800 IU per day for 70+),[8] but these numbers have been severely criticized by scientists who specialize in vitamin D research.[9] They call attention to the over 125 peer-reviewed studies that indicate such recommendations are too low and are likely to lead to vitamin D deficiencies.

A committee of the U.S. Endocrine Society recently convened to review the evidence and concluded that between 600 and 1,000 IU per day is adequate for ages 1 to 18, and between 1,500 and 2,000 IU per day is adequate for ages 19+.[10]

According to Dr. Michael Holick, however, even 2,000 IU per day is suboptimal. Research shows that 2,000 IU per day is the minimum needed to maintain vitamin D sufficiency (30 milligrams per milliliter), but Dr. Holick maintains that optimal vitamin D status is between 50 and 80 milligrams per milliliter, which would call for a daily intake closer to 5,000 IU.[11]

So, I recommend that you start at 2,000 IU per day and then get blood tested for your 25-hydroxyvitamin D levels (the usable form of vitamin D your body creates) to ascertain your vitamin D status. Chances are, you'll come in below 50 to 80 milligrams per milliliter.

Research shows that you need to increase intake of vitamin D by 100 IU to increase blood concentration by 1 milligram per milliliter, so you can then calculate how much additional vitamin D you'll need to take to reach optimal levels.[12] For instance, if your test came back at 30 milligrams per milliliter and you wanted to raise it to 50 milligrams per milliliter, you would need to increase your current intake by 2,000 IU.

PROTEIN SUPPLEMENTS

Using protein supplements such as whey, egg, and casein powders (your three best options) isn't necessary, but it is convenient.

As you know, whey protein is a fantastic source of protein, and there are three forms you can buy it in: *concentrate*, *isolate*, and *hydrolysate*.

Whey concentrate is the least processed form and the cheapest to manufacture, and it contains some fat and lactose. Whey concentrates range from 35 to 80 percent protein by weight, depending on quality.[13]

Whey isolate is a form of whey protein processed to remove the fat and lactose. Isolates are 90+ percent protein by weight, and as they're more expensive to manufacture than whey concentrate, they're more expensive for consumers too.[14]

Whey hydrolysate is a predigested form of whey protein that's easily absorbed by the body and free of allergenic substances found in milk products.[15] Research indicates that the hydrolysis process improves solubility and digestibility, but you pay dearly for these benefits: whey hydrolysate is the most expensive of the three options.[16]

So which should you buy? Well, when choosing a whey protein product, you have a few things to consider.

While isolates and hydrolysates are pushed as superior to concentrates due to purity and higher protein concentrations per scoop, there's insufficient evidence to support claims that they are superior to concentrates in terms of meeting daily protein needs.

That said, choosing the cheapest whey you can find, which will always be a concentrate, isn't a good idea, either. A quality whey concentrate is somewhere around 80 percent protein by weight, but inferior concentrates can be as low as 30 percent.

What else is in there, then?

Unfortunately we can only wonder, as adulteration (the addition of fillers like maltodextrin and flour) is startlingly rampant in this industry.[17] In many cases, you'll get what you pay for. If the product costs a lot less than the going rate for whey, it's probably because it's made with inferior ingredients.

High prices aren't always indicative of high quality, though. Disreputable supplement companies also pull other tricks, such as starting with a low-quality concentrate, adding small amounts of isolate and hydrolysate to create a "blend," and then calling attention to just the isolate and hydrolysate in their marketing and packaging.

To protect yourself as a consumer, always check ingredient lists, serving sizes, and amounts of protein per serving before buying protein powder.

Specifically, you're going to want to look at the order in which the ingredients are listed (ingredients are listed in descending order according to predominance by weight) and the amount of protein per scoop relative to the scoop size.

For instance…

- If a product has maltodextrin (a filler) or any other ingredient listed before the protein powder itself, don't buy it. That means there's more maltodextrin, creatine, or other fillers in it than protein powder.

- If a scoop is 40 grams but there are only 22 grams of protein per serving, don't buy it unless you know that the other 18 grams are made up of stuff you want (weight gainers have quite a few carbs per scoop, for instance).

A high-quality whey protein is easy to spot: whey concentrate, isolate, or hydrolysate will be listed as the first ingredient(s) and the scoop size will be relatively close to the amount of protein per scoop. (It'll never match because there is at least sweetener and flavoring along with the protein powder in every serving.)

Fortunately, there isn't as much to worry about with casein and egg supplements. Stick with a casein product that uses micellar casein (the highest quality available), and most egg products are comparable, but I prefer one company specifically, which you'll find in the bonus report.

WEIGHT GAINERS

Weight gainers are popular among "hardgainers" who struggle with gaining weight, but I'm not a fan of them because they're almost always full of junk calories. I much prefer to see guys eating real food with nutrition.

My general recommendation to people struggling to eat enough is to stick mainly to calorie-dense foods like the following…

- red meat,

- grains like brown rice and quinoa,

- oils like coconut oil and olive oil,

- avocado,

- whole-fat dairy,

- multigrain pasta and bread,

- almonds and almond butter,

- bananas, and

- white and sweet potatoes.

If you focus on these types of foods in your meal planning, you should have no trouble reaching your daily caloric needs without having to resort to weight gainers.

BRANCHED-CHAIN AMINO ACIDS (BCAAS)

You know that gallon of pink liquid the hardcore bodybuilder in your gym lugs around from machine to machine? Chances are that it's a cocktail of branched-chain amino acids (BCAAs) and that he'll swear by its muscle-building powers.

If you listen to the hype, BCAA supplements sound damn near as effective as steroids in their ability to help you build muscle and strength. But, as is the case with many supplements, you're not being told the whole story. Simply put, while BCAAs do have a valid use (which we'll talk about), they're not *nearly* as effective as they're sold to be.

We'll break down why, but let's start at the beginning: what exactly are BCAAs, anyway?

BCAAs are a group of three essential amino acids (amino acids that your body must get from your diet):

- leucine,

- isoleucine, and

- valine.

Leucine is the star of the trio, as it directly stimulates protein synthesis via the activation of an enzyme responsible for cell growth known as the mammalian target of rapamycin, or *mTOR*.[18]

Isoleucine is the number two act on the list, as it improves glucose metabolism and increases muscular uptake.[19]

Valine is a distant third as it doesn't seem to do much of anything when compared to leucine and isoleucine.[20]

You find high amounts of these amino acids in quality proteins such as meat, eggs, and dairy products, with whey protein isolate being particularly high.

If I wanted to sell you a BCAA supplement, it wouldn't be too hard. I could cite a variety of scientifically validated benefits, such as…

- improved immune function,[21]

- reduced fatigue,[22]

- reduced levels of exercise-induced muscle damage,[23]

- increased levels of post-exercise muscle growth,[24]

- and more…

Basically, I could just tell the same story that just about every supplement company selling BCAAs tells, and it would be hard to refute at first glance.

But there are two important points you're *not* told about BCAA research:

Research commonly cited that demonstrates muscle-related benefits of BCAA supplementation was done with subjects who didn't eat enough protein.

For example, a study conducted by researchers at the Centre for Studies and Research of Aerospace Medicine (France) is one of the poster boys for selling BCAAs.[25] Scientists examined the effects of BCAA supplementation on a group of elite wrestlers in a calorie deficit, and after three weeks, the supplement group, who ingested an additional 52 grams of BCAAs per day, preserved more muscle and lost a bit more fat than the control group (who didn't supplement at all).

Sounds pretty cool, right? Well, what you won't hear is that subjects, whose average weight was about 150 pounds, were eating a paltry ~80 grams of protein per day. As you know, based on research on the protein needs of athletes in a calorie restriction, they should have been eating *double* that amount of protein to preserve lean mass.

So all that study tells us is that if we feel like eating half the amount of protein we should be eating, a BCAA supplement can help mitigate the damage. Not too exciting.

Other studies that demonstrate various muscle-related benefits of BCAA supplementation have promising abstracts, but they are almost always hampered by a lack of dietary control and/or a low protein intake.[26] Furthermore, in almost all cases, the subjects are training fasted, which is an important point we'll talk more about in a minute.

You can get all the BCAAs your body needs from food instead, which is cheaper and far more satisfying.

Research that demonstrates the anabolic effects of BCAA supplementation before, during, and after exercise is often used to sell the powders.[27] But this misses the forest for the trees.

What such research tells us is that acutely raising BCAA levels (and leucine in particular) before and after exercise helps us build more muscle.[28] There is *no* evidence that doing it through the ingestion of a BCAA supplement is more effective than food, however.

In fact, there's research to the contrary: food, and whey protein specifically, may be even more effective than amino acid drinks.[29] Most whole-food proteins are made up of about 15 percent BCAAs, and most protein supplements have BCAAs added, so when you're eating enough protein, especially if you're using protein supplements with BCAAs added, you're getting more than enough BCAAs to meet your body's demands.[30]

This is why I recommend that you eat 30 to 40 grams of protein before and after working out and why I use whey protein for these meals. It's cheaper than BCAA powders, tastes better, and is likely more effective.

So that's how things currently look when we strip away the hype and marketing angles. But before I move onto one legitimate use for BCAAs, I want to address a question that may have occurred to you:

Isn't there a study that had resistance-trained subjects lift weights and supplement with BCAAs while also on a high-protein diet? I wish, because that would lend great insight into the controversy.

All we currently have is an unpublished study paid for by Scivation—the creator of the popular *Xtend* BCAA supplement—and headed up by Jim Stoppani, that…cough … demonstrated?…some remarkable results[31]:

Daily intraworkout BCAA supplementation was *twice* as effective as intraworkout whey protein supplementation and resulted in a whopping 9 pounds of muscle growth *and* a 2 percent reduction in body fat in just eight weeks…in strength-trained men with at least two years of weightlifting experience…who were eating 2.2 to 2.4 grams of protein per kilogram of body weight…and were in a calorie surplus…

Wait…what? If I take BCAAs—no sorry, not just any BCAAs but *Xtend*—while I work out I can be in a calorie surplus and achieve steroid-level muscle growth *and* get leaner? Wow! Shut up and take all my money, Scivation!

Not. Color me skeptical here. To quote the popular fitness researcher and author Alan Aragon in his monthly research review:

"The skeptic in me is tempted to chalk up some of the results to not just funding source (Scivation), but also the longstanding friendship[32] [footnote added] between Jim Stoppani and the Scivation staff. The fact is, there's no way to quantify the degree of commercial bias inherent in this trial—or any other for that matter."[33]

Okay then, so BCAAs don't look to be nearly as exciting as the supplement companies say.

If you were on the fence about buying a BCAA supplement for general use, you're probably off it now. It turns out, however, that this supplement does have one scientifically supported use, and it relates to *fasted training.*

People usually think "fasted training" means "training on an empty stomach," but it's a bit different.

Fasted training means training in a "fasted state," and this has to do with insulin levels in your blood. As you know, when you eat food, it gets broken down into various molecules that your cells can use, and these molecules are released into your blood. Insulin is released as well, and its job is to shuttle these molecules into cells.

Your body enters a "fasted" state when it has finished absorbing all nutrients from the food you've eaten and insulin levels return to their normal, low "baseline" levels. When you exercise your body in this state, fat loss is accelerated (and weightlifting in a fasted state is particularly effective in this regard).[34]

There is a downside to fasted training, however, and this is where we get to BCAAs: when you exercise in a fasted state, muscle breakdown is dramatically increased.[35] This is bad simply because too much muscle breakdown impairs total muscle growth over time.

Preventing this is simple, though, and it involves taking BCAAs.

How to Take BCAAs

All you have to do is take 10 grams of BCAAs or 3 to 5 grams of leucine (warning: it tastes bad) 10 to 15 minutes before fasted training.

This suppresses muscle breakdown during your workout with a minimal impact on insulin levels, thus keeping you in a fasted state.[36]

PRE-WORKOUT SUPPLEMENTS

Advertisements for popular pre-workout products are some of the most exaggerated in the industry. If we're to believe what we're told, just a few scoops of powder will basically turn us into superheroes for an hour. I mean, the monstrous bodybuilders who look like they're about to die of a heart attack wouldn't lie, right?

Well, pre-workout supplements are notorious for a few deceitful practices:

- Including small amounts of cheap, ineffective ingredients to make long, impressive ingredient lists and using (and often misinterpreting) cherry-picked, flawed, or biased studies to convince you why the formulation is awesome.

- Underdosing effective ingredients to save money and hiding behind the "proprietary blend" labeling loophole that allows companies to not disclose the dosage of each part of the blend.[37]

- Using chemical names of everyday compounds to mislead you into thinking the products have special ingredients. For instance, *epigallo-3-catechin-3-O-b-gallate* is just green tea extract, and *1,3,7-trimethylxanthine* is just caffeine.

Why do these things?

Because it's *extremely* profitable.

You see, here's the game: When Shady Supplements, Inc. is looking to create a pre-workout supplement, it believes that two things are key for sales:

1. including a few ingredients that have been clinically proven as safe and effective so marketing claims can be defended and

2. including a bunch of other unproven junk to give you the impression that you're getting a lot for your money.

There's a problem though, and it relates to cost.

You see, using clinically effective dosages of worthwhile ingredients gets really expensive, really fast. Shady Supplement's business model revolves around spending as little on production as possible and pouring tons of cash into its marketing and its greedy owner's pockets, so it just can't afford to make a good product.

What to do instead? Simple.

Include small amounts of these key ingredients—much smaller than the dosages used in the actual research proving them to be effective—then pad the ingredients list with tiny amounts of a bunch of junk for good measure.

These companies don't want you to know how much of each ingredient is in the product, however, as you might get suspicious. Again, the solution is simple: use the proprietary blend, which allows them to list just the weight of everything in the blend, not of the individual ingredients themselves.

Because ingredients in proprietary blends are listed in descending order according to predominance by weight, when the first ingredient is something cheap, let's say maltodextrin (a sweet, or sometimes tasteless, filler) or creatine monohydrate, it could be (and often is) 90+ percent of the actual product.

No matter how many other ingredients are listed after the first, they could altogether only constitute a small percentage of the actual blend.

Next, Shady Supplement's marketing department gets a hold of the product and lists all the benefits it can find for higher dosages of the underdosed ingredients, often stretching these to the point of absurdity, and then it adds a few more claims based on nothing to round it out.

In the end, this means you pay $30 to $50 for a product that cost Shady Supplements $2 to $5 to manufacture and that would've cost $30 to create if the junk were dropped and proper dosages were used for the worthwhile ingredients.

If you want to help put an end to all of this chicanery, the first thing you should demand as a consumer is no proprietary blends. There's absolutely no reason to use them for anything other than deception and fraud. All the science behind effective ingredients is publicly available. Everyone knows what works and doesn't and in what dosages. Claims of "trade secrets" or proprietary research are bogus.

You should also know that the inclusion of more ingredients doesn't necessarily mean a better product. In fact, you won't find a legitimate pre-workout product with 30 ingredients because it's not financially feasible to include so many ingredients at clinically effective dosages (and you would be hard-pressed to even find 30 ingredients worth using, period).

By choosing your purchases wisely, you can force the changes that need to happen: the death of the proprietary blend and the use of only scientifically validated ingredients at clinically effective dosages with the elimination of ineffective "label filler" ingredients.

So, then, this brings us to the million-dollar question: are any pre-workout supplements worth using, or should we just stick to our trusty friend caffeine?

Well, caffeine is a useful pre-workout stimulant that can increase muscle endurance and strength, but the fact is there are several other safe, natural substances that can further improve your performance... *if* they're dosed properly.

So, all things considered, a *good* pre-workout supplement is worth the investment, in my opinion. It will give you a kick of energy, more focus, a good pump, and increased muscle endurance.

One thing you should know about pre-workout drinks, however, is that most contain quite a bit of caffeine per serving (anywhere from 100 to 300 milligrams). If your body is sensitive to caffeine, you might want to try one with little or no caffeine.

CREATINE

Creatine is a substance found naturally in the body and in foods like red meat. It is perhaps the most researched dietary supplement in the world of sports nutrition; it has been the subject of more than 200 studies.

Research shows that supplementation with creatine builds muscle and improves strength, increases anaerobic endurance, and reduces muscle damage and soreness from exercise.[38]

And in case you're worried that creatine is bad for your kidneys, these claims have been categorically and repeatedly disproven.[39] In healthy subjects, creatine has been shown to have no harmful side effects, in both short- and long-term usage.[40] People with kidney disease are not advised to supplement with creatine, however.[41]

Thus, creatine is one of the supplements I highly recommend that you take. There are different forms available though. Which is the best?

Well, the monohydrate form has been the subject of the vast majority of studies done on the creatine molecule and is a proven winner, but the marketing machines of supplement companies are constantly pumping up fancy-sounding stuff like creatine citrate, creatine ethyl ester, liquid creatine, creatine nitrate, buffered creatine, creatine hydrochloride, and others.

These variations are certainly more expensive than creatine monohydrate, but they're no more effective. Certain forms of creatine are more water soluble, such as creatine citrate, nitrate, and hydrochloride, but this doesn't make them more effective in your body.[42]

Don't overpay for overhyped forms of creatine pushed by million-dollar ad campaigns and sold in fancy bottles. Creatine monohydrate is the best bang for your buck and is the standard by which all other forms of creatine are still judged.

If plain ol' creatine monohydrate bothers your stomach, try a more water-soluble form of creatine, such as micronized creatine monohydrate or creatine citrate, nitrate, or hydrochloride.

How to Take Creatine

The most common method of creatine supplementation found in the literature is a "loading" period of 20 grams per day for five to seven days, followed by a maintenance dosage of 5 grams per day.[43]

You don't *have* to load creatine if you're just starting with supplementation (you can just start with 5 grams per day), but loading does cause the creatine to accumulate faster in the muscles and thus causes the benefits to "kick in" faster.

Research shows that co-ingesting creatine with carbohydrates increases creatine accumulation in the muscles.[44] As this effect is mainly a result of elevated insulin levels, protein intake can contribute as well.[45] In fact, one study conducted by researchers at the University of Nottingham demonstrated that 50 grams of protein and carbohydrates were equally effective as 100 grams of carbohydrates in augmenting muscular creatine accumulation.[46]

So, based on this research, you should take creatine with a good-sized meal to maximize its effects.

Furthermore, there's research that indicates that creatine taken after a workout is more effective than creatine taken before one, which is why I take my creatine with my post-workout meal consisting of about 50 grams of protein and 75 to 125 grams of carbs.[47]

Do You Have to Cycle Creatine?

No, there's no scientific evidence that long-term creatine usage is harmful, so no, there's no reason to cycle on and off it. It's not a steroid.

Does Caffeine Interfere with Creatine's Effects?

Maybe.

One study conducted by researchers at the University of Leuven demonstrated that ingesting caffeine with creatine monohydrate decreases muscular force production when compared to ingesting just creatine monohydrate alone, but this isn't enough evidence to close the case.[48]

That's especially true considering the fact that a study conducted by researchers at University of Luton demonstrated that caffeine and creatine monohydrate taken together were more effective than just creatine monohydrate in improving the performance of high-intensity interval cardio.[49] Similar results were seen in a study conducted by researchers at Yu Da University (Taiwan) as well.[50]

Based on the evidence, I like to play it safe and take my creatine and caffeine separately, not together like what you find in most pre-workout drinks.

DOES CREATINE MAKE YOU BLOATED?

This used to be a problem, but in the last decade or so, processing has improved greatly and it's a nonissue now.

It's unlikely that you'll notice any difference in subcutaneous water retention when you take creatine, even if you're quite lean.

SHOULD YOU TAKE CREATINE WHILE DIETING FOR FAT LOSS?

Yes.

Creatine works equally well when you're in a calorie deficit, which means you'll retain more strength and thus lean mass while cutting.[51]

TESTOSTERONE BOOSTERS

While studies have shown that you can increase testosterone levels by handling deficiencies in certain vitamins such as D and C and minerals such as zinc, calcium, and magnesium, the flashy "test boosters" sold in your local supplement store are generally just a waste of money.[52]

Some go to town with their ingredients, but most rely on one or more of the following: *Tribulus terrestris*, ZMA, or D-aspartic acid.

Multiple studies have proven that supplementation with *Tribulus terrestris* has no effect on testosterone levels, body composition, or exercise performance.[53]

Research has shown that supplementation with ZMA does not affect testosterone levels if you're not zinc deficient.[54]

And while research has shown that supplementation with D-aspartic acid can increase testosterone levels in both humans and rats, the effect is usually slight and temporary.[55] If you want to try it, however, just buy the amino itself and take 3 grams per day.

The bottom line is that supplements that aim to handle vitamin and mineral deficiencies that suppress testosterone levels can be worthwhile, but these are rarely marketed as "test boosters" and fall under the less sexy category of "male health" instead.

HUMAN GROWTH HORMONE BOOSTERS

Simply put, natural human growth hormone boosters are a complete waste of money. They're usually full of amino acids that do provide various benefits when dosed properly but not an increase in levels of growth hormone associated with muscle growth.

You see, there are more than 100 forms of growth hormone in your body, and all perform different functions. When you're told that something like gamma aminobutyric acid, or GABA, has been proven to elevate resting and post-exercise growth hormone levels, what you're not told is that the form of growth hormone that it stimulates the production of hasn't been proven to contribute to muscle growth.[56]

Save your money and skip the human growth hormone boosters.

GLUTAMINE

Glutamine is the most abundant amino acid in the body and is heavily depleted by intense, prolonged exercise.[57]

Research has shown that supplementation with glutamine can…

- reduce the negative effects of prolonged exercise on the immune system (research has shown that exercise depletes glutamine levels in the body, which in turn can impair immune function),

- improve your endurance and reduce fatigue in prolonged exercise, and

- help your body better deal with the systemic stress of prolonged exercise.[58]

While supplementation with glutamine clearly has its benefits, it can't deliver on the claims commonly used to sell it, which revolve around building more muscle.

These claims usually cite research that has shown that intramuscular glutamine levels play an important role in protein synthesis and the prevention of muscle breakdown, and that glutamine improves the body's ability to use leucine.[59]

The rest of the story, however, is that there are no studies to indicate that supplementation with glutamine helps healthy, well-fed adults build more muscle. You only see these effects in diseased or underfed people and animals.

To the contrary, in fact, several studies conducted with healthy adults show that supplementation with glutamine has no effect on protein synthesis rates, muscle performance, body composition, or the prevention of muscle breakdown.[60]

So, while supplementation with glutamine may not provide an anabolic boost, its anti-stress and anti-fatigue benefits make it a worthwhile buy if you're exercising regularly, intensely, and for prolonged periods.

How to Take Glutamine

Studies have shown that 100 to 200 milligrams per kilogram of body weight of glutamine each day is sufficient for athletes and that chronic usage is important.[61]

NITRIC OXIDE SUPPLEMENTS

These supplements often consist of a form of the amino acids *arginine* and *citrulline* and the substance *agmatine*. They claim to increase the body's production of a substance called nitric oxide. Nitric oxide widens blood vessels and thus enables more oxygen and nutrients to get to the muscles, which can improve performance.

While this sounds like just another dubious marketing pitch, there are studies to support some of these ingredients and claims, but again the problem comes back to dosages.[62] You'll often find nitric oxide-boosting molecules in pre-workout products, but in amounts too small to matter.

That said, when dosed properly (about 8 grams), I've noticed that citrulline in particular improves workout pump and performance.

MULTIVITAMINS

As with most supplements, multivitamins are aggressively overhyped and oversold. Advertisements loudly proclaim that just a few pills per day will ward off disease, optimize hormones, support the gut, enhance cognitive function, and increase energy levels. Some are even bolder, claiming their multivitamins will also help you build muscle, get stronger, and lose fat.

On the other side of the coin, however, are the people claiming that multivitamins are a complete waste of money and offer absolutely no health benefits whatsoever or are even dangerous to our health.

Well, the truth lies somewhere in the middle.

Why a Multivitamin Is Great . . . in Theory

Your body needs a wide spectrum of vitamins and minerals to carry out the millions of sophisticated functions it performs every day. You want to maintain an adequate supply of vitamins and minerals to support every growth and repair process that occurs.

Ideally, we'd get all of the vitamins and minerals we need from the food we eat. Due to the nature of the average Western diet, however, we tend to be deficient in certain vitamins and minerals.

For example, according to research conducted by scientists at Colorado State University published in 2005, at least half the U.S. population fails to meet the recommended dietary allowance (RDA) for vitamin B-6, vitamin A, magnesium, calcium, and zinc, and 33 percent of the population does not meet the RDA for folate.[63] Research also shows that average vitamin K and D intake levels may be suboptimal as well.[64]

What to do, then? How can we easily ensure our bodies get enough of all of the essential vitamins and minerals?

Enter the multivitamin supplement.

The idea of taking a supplement that can cover any possible nutritional deficiencies in our diets and mitigate the harmful effects of some of our less-than-healthy habits is a great concept. It would create a "safety buffer" for our health.

That's the *least* you should expect from a multivitamin, in reality: the right combination of vitamins and minerals and the right dosages. This would at least plug any dietary holes and ensure your body is getting adequate micronutrients.

I think it should do more, though. Namely, there are scores of natural substances that have been scientifically proven to ward off disease and improve health and performance, and I think a multivitamin should include an array of them at clinically effective dosages.

Many companies think differently, though. They would rather play the game we've already talked about in detail: spend very little on production, exaggerate and even invent benefit claims, and enjoy the large profit margins.

The bottom line is that most supplement companies are hoping you won't look into their multivitamins' ingredients lists, because if you did, you would quickly discover several things…

The Failings of the Average Multivitamin

There are two major reasons why multivitamins in general have been attacked over the years.

Multivitamins are often stuffed with all kinds of micronutrients, regardless of whether we need to supplement with them, and in unjustifiably high or low dosages.

If you're not deficient in the vitamins and minerals contained in the multivitamin, you're not going to notice anything by supplementing with more. And in many cases, multivitamins are quite high in vitamins and minerals that most people aren't deficient in and low in what we need.

For example, calcium supplementation is known to be beneficial as individuals with a low dairy and vegetable intake (including vegetarians and vegans who don't eat additional servings of vegetables to compensate) tend to be somewhat deficient, which only increases in frequency with age.[65]

However, athletes tend to have excess levels of calcium due to high-protein dieting (one scoop of casein protein provides 60 percent of the RDA!). While this doesn't pose an acute health risk, excess calcium levels can reduce the absorption of the minerals we care about (zinc and magnesium). Thus, a multivitamin specifically for athletes can safely omit calcium.

Supplying superdoses of various micronutrients via poorly formulated supplements will not only fail to provide any benefits, but it can even be harmful.

For example, vitamin A (retinol) was traditionally added because it is a vitamin, but it was later discovered that high dosages of retinol could actively harm the liver by cutting off the blood supply to its cells.[66]

Due to this, the plant pigment ß-carotene is often used instead of retinol because it turns into retinol when needed and thus is safer, but it's also abundant in most people's diets. A better option would be carotenoids (plant pigments) that tend to be lacking in the average Western diet, such as the sea-based fucoxanthin or the egg-based lutein and zeaxanthin.

The vitamin E found in many multivitamins can also be harmful. It's often surprisingly overdosed on the assumption that including more antioxidants is better and, because it and vitamin C are cheap, both are usually included at high dosages.

Unfortunately, not all antioxidants are similar, and regular supplementation of vitamin E above 400 IU per day is now suspected to increase the risk of all-cause mortality.[67] More is not always better.

In many cases, supplement companies don't bother determining optimal dosages of the essential vitamins and minerals for their target publics and simply choose the cheapest forms available. They also may choose needlessly expensive forms that sound nice in marketing copy but don't confer additional benefits over cheaper forms.

Going the cheap route provides higher profit margins, and going the unnecessarily expensive route adds needless expense to both the manufacturer and customer and results in a product that is ultimately less beneficial than it would be if the manufacturing budget were spent more intelligently.

Another little gimmick to look for is the use of several forms of the same vitamin or mineral, which makes the product look more impressive (in many customers' minds, more and fancier-sounding ingredients means a better product).

For instance, using four different types of magnesium and calling it the "Magnesium Maximization Blend" looks impressive to the customer but means absolutely nothing in terms of effectiveness.

And while we're on the subject of forms of vitamins and minerals, let's look at the controversial subject of natural vs. artificial.

Many people believe that if something comes from nature, it must be better than something synthetically made. Hence, the all-too-common (and meaningless) marketing claims of "all natural" that we find on all kinds of food products.

When it comes to vitamin supplements, it's often assumed the natural forms of vitamins, including whole-food sources, are automatically better than their synthetic counterparts. Some supplement companies even claim that synthetic vitamins are harmful to sell you on their naturally sourced products.

There is some truth to these claims, but they don't apply equally to all molecules. Not all natural vitamins are better than synthetic forms, and not all synthetic forms are harmful.

There are notable examples of natural vitamins having unique properties that synthetic forms do not, such as vitamin E, and notable examples of synthetic vitamins outperforming the natural ones, such as synthetic folic acid being better absorbed than folate from natural sources.[68]

Supplements that brag about only using natural vitamins are preying on our tendency to assume they're automatically healthier or better, and those that also demonize all synthetic vitamins are simply lying and hoping you don't know any better.

Multivitamins often offer little more than the poorly formulated collection of essential micronutrients.

In some cases, multivitamins include nothing else at all in terms of ingredients, but many multivitamins do include additional substances beyond just vitamins and minerals. The normal practice, however, is to jam each serving with proprietary blends of as much stuff as possible to create a long, "impressive" nutrition facts panel.

These extras are often claimed to do all kinds of things like increase anabolism; optimize hormones; provide the body with vital antioxidants; aid in digestion and nutrient absorption; support the liver, immune system, and bones and joints; improve cognitive abilities; and more.

While all of these things *sound* great, and we'd love to believe they're true, when you look into the ingredients and dosages, they tell another story—a story you're well familiar with by now.

In some cases, there's little or no scientific evidence that such substances can confer the benefits claimed, and in others, there's good science to support the substances used but the dosages administered in the clinical research were 5, 10, or even 15 to 20 times higher than what's in the products.

It's the same old scam.

The truth is that for many, multivitamins are just an extremely unscrutinized "faith buy," which is something that does not have any noticeable benefits over the short term. If any noticeable benefits do occur over the long term, it's hard to attribute them to the supplement.

While you *know* that caffeine works soon after ingesting it, something like *Bacopa monnieri* has no acute benefits, and you just have to trust that the benefits seen in scientific studies will occur over time.

The collective marketing machine of the supplement industry has done a good job making the multivitamin a staple, both in our diets and in its revenue sources. While people will be concerned with the benefits of something like a pre-workout drink or sleep supplement, they will take a multivitamin "because it's a multivitamin" and simply have faith that it will benefit them…usually without compelling evidence to prove it.

The bottom line is that if you eat a substantial amount of a wide variety of nutritious foods every day, you may get everything you need in the way of vitamins and minerals. But many people aren't, and supplementation can help provide what's missing.

Furthermore, a good multivitamin contains other substances known to improve health and performance that are difficult or basically impossible to get in adequate amounts through diet alone.

I take a multivitamin every day for these reasons, and I recommend that you do too.

FAT BURNERS

With the weight-loss market valued at a staggering $60.5 billion and more than one-third of U.S. adults obese, it's no surprise that there's a glut of "fat burners" for sale these days.[69]

By the same token, it's also no surprise that fat burners are some of the most expensive supplements on the shelves and come with some of the largest profit margins and loudest marketing claims.

How well do these products work, though? Enough to warrant the significant expense?

Let's find out.

WHY A "FAT BURNER" CAN BE FUNDAMENTALLY MISLEADING

One of the reasons fat burners sell so well is the moniker itself: when you're trying to lose fat as efficiently as possible, a "fat burner" sounds like a perfect addition to your regimen. Anything that "burns fat" is worth a go, no?

It's not that simple, though. No natural substance can just "burn fat" outright, regardless of how complex or pseudo-scientific the marketing claims are.

You see, to sell you on their fat burners, supplement companies will often talk about increasing fat oxidation rates, preserving lean mass, supporting the thyroid, inducing thermogenesis, inhibiting enzymes related to fat storage, inducing enzymes that cause fat loss, manipulating hormone and neurotransmitter levels, reducing water retention, improving nutrient partitioning, and more.

Well, the truth is that these are all aspects of fat loss, but this type of salesmanship is little more than an attempt to dazzle you with terminology and scientific half-truths in hopes that you just accept the claimed benefits at face value.

When you take a cold, hard look at the science of fat loss, there are only three ways to appreciably speed it up:

You can speed up your basal metabolic rate.

While there are many, many ways to increase metabolic rate, they ultimately rely on one or both of the following mechanisms:

1. encourage a cell to produce more energy from carbohydrates and fatty acids, or

2. reduce the efficiency of the process through which cellular energy is produced, thus increasing the "energy cost" of meeting the body's needs.

There *are* ways to manipulate those mechanisms through supplementation, and we'll get to them in a minute, but they're not as numerous or powerful as some supplement companies would have you believe.

You can prevent hunger or cravings from ruining your plans.

A major reason even good diets fail is people just aren't able to stick to them long enough. Wishes turn into cravings and ultimately binges, which can undo days or even weeks of hard work.

While some people have an easier time dieting than others, almost everyone has to deal with hunger and cravings at some point, to one degree or another.

Some natural compounds are known to reduce hunger and others are known to increase the sensation of fullness you get from a meal, and a combination of proven molecules can be used to successfully reduce hunger and cravings and derive the maximum benefits from your dieting.

You can make the overall experience of dieting more enjoyable.

Make no mistake: while changing your body with diet, exercise, and supplementation can dramatically change your life for the better, it's not easy.

No amount of powders or pills is going to get you there. It takes hard work, and it takes time. And this is another major reason why diets fail: people don't want to go through the discomfort of it all.

Well, like reducing hunger and cravings, making the process of dieting more enjoyable, primarily by increasing the overall feeling of well-being, makes it easy to stick to the plan and see it through.

WHAT MAKES A GOOD "FAT BURNER"?

Although the physiological machinery involved in fat loss is vast and complex, the practical application remains simple.

Contrary to what many supplement companies would lead you to believe, directly stimulating any of the thousands of proteins and enzymes involved in fat loss either doesn't work or is uninvestigated.

Remember, fat loss is a whole-body process. For a fat burner to be truly based on good science and noticeably affect fat loss, it should focus on simple, key, and proven targets because then everything else activates and functions accordingly.

Thus, a good "fat burner" would achieve the three targets above: increase our basal metabolic rate, reduce hunger and cravings, and increase satiety and feelings of overall well-being.

Let's look at some of the stuff most commonly found in fat burners that can and can't get the job done.

Caffeine

Caffeine helps you lose fat by simply increasing your body's daily energy expenditure and has other benefits for us fitness folk: it improves strength, muscle endurance, and anaerobic performance, and it also reverses the "morning weakness" experienced by many weightlifters.[70]

How to Use Caffeine for Weight Loss

To maximize caffeine's effectiveness, you want to prevent your body from building up too much of a tolerance to it.

The best way to do this is to limit intake. Here's what I recommend:

1. Before training, supplement with 3 to 6 milligrams of caffeine per kilogram of body weight. f you're not sure of your caffeine sensitivity, start with 3 milligrams per kilogram and work up from there.

2. Keep your daily intake at or below 6 milligrams per kilogram of body weight. Don't take 6 milligrams per kilogram before training and then drink a couple of coffees throughout the day as well.

3. Do one or two low-caffeine days per week and one no-caffeine day per week. A low day should be half your normal intake, and a no day means less than 50 milligrams of caffeine (you can have a cup or two of tea or a small cup of coffee, but no pre-workout, caffeine pills, etc.)

Raspberry Ketones

Raspberry ketones are the primary aroma compound of the red raspberry (it gives the raspberry its smell), and they're also found in other fruits like the blackberry and cranberry.

How did such a seemingly random compound find its way into weight-loss products?

Well, it started with a couple of animal studies that demonstrated that raspberry ketone supplementation prevented weight gain by increasing lipolysis and fat oxidation rates.[71] That might sound promising, but there are good reasons to be skeptical.

First, animal research cannot be used as proof of human effectiveness. The bodies of humans and rats just aren't similar enough, and this is especially true when talking about metabolic functions.

Second, one of the rat studies was in vitro research.[72] This means parts of living rats were removed to be studied in isolation as opposed to research done with living, intact organisms (*in vivo* research). In vitro research is less definitive than in vivo because living organisms are incredibly complex, and sometimes in vitro findings just don't pan out in vivo.

Third, the in vivo rat study that demonstrated weight-gain prevention used a massive oral dose: up to *20 grams per kilogram* of body weight, or *4,761* times greater than the average human intake.[73]

Fourth, there is just one human trial I know of that is commonly cited as evidence of raspberry ketone's effectiveness for weight loss.[74] The problem with this study, however, is the compound was paired with caffeine, capsaicin, garlic, ginger, and citrus aurantium as a source of synephrine. It's impossible to know whether the raspberry ketone did anything.

Considering the evidence currently available, there is insufficient evidence to support the use of low oral doses of raspberry ketone for fat-loss purposes. It has no place in a fat-burner supplement.

Synephrine

Synephrine is a chemical compound found in certain types of citrus fruits (particularly the bitter variety).

It's chemically similar to ephedrine and catecholamines, and although less potent, it induces similar effects in the body.

Research shows that supplementation with synephrine increases both basal metabolic rate and lipolysis, inhibits the activity of certain types of fat cell receptors that prevent fat mobilization, and increases the thermic effect of food (which, in case you don't remember, is the "energy cost" of metabolizing food).[75]

Furthermore, research shows that synephrine works synergistically with caffeine to enhance both caffeine's and its own fat-loss properties.[76] The synergism noted in a standard "ECA" (ephedrine, caffeine, and aspirin) stack also applies to synephrine.

Additionally, anything that has the ability to increase catecholamine activity can also suppress hunger between meals (a component of the fight or flight response), and thus synephrine is generally considered to be an effective appetite suppressant as well.

How to Use Synephrine for Weight Loss

Clinically effective dosages of synephrine range from 25 to 50 milligrams and can be taken anywhere from one to three times daily, depending on individual tolerance.

Garcinia Cambogia

Garcinia cambogia is a small fruit often used in Indian and Asian cuisine to impart a sour flavor. It's a good natural source of *hydroxycitric acid* and has received a lot of media attention recently as a weight-loss aid.

These claims are unfounded, however.

Like many fad supplements, Garcinia cambogia has some animal research on its side, but human research is contradictory and hard to interpret.

A couple of rat studies have demonstrated that Garcinia cambogia can reduce weight gain during a period of overfeeding by suppressing the synthesis of fatty acids in the liver (it reduced the amount of fat the rats could make from the excess calories).[77]

The human research bursts that bubble, though.

A meta-analysis of 12 randomized clinical trials of Garcinia cambogia found the following[78]:

- Three studies with small sample sizes reported statistically significant, albeit small, decreases in fat mass over the placebo groups.

- (In case you were wondering, the best result was 1.3 kilograms more weight lost than the placebo group over a three-month period.)

- Two studies found no difference in weight loss between the Garcinia cambogia and placebo groups, including the largest and most rigorous study reviewed.

- The results of the remaining studies reviewed were marred by serious design and/or execution flaws.

As you can see, the research currently available says that, despite its current popularity, Garcinia cambogia probably won't help you lose weight and thus isn't worth including in a fat-burner supplement.

Green Tea Extract

Green tea extract is an herbal product derived from green tea leaves. It contains a large amount of a substance known as a *catechin*, which is responsible for many of tea's health benefits, one of which relates to weight loss.[79]

Research has shown that supplementation with green tea extract reduces total fat mass, accelerates exercise-induced fat loss, and can reduce abdominal fat, in particular.[80] The primary mechanism by which it accomplishes this is inhibiting an enzyme that degrades catecholamines.[81]

This also makes green tea extract work synergistically with caffeine: caffeine increases catecholamine levels, and green tea extract extends the amount of time they spend in the blood.[82]

How to Use Green Tea Extract for Weight Loss

If you look at the dosages proven effective in clinical studies, you'll see that 400 to 600 milligrams of catechins per day is the normal range.[83]

When you take green tea extract doesn't matter. Research has shown that absorption is faster when pills are taken in a fasted state, but plasma catechin levels remain elevated for several hours after ingestion, whether fed or fasted.[84]

Acai Berry

The acai berry craze has passed, but it still remains a solid top seller in the world of weight-loss supplements.

I'll keep this short and simple and just quote the National Center for Complementary and Alternative Medicine:

"There is no definitive scientific evidence based on studies in humans to support the use of acai berry for any health-related purpose."

"No independent studies have been published in peer-reviewed journals that substantiate claims that acai supplements alone promote rapid weight loss. Researchers who investigated the safety profile of an acai-fortified juice in animals observed that there were no body weight changes in rats given the juice compared with controls." [85]

Don't waste your money on acai berry products if you're trying to lose weight.

Green Coffee Extract

Green coffee extract is a supplement derived from green coffee beans. It's similar to regular coffee beans, but it has high amounts of a substance known as *chlorogenic acid.*

A recent meta-analysis of the five human trials of green coffee extract available found that high dosages of chlorogenic acid via green coffee extract (400 to 800 milligrams chlorogenic acid per day) may induce fat loss, but researchers noted that the studies demonstrating this had high risks of bias due to funding sources (for-profit companies producing green coffee extract).[86]

Green coffee extract may help you lose weight if taken in high enough dosages, but until more research is done on it—particularly unbiased research—its ultimate value as a fat-loss supplement is uncertain.

Carnitine

Carnitine is a compound that your body produces from the amino acids lysine and methionine, and it plays a vital role in the generation of cellular energy.

While there is scientific evidence that carnitine supplementation can help with muscle recovery after exercise, does it have anything to offer in the way of weight loss?[87]

Well, it does have a mechanism that is of interest: it increases fat oxidation in the muscles.[88] What this means is it appears to increase the rate at which muscle tissue burns fat for fuel instead of glycogen. Theoretically, this could result in additional fat loss while exercising.

Actual research on this mechanism isn't exciting, however.

There's evidence that carnitine can reduce fat mass and increase muscle mass in the elderly, but these effects were not seen when tested with overweight premenopausal women.[89] Animal research has also failed to demonstrate any weight-loss benefits when simply combined with a calorie-restricted diet.[90]

Based on what we currently know, unless your body's ability to oxidize fat is impaired by disease or dysfunction, carnitine's metabolic effects aren't likely to help with fat loss.

5-HTP

The amino acid 5-HTP is found in foods like milk, meat, potatoes, pumpkin, and various greens, and it is converted into serotonin in the brain, which is one of the principal neurotransmitters involved in feelings of happiness.

Research shows that when taken with food, 5-HTP increases feelings of fullness and thus helps you control your food intake.[91] Furthermore, studies have demonstrated that 5-HTP's satiety mechanism can reduce cravings for carbohydrates in particular.[92]

How to Use 5-HTP for Weight Loss

Clinically effective dosages of 5-HTP range from 150 to 500 milligrams, which should be taken with meals. Like synephrine, one to three servings per day is common depending on tolerance.

Forskolin

Forskolin is found in the Indian herb *Coleus forskohlii* and has long been used in Ayurvedic medicine to treat heart and respiratory disorders.

Supplementation with forskolin increases blood plasma and intracellular levels of a molecule known as *cAMP (cyclic adenosine monophosphate)*, which functions as an intracellular "message relayer" vital to various biochemical processes, including the regulation of glycogen, sugar, and lipid metabolism.[93]

cAMP and adenosine triphosphate (ATP—the most basic form of cellular energy in the body—interact in a simple yet powerful way in the cell. When ATP is high, it indicates a plentiful energy state, and the body will aim to store and build tissue. But when cAMP is high, it signifies a lack of ATP and thus initiates a process to make more ATP by burning through energy reserves.

Forskolin activates an enzyme known as *adenyl cyclase*, which converts ATP to cAMP, thereby greatly increasing the ratio in favor of cAMP and initiating the energy-burning process.[94] Furthermore, forskolin's effects are amplified by the effects of synephrine.[95]

This isn't just abstract theory, either: research shows that supplementation with forskolin accelerates fat loss and increases testosterone levels.[96]

How to Use Forskolin for Weight Loss

While a clinically effective range is not known and is likely vast, 25 to 50 milligrams forskolin taken once per day is known to be effective.

Yohimbine

Yohimbine is a substance found in the *Pausinystalia yohimbe* plant, and research shows that it helps block a mechanism in fat cells that prevents weight loss, which in turn speeds up fat loss.[97]

There's a catch, though: you must be in a fasted state for it to work. The insulin spike that occurs after eating a meal completely negates the beneficial effects of yohimbine.[98]

Yohimbine is an effective fat-loss accelerator, but I generally don't like its inclusion in fat-burner supplements because some people experience the jitters from it. Thus, I think it's better sold and taken separately so it can be dropped out if necessary without having to lose the benefits of the rest of the fat burner.

How to Use Yohimbine for Weight Loss

I recommend that you start with 0.1 milligrams per kilogram of body weight to assess tolerance. If you feel fine, then increase to the clinically effective dosage of 0.2 milligrams per kilogram.

As with anything, excess doses of yohimbine can have negative side effects.[99] Don't go crazy with this. Furthermore, yohimbine has been shown to raise blood pressure.[100] If you have high blood pressure, I don't recommend that you use it.

FISH OIL

Fish oil is a great source of "omega-3 fatty acids" (*eicosapentaenoic acid*, or EPA, and *docosahexaenoic acid*, or DHA), which are an essential type of fat, meaning they can't be synthesized by the body and must be obtained from the diet.

Research shows that supplementation with fish oil can…

- increase muscle protein synthesis;

- reduce muscle soreness, inflammation, and anxiety;

- reduce blood pressure, depression, the negative effects of stress, and the risk of kidney and cardiovascular disease, stroke, and metabolic syndrome;

- improve glucose uptake and insulin sensitivity in people with impaired insulin response and metabolism, and preserve it in the metabolically healthy;

- improve memory and cognitive performance;

- help prevent weight gain; and

- speed up fat loss.[101]

As you can see, this is definitely a supplement worth taking, especially considering the fact that the average Western diet is quite low in omega-3 fatty acids.[102]

Not all fish oils are the same, however. There are two important things to consider when choosing one:

You want to know how the oil has been processed.

There are two forms of fish oil on the market today: *triglyceride* and *ethyl ester*.

The triglyceride form is fish oil in its natural state and the ethyl ester form is a processed version of the triglyceride form that includes a molecule of ethanol (alcohol).

While plenty of studies have proven the benefits of supplementation with fatty acid ethyl esters (FAEEs), research has shown that the triglyceride form is better absorbed by the body.[103] One of the reasons for this is the ethyl ester form is much more resistant to the enzymatic process by which the body breaks the oil down for use.[104]

Another downside to the ethyl ester form is during the digestive process, your body converts it back to the triglyceride form, which results in the release of the ethanol molecule. Although the dose is small, those with alcohol sensitivity or addiction can be negatively affected. Furthermore, research has provided evidence of cellular and organic toxicity and injury resulting from the ingestion of FAEEs.[105]

You want to know the EPA/DHA content of each serving.

Because of the varying quality of fish oils on the market, it's important that you look at how many milligrams of EPA and DHA are in each serving.

Lower quality supplements might have as little as 150 to 200 milligrams per 1 gram of fat, which makes them nearly worthless as you have to take far too much every day to get enough omega-3s (you want a minimum of 2 to 3 grams of omega-3s per day).

A high-quality fish oil is quite a bit more money than a low-quality one, but when you look at how much you're getting for that money in terms of omega-3 fatty acids, the price makes more sense.

For example, here's the label from a cheap, low-quality (ethyl ester) fish oil product:

100 Softgels

Serving Size 1 Softgel
Servings Per Container 100

Amount Per Serving	% Daily Value *	
Calories	10	
Calories From Fat	10	
Total Fat	1 g	2%*
Cholesterol	5 mg	2%
Fish Oil	1 g	**
Total Omega-3 Fatty Acids	300 mg	**
Epa (Eicosapentaenoic Acid)		
Dha (Docosahexaenoic Acid)		**

* Percent Daily Values are based on 2,000 calorie diet.
** Daily Value Not Established

Other Ingredients:

Gelatin, Glycerin, Food Glaze, Ethylcellulose, Enteric Coating, (Sodium Alginate, Stearic Acid), Mixed Tocopherols, Vanillin

ALLEREGEN INFORMATION:
CONTAINS FISH (ANCHOVY, MACKEREL, SARDINE) INGREDIENTS.

This product costs about $11 and comes with 100 pills, which means you're getting 30 grams of omega-3 fatty acids per bottle and paying about 37 cents per gram.

Here's the label from a high-quality triglyceride fish oil product:

120 Softgels

Serving Size 2 Softgel
Servings Per Container 60

Amount Per Serving	% Daily Value*	
Calories	18	
Calories From Fat	18	
Total Fat	2 g	3%
Saturated Fat	0.1 g	1%
Trans Fat	0 g	†
Vitamin E	30 IU	100%

Weight	Volume %	
Omega-3s		
EPA (Eicosapentaenoic Acid)	650 mg	35%
DHA (Docosahexaenoic Acid)	450 mg	25%
Other Omega-3s	180 mg	10%
Total Omega-3s	1280 mg	70%
Oleic Acid (Omega-9)	56 mg	3%

* Percent Daily Values are based on a 2,000 calorie diet
† Daily Value not established
Less Than 5 Mg Of Cholesterol Per Serving.

Other Ingredients

Purified Deep Sea Fish Oil (From Anchovies And Sardines), Soft Gel Capsule (Gelatin, Water, Glycerin, Natural Lemon Oil), Natural Lemon Oil, D-Alpha Tocopherol, Rosemary Extract.

No Gluten, Yeast, Milk Derivatives, Artificial Colors Or Flavors. Contains Vitamin E Derived From Refined Soybean Oil.

This product costs about $40 and comes with 120 pills, which means you're getting about 77 grams of omega-3 fatty acids per bottle and paying about 52 cents per gram.

So, as you can see, the initial price difference of $11 vs. $40 isn't as drastic when you look at what you're getting: 37 cents per gram of low-quality oil that isn't likely to deliver all of the benefits you're looking for vs. 52 cents per gram for the highest-quality oil on the market that will.

Thus, I recommend that you pay a bit more for a high-quality fish oil product. You can see exactly what I use in the bonus report.

How to Use Fish Oil to Improve Performance and Overall Health

Research indicates that 1.3 to 2.7 grams of omega-3 fatty acids per day is ideal for a person eating a normal, 2,000-calorie diet and that just over 6.5 grams per day is the upper recommended limit.[106]

Note that I said grams of *omega 3 fatty acids*, not grams of fish oil. This is an important distinction because 1 gram of fish oil isn't 1 gram of omega-3 fatty acids.

SPIRULINA

Spirulina is a nontoxic, blue-green algae that is a rich in nutrients. Research shows that supplementation with spirulina can…

- reduce muscle damage caused by exercise,

- improve exercise performance,

- increase strength,

- improve cholesterol and triglyceride levels,

- reduce blood pressure,

- improve blood sugar control,

- reduce systemic inflammation,

- improve allergy symptoms, and

- improve insulin sensitivity.[107]

As you can see, it confers similar benefits to fish oil but with a few additional goodies relating directly to exercise and weightlifting in particular.

How to Use Spirulina to Improve Performance and Overall Health

The common dosage seen in studies is 1 to 3 grams per day, although you can find additional benefits up to 10 grams per day, which is the recommended high dosage for humans.

It's worth noting that some people have an allergic reaction to spirulina. If you have any type of negative reaction such as a swollen face, reddening of the skin, or diarrhea, stop the use of spirulina.

CONSISTENCY IS THE KEY

Just like training and diet, the most important aspect of supplementing is *consistency*. You must take your supplements consistently to realize their full benefits.

To keep it simple, just include your supplementation regimen in your daily meal plan so you don't forget.

THE BOTTOM LINE

While we've gone over most of the popular types of supplements, you can always find more on the shelves of your local supplement store. Do your wallet a favor and skip 'em all, and *especially* the fancy-sounding ones.

You can make great gains without any supplements whatsoever, but if you're willing to spend some money to get the most out of your training, then adding the right supplements makes sense.

In case you don't want to throw in for everything I recommend in this chapter (and I totally understand—it's not cheap), here's how I would rank them in overall importance and worthiness:

- Vitamin D

- Multivitamin

- Fish oil

- Protein powder (if necessary to hit your daily protein needs)

- Spirulina

- Creatine

- Pre-workout or NO-booster

- Glutamine

And if you're dieting to lose fat, here's how I would rank the fat-loss supplements:

- Caffeine

- Fat burner (if it's properly formulated, as it will contain much of the below)

- Synephrine

- Yohimbine and BCAAs (if you're training fasted)

- Green tea extract

- Forskolin

- 5-HTP

And again, check out the bonus report if you'd like to see which brands and products I specifically use and recommend.

SECTION VI:

THE BEGINNING

23

FROM HERE, YOUR BODY WILL CHANGE

Your love for what you do and willingness to push yourself where others aren't prepared to go is what will make you great.
—LAURENCE SHAHLAEI

SO…I GUESS THIS IS IT, RIGHT? We've reached the end…

No way.

You're in a process now—and yup, it has already begun—of proving to yourself that you can transform your body faster than you ever believed. Within your first three to four months of training, you're going to know with *absolute certainty* that you can follow what you've learned in this book to build the body of your dreams.

It's pretty cool to realize that you *do* have the power to change your body—to get big, lean, strong, and healthy—and that you are in complete control of how your body looks and performs.

No matter how "ordinary" you might think you are, I promise you that you can not only create an extraordinary physique but an extraordinary life as well. Don't be surprised if the confidence and pride you'll gain from your workouts ripples out to affect other areas of your life, inspiring you to reach for other goals and improve in other ways.

From here, all you have to do is walk the path I've laid out, and in 12 weeks, you'll look in the mirror and think, "I'm glad I did," not "I wish I had."

My goal is to help you reach your goal, and I hope this book helps.

If we work together as a team, we can and will succeed.

So, I'd like you to make a promise as you begin your transformation: Can you promise me—and yourself—that you'll let me know when you've reached your goal?

Here's how we can connect:

Facebook: facebook.com/muscleforlifefitness

Twitter: @muscleforlife

Instagram: instagram.com/muscleforlifefitness

G+: gplus.to/MuscleForLife

And last but not least, my website is www.muscleforlife.com. If you want to write me, my e-mail address is mike@muscleforlife.com. (Keep in mind that I get a lot of e-mails every day and answer everything personally, so if you can keep your message as brief as possible, it helps ensure that I can get back to everyone!)

Thanks again. I hope to hear from you, and I wish you the best!

SECTION VII:

Q & A AND END OF BOOK GOODIES

24

FREQUENTLY ASKED QUESTIONS

In this age, which believes that there is a short cut to everything, the greatest lesson to be learned is that the most difficult way is, in the long run, the easiest.
— HENRY MILLER

Q: I CAN'T FIND TIME TO EXERCISE, BUT I WANT TO GET INTO SHAPE. WHAT CAN I DO?

A: I don't know anybody who can *find* time to exercise. I've never had anyone tell me, "Mike, I have too much free time these days. I think I'll just spend a few hours in the gym every day to get in shape. What should I do while I'm there?"

It's always the opposite: most of us lead busy, hectic lives and feel we don't have time for anything new. But in almost all cases, that just isn't true. As much as some people would like to *think* they're too busy to exercise, if they broke down and rearranged how they spend every waking minute, they could figure it out.

People who have successfully transformed their bodies have the same 24 hours in a day as the rest of us and still have to do everything else they need to do: go to work, enjoy family time, have a social life, and do everything else we have to juggle. They simply made their 45 to 60 minutes of daily exercise important enough to be a part of the plan. Some watch an hour less of TV each night. Others, like me, wake up an hour earlier every day. Others get their spouses to handle their kids for an hour after dinner and even trade off every other day so both can get into shape.

The point is that if you want to carve out an hour to exercise 3 to 5 days per week, I'm positive that you can do it.

Q: I'M IN MY 40S/50S+. CAN I STILL BENEFIT FROM A PROGRAM LIKE THIS?

A: Every week I get e-mailed by at least a few guys who ask whether it's too late to build muscle and get fit.

Most are pleasantly surprised when I explain that it's most definitely *not* too late and that I'm regularly working with guys in their 50s and even 60s who are rapidly building muscle and getting into the best shape of their lives.

How should people in their forties and beyond go about building muscle, though? Certainly they can't train and eat like the 20-year-olds, right? Well, you might be surprised to learn that not nearly as much changes as people think.

One of the first things I show people who are worried about their age squashing their dreams of being fit is a study conducted by researchers from the University of Oklahoma.[1] In this study, 24 college-aged (18 to 22) and 25 middle-aged (35 to 50) men followed the same weightlifting routine for eight weeks.

Researchers used DEXA scans for pre- and post-routine measurements, and they found that the middle-aged men built just as much bone density as their college-aged counterparts! In fact, the middle-aged men built a little *more* on average, but it wasn't enough to be statistically significant.

Strength gains were comparable as well. The middle-aged men gained an average of 14 pounds of strength on the bench press and 40 pounds on the leg press, and the college-aged men gained an average of 7 pounds of strength on the bench press and 55 pounds on the leg press.

People age 60 and beyond aren't left out of the party, either. Research has shown that they too can build significant amounts of muscle and strength and that doing so is a great way to fight the dwindling health spiral normally associated with aging.[2]

These findings agree with my experiences working with hundreds of men and women aged 40 to 70. One for one, they were able to build visible muscle, get lean, and improve their overall health and well-being. The bottom line is you can get into great shape at any age.

If you're middle-aged and excited to learn that it's not too late, you're probably wondering what the best way to go about it is. Fortunately, age doesn't change much in terms of routine, but there are a few points you should know.

While I'm a big proponent of heavy weightlifting, you may need to take it easy.

Heavy, compound lifting is the absolute best way to build muscle and strength. But it also demands a lot from your body, both from your muscles and nervous system.

You shouldn't be *afraid* of heavy weightlifting, even if you're in your fifties or sixties, but if you're not an experienced weightlifter, I recommend that you start your training in the 8- to 10-rep range and stay there until exercises feel very comfortable.

You can then move into 6- to 8-rep range and work with that until it feels completely stable and comfortable. You can then move into the 4- to 6-rep range, but it's not mandatory. You have to see how your body feels.

Furthermore, many middle-aged men find it helpful to rotate through rep ranges in their training. That is, one week they train in the 10- to 12-rep range; the next week, the 6- to 8-rep range; the next, the 4- to 6-rep range; and the next, back to the 10- to 12-rep range.

Don't ignore problems with your back, knees, shoulders, or other body parts.

If you have any lower-back issues, don't deadlift unless instructed to do so by a physical therapist. The same goes for knee issues and squatting as well as for shoulder issues and pressing (both bench and military press).

Work around such limitations: don't try to blast through them, or you may wind up injured and out of the gym for months.

Make sure you get adequate rest.

While age doesn't impair the recovery process nearly as much as some people think, it does slow it down as we get older.[3]

The solution is simple: make sure you get plenty of sleep, eat enough protein, and take a week off the weights every six to seven weeks instead of the normal eight to ten.

That's it for the training side of the game. In terms of diet, I have some good news for you: don't worry about your metabolism—it's fine.

A common worry among middle-aged people is that their metabolisms have slowed to a crawl, making weight loss or muscle growth nearly impossible.

Well, it's true that aging causes some metabolic slowdown, but much of it is caused by the loss of muscle.[4] Muscle burns calories, and as we naturally lose muscle as we age, our bodies burn fewer and fewer calories over time.[5]

The good news, however, is that you can totally reverse this process with regular resistance training. Your metabolism can be just as robust as it was decades ago.

Q: I TRAVEL A LOT. CAN I STILL FOLLOW THIS PROGRAM PROPERLY?

A: Absolutely, but it requires that you *plan*. Stay at hotels that are close to an adequate gym (pretty much all hotel exercise facilities are inadequate for the type of training you'll be doing) and plan when you'll work out. For most travelers, this means early in the morning or after dinner. Bring your supplements with you and just follow your regular routine.

If you're unable to make it to a gym while you're out of town, you can always do a bodyweight routine in your hotel room to help maintain your strength.

Here's what I do:

Push-ups to failure (one-handed if possible)
Rest 60 seconds
Pull-Ups to failure (I bring one of those bars that install in a doorway)
Rest 60 seconds
Squats for 30 seconds (one-legged if possible)
Burpees for 30 seconds
Mountain climbers to failure
Rest 90 seconds
Crunches to failure
Rest 60 seconds
Start over with push-ups

I do this for 20 to 30 minutes and find it effective in maintaining my strength and making the transition back to weightlifting less jarring.

Following a diet can be tougher when traveling, but it can still be done. Before arriving, I find a nearby health food store (like Whole Foods) and plan out what to eat while visiting. When I arrive, I go stock up on what I need.

Q: I DON'T GET AS SORE ON THIS PROGRAM AS I DID ON OTHERS. IS THAT BAD?

A: Most people think that sore muscles are a good sign—that it means their muscles are growing.

Intuitively, this makes sense. We're training to damage our muscles, and muscle damage leads to muscle soreness, so therefore little or no soreness would mean little or no damage and thus little or no gains, right?

It turns out that it's not that simple.

Workouts that create large amounts of muscle soreness won't necessarily result in muscle growth, and workouts that cause little to no soreness can result in significant muscle growth.[6] For instance, if you do an hour of downhill running, your legs are going to be *very* sore the next day, but downhill running is definitely not going to build big, strong legs. The stretching involved in dumbbell flys is likely to cause soreness, but they're a pretty poor movement for adding mass when compared to something like the incline bench press, which is likely to cause less soreness.

To quote researchers from Yokohama City University:

> *"Because of generally poor correlations between DOMS [delayed onset muscle soreness] and other indicators, we conclude that use of DOMS is a poor reflector of eccentric exercise-induced muscle damage and inflammation, and changes in indirect markers of muscle damage and inflammation are not necessarily accompanied with DOMS."* [7]

In other words, damaged muscles won't necessarily hurt, and muscles that hurt aren't necessarily damaged much.

The exact physiology behind this isn't fully understood yet (muscle growth is a *very* complicated process), but one study conducted by researchers at Concordia University demonstrated that at least some of the pain we're feeling in muscle soreness stems from the connective tissue holding muscle fibers together, not from the actual fibers themselves.[8]

We also know that the more often the muscles are exposed to certain types of stimuli, the less sore they become as a result. That doesn't mean they won't grow bigger and stronger, though.

Personally, I only get *really* sore from a workout if I missed it the week prior. When I'm in my normal routine, I only get mildly sore despite working *hard* in the gym.

So, the bottom line with muscle soreness is this: it doesn't tell us much regarding whether we're making gains. Don't think that excessive soreness means major muscle growth, and don't worry if you're not getting sore.

Q: I SHOWED THIS BOOK TO A TRAINER AND HE DIDN'T LIKE IT AND SAID I SHOULD DO SOMETHING ELSE. IS HE RIGHT?

A: I'm sure the trainer's heart is in the right place and he's just trying to help, but unfortunately, most trainers just don't know what they're talking about. Ironically, many aren't even in great shape themselves and don't have much in the way of client successes to share. Many are just teaching whatever they learned in their textbooks without knowing whether it's the most effective way to get fit.

If you follow what I wrote in this book, you *will* make awesome strength and size gains—I guarantee you that. Hundreds of thousands of guys around the world use the principles taught in this book to build muscle, lose fat, and get healthy. The results speak for themselves.

Q: THIS HUGE GUY IN THE GYM RECOMMENDS THAT I WORK IN A HIGHER-REP RANGE. WHAT GIVES?

A: As you know, the science isn't definitive on the "perfect" rep range for hypertrophy (muscle growth). What scientists can agree on is that somewhere between 4 to 8 reps is the sweet spot.

When you see huge guys doing high-rep routines, you're not seeing the whole picture. What's missing? *Drugs.*

That might sound a bit cynical, but it's true, unfortunately. Unless they're training to be powerlifters, guys on steroids do high-rep, low-weight (for them) routines for several reasons.

First, it helps prevent injury, as steroids cause your muscles to grow much stronger than your tendons and ligaments can handle. Thus, you might feel like you can handle a 500-pound bench press or squat, but your tendons and ligaments can't, and a horrible injury can result.

Second, it's easy and they can get away with it. When you're all drugged up, you can just go get a pump every day and grow.

Again, the simplest way to settle this type of internal debate for yourself is to just give my program an honest eight weeks of hard work. I'm positive you'll never look back.

Q: SHOULDN'T YOU TRAIN EACH MUSCLE GROUP TWO OR THREE TIMES PER WEEK TO MAXIMIZE MUSCLE GROWTH?

A: Like "ideal" rep ranges, optimal training frequency is a hotly debated subject. It boils down to workout intensity and volume. The lighter the weights and the fewer the sets, the more often you can train the muscle group.

In the case of *Bigger Leaner Stronger*, you hit your muscles hard, with about 50 to 60 reps per workout, with all reps recruiting maximum muscle fibers (due to the load). Unless you have superhuman recovery, you won't be able to do these workouts more than once every five to seven days, which is why the additional pressing is limited to 3 sets and in the 8- to 10-rep range.

The bottom line is that weekly *intensity* and *volume* are more important than frequency when we look at five- to seven-day training cycles, and *everyone* who follows the program makes rapid strength and size gains. Even long-time lifters.

Q: CAN I DO THIS PROGRAM AT HOME?

A: Yes.

All you need to follow the program is a power cage or multipress rack for squatting and benching, a barbell with plates, a set of dumbbells (I prefer adjustables), and an adjustable bench. You can also get a utility bench for your military press so you can do the exercise seated instead of standing.

With this equipment, the only limitations you have are not being able to do a few things like the lat pulldown, triceps pushdown, dip, leg press, and captain's chair leg raise. You can substitute other "approved" exercises for these though, such as weighted pull-ups, skullcrushers, more dumbbell and barbell pressing, more squatting, and hanging leg raises.

You also have the option of including bodyweight exercises as talked about here:

http://bit.ly/body-weight-training

Q: I HAVE A LOT OF TROUBLE GAINING MUSCLE. WILL THIS PROGRAM WORK FOR ME?

A: Absolutely. I don't believe in the "hardgainer" myth.

In my many years in this game, I've never met a hardgainer who was training and eating properly. In most cases, the hardgainers weren't focusing on heavy, compound lifting and weren't eating enough food (and sometimes this meant they had to eat 4,000 or more calories per day just to gain 0.5 to 1 pound per week!).

So if you're afraid that your body is genetically destined to be small and weak or even "skinny fat," you can lay those fears to rest. Your body contains the same genetic programs as mine that result in muscle growth and fat loss. If I've made better progress than you with my physique, it's only because I have a better understanding of how to put all the pieces of the puzzle together: that is, I know more about proper training, eating, and resting. That's it.

That said, it's true that genetics can make it easier or harder to build muscle and lose fat. Some people have naturally high testosterone and growth hormone levels, which means faster muscle growth and an overall leaner physique. Some people's bodies mobilize fat stores more effectively than others, making fat loss an all-around easier endeavor.

Genetics also plays a role in the shape of your muscles. Not all guys can have that perfect square chest or ridiculous bicep peak, and not all women can have a gravity-defying, perfectly round butt.

But none of these things are real limitations.

Who cares whether you build muscle or lose fat more slowly than someone else? As long as you can see regular improvements and get to where you want to be, the added time is irrelevant. Big deal if you can't have the same "aesthetics" as your favorite fitness cover model. You can still look awesome and feel great, and that's what it's all about.

Regardless of the "quality" of your genetic programming, you can build the body of your dreams in a matter of a few years and maintain it for the rest of your life.

Q: I ONLY HAVE ACCESS TO DUMBBELLS. CAN I STILL DO THE PROGRAM?

A: Working out with only dumbbells is tough because you can't squat or deadlift effectively. While you can press for your chest and shoulders, an optimal routine has you press both dumbbells and barbells.

If I can convince you to get a proper home setup or work out a gym instead, you'll be glad you did. You can find my recommendations for home gym products in the bonus report.

That said, if neither is possible, you can focus on the dumbbell exercises given in the "approved exercises" section of the book. For instance, a chest day would look like this:

Incline Dumbbell Press: Warm up and 6 sets 4 to 6 reps
Flat Dumbbell Press: 3 to 6 sets of 4 to 6 reps

While that might seem redundant and inefficient, it's a great chest workout. I did that for nearly six months a couple of years ago and was pleasantly surprised to see how well my chest responded.

For your leg training, you can work with exercises like dumbbell lunges, goblet squats, and one-legged (pistol) squats, which are challenging even without weight.

For your back, I recommend doing a lot of dumbbell rows and weighted wide- and narrow-grip pull-ups.

You also have the option of working some modified bodyweight exercises into your routine, as discussed here:

http://bit.ly/body-weight-training

Q: SHOULD I TAKE SUPPLEMENTS ON MY OFF DAYS?

A: Yes. Take everything you would normally take except pre-workout products and/or nitric oxide boosters on your off days.

Q: I'M SICK. SHOULD I TRY TO TRAIN ANYWAY?

A: I totally understand the desire to exercise when sick. Once you've established a good exercise routine, you *really* don't like messing with it.

Intense exercise is only going to make the sickness worse, though, because intense exercise temporarily depresses immune function, which gives invaders more time to wreak havoc on your body.[9]

That said, animal research has shown that light exercise (20 to 30 minutes of light jogging on a treadmill) performed while infected with the influenza virus boosts immune function and speeds recovery.[10]

Similar effects have been seen in human studies as well, which is why I recommend no more than three sessions of 20 to 30 minutes of light cardio when you're sick (you shouldn't get too winded to speak).[11]

Q: I HAVE TROUBLE PREPARING HEALTHY MEALS THROUGHOUT THE WEEK. WHAT SHOULD I DO?

A: A simple solution is to prepare your food on one day per week, portion it out, and then bring it to work with you. Pop it in a toaster oven or microwave for a few minutes, and you're good to go.

Q: SHOULD I USE A WEIGHT BELT?

I'm not a fan of weight belts.

They don't prevent injury unless you've injured yourself previously. They just help you lift more weight, and this can be a real problem if you slip on your form.

Q: MY OUT-OF-SHAPE FRIENDS ALWAYS WANT ME TO EAT UNHEALTHY STUFF WITH THEM. WHAT SHOULD I DO?

A: Don't fall into the trap that made them out of shape in the first place. When you eat with people who don't eat well, you should be careful to not use their poor habits as justification to follow suit.

Remember that sticking to your quest for a healthier, better-looking, more energetic body can also inspire them to do the same! Or, if necessary, eat before you meet up or only eat with them when you can have a cheat meal.

Q: DO I NEED TO GO TO FAILURE EVERY SET?

A: You don't have to go to absolute failure every set. I rarely do.

What I shoot for is reaching the point where I struggle to finish a rep and know I wouldn't be able to get another without assistance (the rep before failure).

If you feel you can maybe get it and want to go for it anyway, that's fine, but you don't have to train like this every set.

Q: I'VE BEEN UNABLE TO STICK WITH WORKOUT PROGRAMS. WHY SHOULD I EVEN TRY YOURS?

A: Nothing is more annoying than working your butt off in the gym every day and seeing no results. This is, hands down, the number-one reason why people quit their workout routines. Well, my program works. And, better yet, it works *quickly*.

Imagine that, in three months, you've put on 10 pounds of lean muscle and your friends and family keep commenting on how good you look. Women start turning their heads. Guys you know are asking what in the world you're doing. You feel strong and energetic—better than you have in a long time.

Well, that's totally achievable. All you have to do is get started.

Q: I LIKE ALCOHOL. IS THAT GOING TO BE A PROBLEM?

A: As you know, alcohol blocks fat oxidation, which in turn accelerates the rate at which your body stores dietary fat as body fat.[12]

If you want to be able to drink while dieting and still lose weight, don't drink more than one day per week, and use the following tips to protect yourself from excess fat storage:

- Restrict your dietary fat intake that day, and don't eat any fatty foods while you're drinking.

- Get the vast majority of your calories from lean protein and carbs that day (with most coming from protein).

- Stay away from carb-laden drinks like beer and fruity stuff. Dry wines are a good choice, as are spirits.

By following this advice, you can enjoy a few drinks every week without having to feel guilty or ruining your weight-loss regimen.

BONUS REPORT

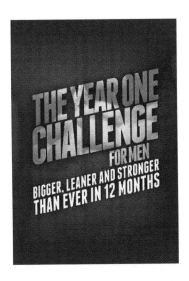

YOU NOW KNOW THINGS THAT MOST guys will never understand about how to build a muscular, strong, and healthy body, but you might feel unsure about how to work out a daily meal plan or how to combine different exercises.

Well, how would you like a full, detailed training program to follow for the next year to ensure that you get bigger, leaner, and stronger than ever?

I've got you covered! I created this totally free bonus report to help you out. In it, I cover things like…

- **What brands of supplements I recommend and why. I've tried pretty much every brand you can name over the years and have found what I feel are the best of the best for each type of supplement that I recommend.**

- The workout equipment that is useful, and the brands that have stood the test of time for me. I've torn through gloves, and I've tried all kinds of crappy straps, every body fat testing device you can buy, and many types of shakers, and I want to save you the money and frustration of buying junk.

- **Complete workout plans for your entire first year of training. All you'll have to do is show up every day and do what I say, and you'll build muscle faster than ever.**

- Twenty delicious recipes from my cookbooks that you can fit into any type of meal plan! No eating boring foods every day allowed!

- And more!

By following this program, you're going to build a physique that you're proud of. It will be a trophy for your unswerving dedication, perseverance, and toughness.

My mission is to help you get to that moment. That's what makes me happiest.

Download this free special report today and make this next year the year where you get bigger, leaner, and stronger than ever!

Visit http://bit.ly/year-one-challenge to get this report now!

If you'd prefer to get a hard-copy version of the *Year One Challenge*, with all workouts included and formatted so you can record every workout and track your progress through each phase of the program, then you can find it on my website, www.muscleforlife.com.

Thanks again for reading my book. If you have any questions or run into any difficulties, shoot me an e-mail and I'll do my best to help!

WOULD YOU DO ME A FAVOR?

THANK YOU FOR BUYING MY BOOK. I'm positive that if you just follow what I've written, you will be on your way to looking and feeling better than you ever have before.

I have a small favor to ask. Would you mind taking a minute to write a blurb on Amazon about this book? I check all my reviews and love to get feedback (that's the real pay for my work—knowing that I'm helping people).

Also, if you have any friends or family who might enjoy this book, spread the love and lend it to them!

Thanks again. I hope to hear from you, and I wish you the best!

Mike

P.S. If you'd like professional help with your meal planning to make sure you reach your fitness goals, turn to the next page!

THE MUSCLE FOR LIFE CUSTOM MEAL PLAN
HOW TO BUILD MUSCLE AND LOSE FAT EATING FOODS YOU LOVE

IF YOU WANT TO TAKE ALL the thought out of dieting and get a meal plan built specifically for you, that is *guaranteed* to work if you simply follow it, then you want to read this page.

The first thing I want you to know is when I say "custom" meal plan, I mean it.

Nothing is more annoying than paying for a meal plan from a ""guru" and receiving a bland, copy-and-paste job that doesn't take into account foods you like, dislike, your schedule, training times, and lifestyle.

That's why we do our custom meal plans differently.

Not only do we build each and every one from scratch, we can work with any and all budgetary and dietary needs as well: vegan vegetarian, Paleo, food availabilities, sensitivities, and allergies, and any other food preferences or restrictions.

What this means is you'll actually *enjoy* your diet. You'll look forward to every meal, every day, which works wonders for compliance. It's easy to stick to a diet full of foods you love!

We don't just shoot you a plan and send you off on your way, either. We're always available to help via email to make sure you actually get results.

HERE'S HOW THE PROCESS WORKS...

Step 1:

You pay and create your account, and then fill out a detailed questionnaire that tells my team about your fitness goals, exercise schedule, food preferences, and everything else we need to make your meal plan.

Step 2:

We use your answers to create your meal plan and upload it to the Website within 5 to 7 days of receiving your completed questionnaire.

Step 3:

You're notified via email that your meal plan is ready and you access your account to download it.

You check it out and let us know if any tweaks are needed. If not, you get rolling.

Step 4:

If, at any time along the way, you run into any issues, we're always available via email to answer any questions you might have and ensure everything goes smoothly for you.

So, how much fat would you like to lose? Or how much muscle would you like to build? Working out isn't enough. Let me show you exactly how to eat to get there!

VISIT <u>WWW.MUSCLEFORLIFE.COM/MP</u> NOW TO GET YOUR CUSTOM MEAL PLAN!

I WANT TO CHANGE THE SUPPLEMENT INDUSTRY. WILL YOU JOIN ME?

THE SUPPLEMENT INDUSTRY COULD BE BEST described by Obi-Wan Kenobi's famous words: a wretched hive of scum and villainy.

Here's the bottom-line truth of this multibillion-dollar industry:

While certain supplements can help, they do *NOT* build great physiques (proper training and nutrition does), and most are a complete waste of money.

Too many products are "proprietary blends" of low-quality ingredients, junk fillers, and unnecessary additives. Key ingredients are horribly underdosed. There's a distinct lack of credible scientific evidence to back up the outrageous claims made on labels and in ads. The list of what's wrong with this industry goes on and on.

And that's why I decided to get into the supplement game.

What gives? Am I just a hypocritical sell-out? Should you grab your pitchfork and run me off the Internet? Well, hear me out for a minute and then decide.

The last thing we need is yet another marketing machine churning out yet another line of hyped-up, flashy products claiming to be more effective than steroids.

I think things should be done differently, and I believe in being the change I want to see. That's why I started LEGION.

You see, I created LEGION not only to bring unique products to the supplement world but also to start a movement. Here's what sets LEGION apart from the rabble:

- **100 percent transparent product formulas.** We don't hide behind proprietary blends, whose only purpose is fraud and deception. You deserve to know exactly what you're buying.

- **100 percent science-based ingredients and dosages.** Every ingredient we use is backed by published scientific literature proving its effectiveness and is included at true clinically effective dosages.

- **100 percent naturally sweetened and flavored.** Research suggests that regular consumption of artificial sweeteners can be harmful to our health, which is why we use stevia, a natural sweetener with proven health benefits.

Not only are LEGION supplements a better value and better for your health...but they also deliver REAL RESULTS you can see and feel.

And as you're a reader of mine, I want to give you a special coupon for 10% off everything in our store. Here it is:

BLS10

Simply enter that code in the coupon field when you check out and you'll save 10% on the entire order.

SHOP NOW AT <u>WWW.LEGIONATHLETICS.COM</u>! AND SAVE 10%!

OTHER BOOKS BY MICHAEL MATTHEWS

VISIT WWW.MUSCLEFORLIFE.COM TO LEARN MORE ABOUT THESE BOOKS!

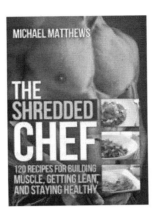

The Shredded Chef: 120 Recipes for Building Muscle, Getting Lean, and Staying Healthy

If you want to know how to forever escape the dreadful experience of "dieting" and learn how to cook nutritious, delicious meals that make building muscle and burning fat easy and enjoyable, then you need to read this book.

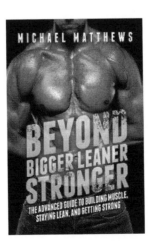

Beyond Bigger Leaner Stronger: The Advanced Guide to Building Muscle, Staying Lean, and Getting Strong

The bestselling sequel to *Bigger Leaner Stronger* that teaches you how to smoothly transition from an "intermediate" to an "advanced" lifter and continue making gains.

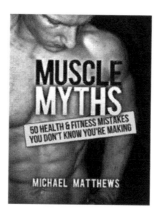

Muscle Myths: 50 Health & Fitness Mistakes You Don't Know You're Making

If you've ever felt lost in the sea of contradictory training and diet advice out there and you just want to know once and for all what works and what doesn't—what's scientifically true and what's false—when it comes to building muscle and getting ripped, then you need to read this book.

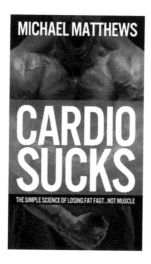

Cardio Sucks! The Simple Science of Losing Fat Fast...Not Muscle

If you're short on time and sick of the same old boring cardio routine and want to kick your fat loss into high gear by working out less and…heaven forbid…have some fun…then you want to read this book.

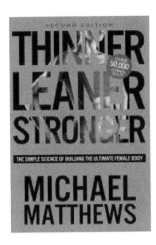

Thinner Leaner Stronger: The Simple Science of Building the Ultimate Female Body

If you want to be toned, lean, and strong as quickly as possible without going on crash diets, needing "good genetics," or wasting ridiculous amounts of time in the gym and money on supplements…*regardless of your age*…then you want to read this book.

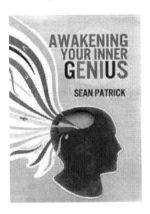

Awakening Your Inner Genius

If you'd like to know what some of history's greatest thinkers and achievers can teach you about awakening your inner genius and how to find, follow, and fulfill your journey to greatness, then you want to read this book today.

(I'm using a pen name for this book as well as for a few other projects not related to health and fitness, but I thought you might enjoy it so I'm including it here.)

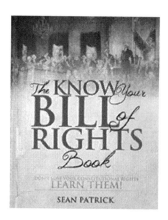

The Know Your Bill of Rights Book

Are you comfortable letting crooked politicians decide what your rights are? I'm not, which is why I wrote this book. It helps you easily reach a deep understanding of the Bill of Rights by walking you through the historical context needed to fully grasp the spirit and importance of key amendments.

RECOMMENDED READING

VISIT WWW.MUSCLEFORLIFE.COM TO LEARN MORE ABOUT THESE BOOKS!

IF YOU WANT TO FURTHER YOUR health and fitness education, I recommend that you check out the following books. I found each extremely helpful and think you will too.

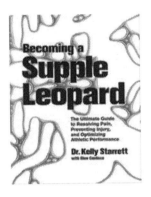

Becoming a Supple Leopard

This book teaches you common movement errors that cause injury and rob you of speed, power, endurance, and strength, and it gives you hundreds of techniques you can use to correct them, and thus optimize your athletic performance.

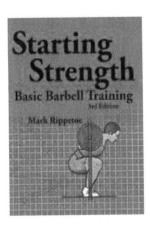

Starting Strength

This is the book that finally fixed my squat, deadlift, and bench press, which enabled me to greatly accelerate my strength and muscle growth over the years. It should be on every serious lifter's shelf.

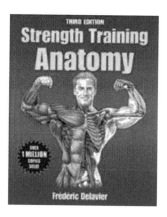

Strength Training Anatomy

Strength Training Anatomy is a great resource for diving into anatomy and the biomechanics of exercise, and it's also a great encyclopedia of exercises.

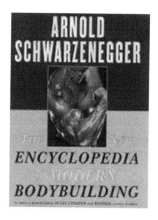

The New Encyclopedia of Modern Bodybuilding

This is a book we should all just own on principle. Arnold truly was a bodybuilding phenomenon.

In all seriousness, this book has several plusses: Arnold's story is truly inspiring, and his take on the history and profession of bodybuilding is good reading; it has a ton of exercises for training various body parts; and it's huge and glossy—it's just a nice product.

REFERENCES

CHAPTER 2
WHAT MOST PEOPLE DON'T KNOW ABOUT HEALTH, NUTRITION, AND FITNESS
PART ONE: PHYSIOLOGY 101

1. Patty W. Siri-Tarino, Qi Sun, Frank B. Hu, and Ronald M. Krauss, "Meta-Analysis of Prospective Cohort Studies Evaluating the Association of Saturated Fat with Cardiovacular Disease," American Journal of Clinical Nutrition, 91 no. 2 (2010): 535-46; Rajiv Chowdhury, Samantha Warnakula, Setor Kunutsor, Francesca Crowe, Heather A. Ward, Laura Johnson, Oscar H. Franco, Adam S. Butterworth, Nita G. Forouhi, Simon G. Thompson, Kay-Tee Khaw, Dariush Mozaffarian, John Danesh, and Emanuele Di Angelantonio, "Association of Dietary, Circulating, and Supplement Fatty Acids with Coronary Risk: A Systematic Review and Meta-Analysis," Annals of Internal Medicine, 160, no. 6 (2014): 398-406. doi:10.7326/M13-1788.

CHAPTER 4
WHAT MOST PEOPLE DON'T KNOW ABOUT HEALTH, NUTRITION, AND FITNESS
PART THREE: GENERAL HEALTH

1. Deepak Bhatnagar, Handrean Soran, and Paul N. Durrington, "Hypercholesterolaemia and Its Management," BMJ 337 (August 21, 2008): a993. doi: 10.1136/bmj.a993.

CHAPTER 5
THE 7 BIGGEST MUSCLE-BUILDING MYTHS AND MISTAKES

1. Shane Schwanbeck, Philip D. Chilibeck, and Gordon Binsted, "A Comparison of Free Weight Squat to Smith Machine Squat Using Electromyography," Journal of Strength and Conditioning Research 23, no. 9 (2009): 2588-91. doi: 10.1519/JSC.0b013e3181b1b181.

2. Schick, Evan E., Jared W. Coburn, Lee E. Brown, Daniel A. Judelson, Andy V. Khamoui, Tai T. Tran, and Brandon P. Uribe. "A comparison of muscle activation between a Smith machine and free weight bench press." The Journal of Strength & Conditioning Research 24, no. 3 (2010): 779-784.

3. Ryan A. Rogers, Robert U. Newton, K. P. McEvoy, Eva M. Popper, Brandon K. Doan, Jae Kun Shim, Lori R. Bolt, Jeff S. Volek, and William J. Kraemer, "The Effect of Supplemental Isolated Weight-Training Exercises on Upper-Arm Size and Upper-Body Strength." Abstract. NSCA Conference (2000): 369.

CHAPTER 6
THE 3 SCIENTIFIC LAWS OF MUSCLE GROWTH

1. Brad J. Schoenfeld, "The Mechanisms of Muscle Hypertrophy and Their Application to Resistance Training," *Journal of Strength and Conditioning Research*, 24, no. 10 (2010): 2857-72. doi: 10.1519/JSC.0b013e3181e840f3.

2. Alfred L. Goldberg, Joseph D. Etlinger, David F. Goldspink, and Charles Jablecki, "Mechanism of Work-Induced Hypertrophy of Skeletal Muscle," *Medicine and Science in Sports* 7, no. 3 (1975): 185-98.

3. Matthew R. Rhea, Brent A. Alvar, Lee N. Burkett, and Stephen D. Ball, "A Meta-Analysis to Determine the Dose Response for Strength Development," *Medicine and Science in Sports and Exercise* 35, no. 3 (2003): 456-64.

4. Schoenfeld, "The Mechanisms of Muscle Hypertrophy and Their Application to Resistance Training," 2857-72.

5. Débora F. Flores, Paulo Gentil, Lee E. Brown, Ronei S. Pinto, Rodrigo L. Carregaro, and Martim Bottaro, "Dissociated Time Course of Recovery between Genders after Resistance Exercise," *Journal of Strength and Conditioning Research* 25, no. 11 (2011): 3039-44. doi: 10.1519/JSC.0b013e318212dea4.

CHAPTER 7
THE 5 BIGGEST FAT LOSS MYTHS AND MISTAKES

1. Frank M. Sacks, George A. Bray, Vincent J. Carey, Steven R. Smith, Donna H. Ryan, Stephen D. Anton, Katherine McManus, Catherine M. Champagne, Louise M. Bishop, Nancy Laranjo, Meryl S. Leboff, Jennifer C. Rood, Lilian de Jonge, Frank L. Greenway, Catherine M. Loria, Eva Obarzanek, and Donald A. Williamson, "Comparison of Weight-Loss Diets with Different Compositions of Fat, Protein, and Carbohydrates," *New England Journal of Medicine* 360 (Feb. 26, 2009): 859-73. doi: 10.1056/NEJMoa0804748.

2. Amy M. Knab, R. Andrew Shanely, Karen D. Corbin, Fuxia Jin, Wei Sha, and David C. Nieman, "A 45-Minute Vigorous Exercise Bout Increases Metabolic Rate for 14 Hours," *Medicine and Science in Sports and Exercise* 43, no. 9 (2011): 1643-48. doi: 10.1249/MSS.0b013e3182118891.

3. Stefan M. Pasiakos, Lisa M. Vislocky, John W. Carbone, Nicholas Altieri, Karen Konopelski, Hedley C. Freake, Jeffrey M. Anderson, Arny A. Ferrando, Robert R. Wolfe, and Nancy R. Rodriguez, "Acute Energy Deprivation Affects Skeletal Muscle Protein Synthesis and Associated Intracellular Signaling Proteins in Physically Active Adults," *Journal of Nutrition* 140, no. 4 (2010): 745-51. doi: 10.3945/jn.109.118372.

4. William J. Kraemer, Kent Adams, Enzo Cafarelli, Gary A. Dudley, Cathryn Dooly, Matthew S. Feigenbaum, Steven J. Fleck, Barry Franklin, Andrew C. Fry, Jay R. Hoffman, Robert U. Newton, Jeffrey Potteiger, Michael H. Stone, Nicholas A. Ratamess, and Travis Triplett-McBride, "American College of Sports Medicine Position Stand: Progression Models in Resistance Training for Healthy Adults," *Medicine and Science in Sports and Exercise*, 41, no. 3 (2009): 687-708. doi: 10.1249/MSS.0b013e3181915670.

5. Ioannis G. Fatouros, Athanasios Chatzinikolaou, Symeon Tournis, Michalis G. Nikolaidis, Athanasios Z. Jamurtas, Ioannis I. Douroudos, Ioannis Papassotiriou, Petros M. Thomakos, Kyriakos Taxildaris, George Mastorakos, and Asimina Mitrakou, "Intensity of Resistance Exercise Determines Adipokine and Resting Energy Expenditure Responses in Overweight Elderly Individuals," *Diabetes Care* 32, no. 12 (2009): 2161-67. doi: 10.2337/dc08-1994.

6. Paulo T. V. Farinatti and Antonio G. C. Neto, "The Effect of Between-Set Rest Intervals on the Oxygen Uptake during and after Resistance Exercise Sessions Performed with Large- and Small-Muscle Mass," *Journal of Strength and Conditioning Research* 25, no. 11 (2011): 3181-90. doi: 10.1519/JSC.0b013e318212e415.

7. Bente Stallknecht, Flemming Dela, and Jørn W. Helge, "Are Blood Flow and Lipolysis in Subcutaneous Adipose Tissue Influenced by Contractions in Adjacent Muscles in Humans?" *American Journal of Physiology—Endocrinology and Metabolism* 292, no. 2 (2007): E394-99. doi: 10.1152/ajpendo.00215.2006.

8. Matthew A. Kostek, Linda S. Pescatello, Richard L. Seip, Theodore J. Angelopoulos, Priscilla M. Clarkson, Paul M. Gordon, Niall M. Moyna, Paul S. Visich, Robert F. Zoeller, Paul D. Thompson, Eric P. Hoffman, and Thomas B. Price, "Subcutaneous Fat Alterations Resulting from an Upper-Body Resistance Training Program," *Medicine and Science of Sports and Exercise* 39, no. 7 (2007): 1177-85. 10.1249/mss.0b0138058a5cb.

9. Sachin Vispute, John Smith, James LeCheminant, and Kimberly S. Hurley, "The Effect of Abdominal Exercise on Abdominal Fat," *Journal of Strength and Conditioning Research* 25, no. 9 (2011): 2559-64. doi: 10.1519/JSC.0b013e3181fb4a46.

CHAPTER 8
THE 4 SCIENTIFIC LAWS OF HEALTHY FAT LOSS

1. Corby K. Martin, Leonie K. Heilbronn, Lilian de Jonge, James P. DeLany, Julia Volaufova, Stephen D. Anton, Leanne M. Redman, Steven R. Smith, and Eric Ravussin, "Effect of Calorie Restriction on Resting Metabolic Rate and Spontaneous Physical Activity," *Obesity* 15, no. 12 (2007): 2964-73. doi: 10.1038/oby.2007.354.

2. Leanne M. Redman, Leonie K. Heilbronn, Corby K. Martin, Lilian de Jonge, Donald A. Williamson, James P. Delany, and Eric Ravussin, "Metabolic and Behavioral Compensations in Response to Caloric Restriction: Implications for the Maintenance of Weight Loss," *PLOS One*, 4, no. 2 (2009): e4377. doi: 10.1371/journal.pone.0004377.

3. Merril L. Durrant, J. S. Garrow, P. Royston, Susan F. Stalley, Shirley Sunkin, and Penelope M. Warwick, "Factors Influencing the Composition of the Weight Lost by Obese Patients on a Reducing Diet," *British Journal of Nutrition* 44, no. 3 (1980): 275-85. doi: 10.1079/BJN19800042; Robert R. Wolfe, "The Underappreciated Role of Muscle in Health and Disease," *American Journal of Clinical Nutrition* 84, no. 3 (2006): 475-82.

4. Roberto Cangemi, Alberto J. Friedmann, John O. Holloszy, and Luigi Fontana, "Long-Term Effects of Calorie Restriction on Serum Sex-Hormone Concentrations in Men," *Aging Cell* 9, no. 2 (2010): 236-42. doi: 10.1111/j.1474-9726.2010.00553.x; A. Janet Tomiyama, Traci Mann, Danielle Vinas, Jeffrey M. Hunger, Jill DeJager, and Shelley E. Taylor, "Low Calorie Dieting Increases Cortisol," *Psychosomatic Medicine* 72, no. 4 (2010): 357-64. doi: 10.1097/PSY.0b013e3181d9523c.

5. Eating Disorders Network, *Effects of Semi-Starvation on Behaviour and Physical Health*, accessed October 17, 2014, http://www.ednses.com/downloads/effects_of_semi-starvation.pdf.

6. http://www.cnn.com/2010/HEALTH/11/08/twinkie.diet.professor/

7. France Bellisle, Regina McDevitt, and Andrew M. Prentice, "Meal Frequency and Energy Balance," *British Journal of Nutrition* 77, no. S1 (1997): S57-S70.

8. Abdul G. Dulloo, Jean Jacquet, and Jean-Pierre Montani, "How Dieting Makes Some Fatter: From a Perspective of Human Body Composition Autoregulation Proceedings of the Nutrition Society," *Proceedings of the Nutrition Society* 71, no. 3 (2012): 379-89. doi: 10.1017/S002966511200022.

9. Stefan M. Pasiakos, Jay J. Cao, Lee M. Margolis, Edward R. Sauter, Leah D. Whigham, James P. McClung, Jennifer C. Rood, John W. Carbone, Gerald F. Combs Jr., and Andrew J. Young, "Effects of High-Protein Diets on Fat-Free Mass and Muscle Protein Synthesis Following Weight Loss: A Randomized Controlled Trial," *FASEB Journal*, vol. 27 no. 9 (2013): 3837-47. doi: 10.1096/fj.13-230227.

10. Amy R. Lane, Joseph W. Duke, and Anthony C. Hackney, "Influence of Dietary Carbohydrate Intake on the Free Testosterone: Cortisol Ratio Responses to Short-Term Intensive Exercise Training," *European Journal of Applied Physiology* 108, no. 6 (2009): 1125-31. doi: 10.1007/s00421-009-1220-5.

11. Joanne F. Dorgan, Joseph T. Judd, Christopher Longcope, Charles Brown, Arthur Schatzkin, Beverly A. Clevidence, William S. Campbell, Padmanabhan P. Nair, Charlene Franz, Lisa Kahle, and Philip R. Taylor, "Effects of Dietary Fat and Fiber on Plasma and Urine Androgens and Estrogens in Men: A Controlled Feeding," *American Journal of Clinical Nutrition* 64, no. 6 (1996): 850-55.

12. Bellisle, McDevitt, and Prentice, "Meal Frequency and Energy Balance," S57-S70.

13. Jameason D. Cameron, Marie-Josée Cyr, and Éric Doucet, "Increased Meal Frequency Does Not Promote Greater Weight Loss in Subjects Who Were Prescribed an 8-Week Equi-Energetic Energy-Restricted Diet," *British Journal of Nutrition* 103, no. 8 (2010): 1098-101. doi: 10.1017/S0007114509992984.

14. Heather J. Leidy, Minghua Tang, Cheryl L. H. Armstrong, Carmen B. Martin, and Wayne W. Campbell, "The Effects of Consuming Frequent, Higher Protein Meals on Appetite and Satiety during Weight Loss in Overweight/Obese Men," *Obesity* 19, no. 4 (2011): 818-24. doi: 10.1038/oby.2010.203.

15. Heather J. Leidy, Cheryl L. H. Armstrong, Minghua Tang, Richard D. Mattes, and Wayne W. Campbell, "The Influence of Higher Protein Intake and Greater Eating Frequency on Appetite Control in Overweight and Obese Men," *Obesity* 18, no. 9 (2010): 1725-32. doi: 10.1038/oby.2010.45.

16. Heather J. Leidy and Wayne W. Campbell, "The Effect of Eating Frequency on Appetite Control and Food Intake: Brief Synopsis of Controlled Feeding Studies," *Journal of Nutrition* 141, no. 1 (2010): 154-57. doi: 10.3945/jn.109.114389.

17. Joseph LeSauter, Nawshin Hoque, Michael Weintraub, Donald W. Pfaff, and Rae Silvera, "Stomach Ghrelin-Secreting Cells as Food-Entrainable Circadian Clocks," *Proceedings of the National Academy of Science* 106, no. 32 (2009): 13582-87. doi: 10.1073/pnas.0906426106.

18. S. Sensi and F. Capani, "Chronobiological Aspects of Weight Loss in Obesity: Effects of Different Meal Timing Regimens," *Chronobiology International* 4, no. 2 (1987):251-61.

19. David G. Schlundt, James O. Hill, Tracy Sbrocco, Jamie Pope-Cordle, and Teresa Sharp, "The Role of Breakfast in the Treatment of Obesity: A Randomized Clinical Trial," *American Journal of Clinical Nutrition* 55, no. 3 (1992): 645-51.

20. Carla Barbosa Nonino-Borges, Ricardo Martins Borges, Marinella Bavaresco, Vivian M. M. Suen, Ayrton Custódio Moreira, and Júlio Sérgio Marchini, "Influence of Meal Time on Salivary Circadian Cortisol Rhythms and Weight Loss in Obese Women," *Nutrition* 23, no. 5 (2007): 385-91. doi: 10.1016/j.nut.2007.02.007.

21. Groen, Bart, B. A. R. T. Pennings, Milou Beelen, Gareth A. Wallis, ANNEMIE P. Gijsen, J. M. Senden, and L. J. Van Loon. "Protein ingestion before sleep improves postexercise overnight recovery." Medicine and science in sports and exercise 44, no. 8 (2012): 1560-1569.

22. Randy W. Bryner, Irma H. Ullrich, Janine Sauers, David Donley, Guyton Hornsby, Maria Kolar, and Rachel Yeater, "Effects of Resistance vs. Aerobic Training Combined with an 800 Calorie Liquid Diet on Lean Body Mass and Resting Metabolic Rate," *Journal of the American College of Nutrition* 18, no. 2 (1999): 115-21.

23. Ioannis G. Fatouros, Athanasios Chatzinikolaou, Symeon Tournis, Michalis G. Nikolaidis, Athanasios Z. Jamurtas, Ioannis I. Douroudos, Ioannis Papassotiriou, Petros M. Thomakos, Kyriakos Taxildaris, George Mastorakos, and Asimina Mitrakou, "Intensity of Resistance Exercise Determines Adipokine and Resting Energy Expenditure Responses in Overweight Elderly Individuals," *Diabetes Care* 32, no. 12 (2009): 2161-67. doi: 10.2337/dc08-1994.

CHAPTER 10
HOW TO BECOME YOUR OWN MASTER THE SIMPLE SCIENCE OF WILLPOWER AND SELF-CONTROL

1. *American Psychological Association*, "APA: Americans Report Willpower and Stress as Key Obstacles to Meeting Health-Related Resolutions," news release, March 29, 2010, http://www.apa.org/news/press/releases/2010/03/lifestyle-changes.aspx.

2. Angela L. Duckworth and Martin E.P. Seligman, "Self-Discipline Outdoes IQ in Predicting Academic Performance of Adolescents," *Psychological Science* 16, no. 12 (2005): 939-44. doi: 10.1111/j.1467-9280.2005.01641.x; June P. Tangney, Roy F. Baumeister, and Angie Luzio Boone, "High Self-Control Predicts Good Adjustment, Less Pathology, Better Grades, and Interpersonal Success," *Journal of Personality* 72, no. 2 (2004): 271-324. doi: 10.1111/j.0022-3506.2004.00263.x; Shelley A. Kirkpatrick and Edwin A. Locke, "Leadership: Do Traits Matter?" *The Executive* 5, no. 2 (1991): 48-60.

3. Joan S. Tucker, Nancy R. Kressin, Avron Spiro III, and John Ruscio, "Intrapersonal Characteristics and the Timing of Divorce: A Prospective Investigation," *Journal of Social and Personal Relationships* 15, no. 2 (1998): 211-25. doi: 10.1177/0265407598152005; Margaret L. Kern and Howard S. Friedman, "Do Conscientious Individuals Live Longer? A Quantitative Review," *Health Psychology* 27 no. 5 (2008): 505-12. doi:10.1037/0278-6133.27.5.505.

4. Kent C. Berridge, "The Debate over Dopamine's Role in Reward: The Case for Incentive Salience," *Psychopharmacology* 191, no. 3 (2007): 391-431.

5. Xiao Tian Wang and Robert D. Dvorak, "Sweet Future: Fluctuating Blood Glucose Levels Affect Future Discounting," *Psychological Science* 21 no. 2 (2010): 183-88. doi: 10.1177/0956797609358096.

6. Kent C. Berridge, "Wanting and Liking: Observations from the Neuroscience and Psychology Laboratory," *Psychological Science* 21, no. 2 (2010): 183-88. doi: 10.1177/0956797609358096.

7. Berridge, "The Debate over Dopamine's Role in Reward," 391-431.

8. Thomas L. Kash, William P. Nobis, Robert T. Matthews, and Danny G. Winder, "Dopamine Enhances Fast Excitatory Synaptic Transmission in the Extended Amygdala by a CRF-R1-Dependent Process," *Journal of Neuroscience* 28, no. 51 (2008): 13856-65. doi: 10.1523/JNEUROSCI.4715-08.2008.

9. Brian Knutson, G. Elliott Wimmer, Camelia M. Kuhnen, and Piotr Winkielman, "Nucleus Accumbens Activation Mediates the Influence of Reward Cues on Financial Risk Taking," *Neuroreport* 19, no. 5 (2008): 509-13. doi: 10.1097/WNR.0b013e3282f85c01.

10. Barbara Briers, Mario Pandelaere, Siegfried Dewitte, and Luk Warlop, "Hungry for Money: The Desire for Caloric Resources Increases the Desire for Financial Resources and Vice Versa," *Psychological Science* 17, no. 11 (2006): 939-43. doi: 10.1111/j.1467-9280.2006.01808.x.

11. Matthias J. Koepp, Roger N. Gunn, Andrew D. Lawrence, Vincent J. Cunningham, Alain Dagher, Terry Jones, David J. Brooks, Christopher J. Bench, and Paul M. Grasby, "Evidence for Striatal Dopamine Release during a Video Game," *Nature* 393, no. 6682 (1998): 266-68. doi:10.1038/30498.

12. David T. Neal, Wendy Wood, and Aimee Drolet, "How Do People Adhere to Goals When Willpower Is Low? The Profits (and Pitfalls) of Strong Habits," *Journal of Personality and Social Psychology* 104, no. 6 (2013): 959-75. doi: 10.1037/a0032626.

13. Julian F. Thayer, Anita L. Hansen, Evelyn Saus-Rose, and Bjorn Helge Johnsen, "Heart Rate Variability, Prefrontal Neural Function, and Cognitive Performance: The Neurovisceral Integration Perspective on Self-regulation, Adaptation, and Health," *Annals of Behavioral Medicine* 37, no. 2 (2009): 141-53. doi: 10.1007/s12160-009-9101-z.

14. Suzanne C. Segerstrom and Lise Solberg Nes, "Heart Rate Variability Reflects Self-Regulatory Strength, Effort, and Fatigue," *Psychological Science* 18, no. 3 (2007): 275-81. doi: 10.1111/j.1467-9280.2007.01888.x; C. Barr Taylor, "Depression, Heart Rate Related Variables and Cardiovascular Disease," *International Journal of Psychophysiology* 78 no. 1 (2010): 80-88. doi: 10.1016/j.ijpsycho.2010.04.006.

15. American Psychological Association, *Stress in America: Are Teens Adopting Adults' Stress Habits?* February 11, 2014, http://www.apa.org/news/press/releases/stress/2013/stress-report.pdf.

16. Emma Childs, Sean O'Connor, and Harriet de Wit, "Bidirectional Interactions between Acute Psychosocial Stress and Acute Intravenous Alcohol in Healthy Men," *Alcoholism: Clinical and Experimental Research* 35, no. 10 (2011): 1794–1803. doi: 10.1111/j.1530-0277.2011.01522.x; Leonard Reinecke, Tilo Hartmann, and Allison Eden, "The Guilty Couch Potato: The Role of Ego Depletion in Reducing Recovery through Media Use," *Journal of Communication* 64, no. 4 (2014): 569-89. doi: 10.1111/jcom.12107.

17. Wang and Dvorak, "Sweet Future: Fluctuating Blood Glucose Levels Affect Future Discounting," 183-88.

18. Matthew T. Gailliot, Roy F. Baumeister, C. Nathan DeWall, Jon K. Maner, E. Ashby Plant, Dianne M. Tice, Lauren E. Brewer, and Brandon J. Schmeichel, "Self-Control Relies on Glucose as a Limited Energy Source: Willpower Is More Than a Metaphor," *Journal of Personality and Social Psychology* 92, no. 2 (2007): 325-36. doi: 10.1037/0022-3514.92.2.325; C. Nathan DeWall, Timothy Deckman, Matthew T. Gailliot, and Brad J. Bushman, "Sweetened Blood Cools Hot Tempers: Physiological Self-Control and Aggression," *Aggressive Behavior* 37, no. 1 (2011): 73-80. doi: 10.1002/ab.20366; Matthew T. Gailliot, B. Michelle Peruche, E. Ashby Plant, and Roy F. Baumeister, "Stereotypes and Prejudice in the Blood: Sucrose Drinks Reduce Prejudice and Stereotyping," *Journal of Experimental Social Psychology* 45, no. 1 (2009): 288-90. doi: 10.1016/j.jesp.2008.09.003; C. Nathan DeWall, Roy F. Baumeister, Matthew T. Gailliot, and Jon K. Maner, "Depletion Makes the Heart Grow Less Helpful: Helping as a Function of Self-Regulatory Energy and Genetic Relatedness," *Personality and Social Psychology Bulletin* 34, no. 12: 1653-62. doi: 10.1177/0146167208323981.

19. Hye-Sue Song and Paul M. Lehrer, "The Effects of Specific Respiratory Rates on Heart Rate and Heart Rate Variability," *Applied Psychophysiology and Biofeedback* 28, no. 1 (2003): 13-23. doi: 10.1023/A:1022312815649; Terri L. Zucker, Kristin W. Samuelson, Frederick Muench, Melanie A. Greenberg, and Richard N. Gevirtz, "The Effects of Respiratory Sinus Arrhythmia Biofeedback on Heart Rate Variability and Posttraumatic Stress Disorder Symptoms: A Pilot Study," *Applied Psychophysiology and Biofeedback* 34, no. 2 (2009): 135-43. doi: 10.1007/s10484-009-9085-2; Daniele Martarelli, Mario Cocchioni, Stefania Scuri, and Pierluigi Pompei, "Diaphragmatic Breathing Reduces Exercise-Induced Oxidative Stress," *Evidence-Based Complementary and Alternative Medicine* 2011 (2011). doi: 10.1093/ecam/nep169.

20. Janice K. Kiecolt-Glaser, Lisa Christian, Heather Preston, Carrie R. Houts, William B. Malarkey, Charles F. Emery, and Ronald Glaser, "Stress, Inflammation, and Yoga Practice," *Psychosomatic Medicine* 72, no. 2 (2010): 113-21. doi: 10.1097/PSY.0b013e3181cb9377; Herbert Benson, *The Relaxation Response* (New York: Morrow, 1975).

21. Jo Barton and Jules Pretty, "What Is the Best Dose of Nature and Green Exercise for Improving Mental Health? A Multi-Study Analysis," *Environmental Science and Technology* 44, no. 10 (2010): 3947-55. doi: 10.1021/es903183r; "Reading 'Can Help Reduce Stress,'" *The Telegraph*, March 30, 2009, http://www.telegraph.co.uk/health/

healthnews/5070874/Reading-can-help-reduce-stress.html; Kathi J. Kemper and Suzanne C. Danhauer, "Music as Therapy," *Southern Medical Journal* 98, no. 3 (2005): 282-88. doi: 10.1097/01.SMJ.0000154773.11986.39; Amber W. Li and Carroll-Ann W. Goldsmith, "The Effects of Yoga on Anxiety and Stress," *Alternative Medicine Review* 17, no. 1 (2012): 21-35; Agnes E. Van Den Berg and Mariette H. Custers, "Gardening Promotes Neuroendocrine and Affective Restoration from Stress," *Journal of Health Psychology* 16, no. 1 (2011): 3-11. doi: 10.1177/1359105310365577.

22. Avis R. Brennan and Amy F. T. Arnsten, "Neuronal Mechanisms Underlying Attention Deficit Hyperactivity Disorder," *Annals of the New York Academy of Sciences* 1129: 236-45. doi: 10.1196/annals.1417.007.

23. Naomi Mandel and Dirk Smeesters, "The Sweet Escape: Effects of Mortality Salience on Consumption Quantities for High- and Low-Self-Esteem Consumers," *Journal of Consumer Research* 35, no. 2 (2008): 309-23; Naomi Mandel and Steven J. Heine, "Terror Management and Marketing: He Who Dies With the Most Toys Wins," in *NA—Association for Consumer Research Volume 26*, eds. Eric J. Arnould and Linda M. Scott (1999): 527-32; Brian L. Burke, Andy Martens, and Erik H. Faucher, "Two Decades of Terror Management Theory: A Meta-Analysis of Mortality Salience Research," *Personality and Social Psychology Review* 14, no. 2 (2010): 155-95. doi: 10.1177/1088868309352321.

24. Kate Janse Van Rensburg, Adrian Taylor, and Tim Hodgson, "The Effects of Acute Exercise on Attentional Bias towards Smoking-Related Stimuli during Temporary Abstinence from Smoking," *Addiction* 104, no. 11 (2009): 1910-17. doi: 10.1111/j.1360-0443.2009.02692.x; Anita Lill Hansen, Bjørn Helge Johnsen, John J. Sollers III, Kjetil Stenvik, and Julian F. Thayer, "Heart Rate Variability and Its Relation to Prefrontal Cognitive Function: The Effects of Training and Detraining," *European Journal of Applied Physiology* 93, no. 3 (2004): 263-72. doi: 10.1007/s00421-004-1208-0; Chanudda Nabkasorn, Nobuyuki Miyai, Anek Sootmongkol, Suwanna Junprasert, Hiroichi Yamamoto, Mikio Arita, and Kazuhisa Miyashita, "Effects of Physical Exercise on Depression, Neuroendocrine Stress Hormones and Physiological Fitness in Adolescent Females with Depressive Symptoms," *European Journal of Public Health* 16 no. 2 (2006): 179-84. doi: 10.1093/eurpub/cki159; Charles H. Hillman, Kirk I. Erickson, and Arthur F. Kramer, "Be Smart, Exercise Your Heart: Exercise Effects on Brain and Cognition," *Nature Review Neuroscience* 9, no. 1 (2008): 58-65. doi:10.1038/nrn2298.

25. Megan Oaten and Ken Cheng, "Longitudinal Gains in Self-Regulation from Regular Physical Exercise," *British Journal of Health Psychology* 11 (2006): 717-33.

26. Jo Barton and Jules Pretty, "What Is the Best Dose of Nature and Green Exercise for Improving Mental Health? A Multi-Study Analysis," *Environmental Science and Technology* 44, no. 10 (2010): 3947-55. doi: 10.1021/es903183r.

27. Shinsuke Ikeda, Myong-Il Kang, and Fumio Ohtake, "Hyperbolic Discounting, the Sign Effect, and the Body Mass Index," *Journal of Health Economics* 29, no. 2 (2010): 268-84. doi: 10.1016/j.jhealeco.2010.01.002; Kris N. Kirby, Nancy M. Petrie, and Warren K. Bickel, "Heroin Addicts Have Higher Discount Rates for Delayed Rewards Than Non-Drug-Using Controls," *Journal of Experimental Psychology* 128, no. 1 (1999): 78-87. doi: 10.1037/0096-3445.128.1.78; Sheila M. Alessi and Nancy M. Perry, "Pathological Gambling Severity Is Associated with Impulsivity in a Delay Discounting Procedure," *Behavioural Processes* 64, no. 3 (2003): 345-54. doi: 10.1016/S0376-6357(03)00150-5.

28. Elke U. Weber, Eric J. Johnson, Kerry F. Milch, Hanna Chang, Jeffrey C. Brodscholl, and Dan Goldstein, "Asymmetric Discounting in Intertemporal Choice: A Query-Theory Account," *Psychological Science* 18, no. 6: 516-23. doi: 10.1111/j.1467-9280.2007.01932.x.

29. Damon Centola, "The Spread of Behavior in an Online Social Network Experiment," *Science* 329, no. 5996 (2010): 1194-97. doi: 10.1126/science.1185231.

30. Dylan D. Wagner, Sonya Dal Cin, James D. Sargent, William M. Kelley, and Todd F. Heatherton, "Spontaneous Action Representation in Smokers When Watching Movie Characters Smoke," *Journal of Neuroscience* 31, no. 3 (2011): 894-98. doi: 10.1523/JNEUROSCI.5174-10.2011.

31. James H. Fowler and Nicholas A. Christakis, "Estimating Peer Effects on Health in Social Networks: A Response to Cohen-Cole and Fletcher; and Trogdon, Nonnemaker, and Pais," *Journal of Health Economics* 27, no. 5 (2008): 1400-05. doi: 10.1016/j.jhealeco.2008.07.001; James H. Fowler and Nicholas A. Christakis, "The Spread of Obesity in a Large Social Network Over 32 Years," *New England Journal of Medicine* 357, no. 4 (2007): 370-79. doi: 10.1056/NEJMsa066082.

32. Donald L. McCabe, Linda Klebe Treviño, and Kenneth D. Butterfield, "Honor Codes and Other Contextual Influences on Academic Integrity: A Replication and Extension to Modified Honor Code Settings," *Research in Higher Education* 43, no. 3 (2002): 357-78. doi: 10.1023/A:1014893102151.

33. Michael Wenzel, "Misperceptions of Social Norms about Tax Compliance: From Theory to Intervention," *Journal of Economic Psychology* 26, no. 6 (2005): 862-83. doi: 10.1016/j.joep.2005.02.002.

34. J. Niels Rosenquist, Joanne Murabito, James H. Fowler, and Nicholas A. Christakis, "The Spread of Alcohol Consumption Behavior in a Large Social Network," *Annals of Internal Medicine* no. 152, no. 7 (2010): 426-W141; Nicholas A. Christakis and James H. Fowler, "The Collective Dynamics of Smoking in a Large Social Network," *New England Journal of Medicine* 358 (May 22, 2008): 2249-2258. doi: 10.1056/NEJMsa0706154; Sara C. Mednick, Nicholas A. Christakis, and James H. Fowler, "The Spread of Sleep Loss Influences Drug Use in Adolescent Social Networks," *PlOS One* 5, no. 3 (2010): e9775. doi: 10.1371/journal.pone.0009775; John T. Cacioppo, James H. Fowler, and Nicholas A. Christakis, "Alone in the Crowd: The Structure and Spread of Loneliness in a Large Social Network," *Journal of Personality and Social Psychology* 97, no. 6 (2009): 977-91. doi: 10.1037/a0016076; J. Niels Rosenquist, James H. Fowler, and Nicholas A. Christakis, "Social Network Determinants of Depression," *Molecular Psychiatry* 16 (2011): 273-81. doi: 10.1038/mp.2010.13.

35. Kees Keizer, Siegwart Lindenberg, and Linda Steg, "The Spreading of Disorder," *Science* 322, no. 5908: 1681-85. doi: 10.1126/science.1161405.

36. James H. Fowler and Nicholas A. Christakis, "Dynamic Spread of Happiness in a Large Social Network: Longitudinal Analysis Over 20 Years in the Framingham Heart Study," *BMJ* 337 (2008): a2338. doi: 10.1136/bmj.a2338; Henk Aarts, Peter M. Gollwitzer, and Ran R. Hassin, "Goal Contagion: Perceiving Is for Pursuing," *Journal of Personality and Social Psychology* 87, no. 1 (2004): 23-37. doi: 10.1037/0022-3514.87.1.23.

37. Michelle R. van Dellen and Rick H. Hoyle, "Regulatory Accessibility and Social Influences on State Self-Control," *Personality and Social Psychology Bulletin* 36, no. 2 (2010): 251-63. doi: 10.1177/0146167209356302.

38. Ayelet Fishbach and Yaacov Trope, "Implicit and Explicit Counteractive Self-Control," in *Handbook of Motivation Science*, eds. James Y. Shah and Wendi L. Gardner (New York: Guilford, 2008), 281-94.

39. Peter M. Gollwitzer and Gabrielle Oettingen, "Planning Promotes Goal Striving," in *Handbook of Self-Regulation: Research, Theory, and Applications*, eds. Kathleen D. Vohs and Roy F. Baumeister (New York: Guilford, 2011), 162-85.

40. Anirban Mukhopadhyay, "Indulgence as Self-Reward for Prior Shopping Restraint: A Justification-Based Mechanism," *Journal of Consumer Psychology* 19, no. 3 (2009): 334-45. doi: 10.1016/j.jcps.2009.02.016.

41. Sonya Sachdeva, Rumen Iliev, and Douglas L. Medin, "Sinning Saints and Saintly Sinners: The Paradox of Moral Self-Regulation," *Psychological Science* 20, no. 4 (2009): 523-28. doi: 10.1111/j.1467-9280.2009.02326.x.

42. Uzma Khan and Ravi Dhar, "Licensing Effect in Consumer Choice," *Journal of Marketing Research* 43, no. 2 (2006): 259-66. doi: 10.1509/jmkr.43.2.259.

43. Keith Wilcox, Beth Vallen, Lauren Block, and Gavan J. Fitzimons, "Vicarious Goal Fulfillment: When the Mere Presence of a Healthy Option Leads to an Ironically Indulgent Decision," *Journal of Consumer Research* 36, no. 3 (2009): 380-93.

44. Pierre Chandon and Brian Wansink, "The Biasing Health Halos of Fast Food Restaurant Health Claims: Lower Calorie Estimates and Higher Side-Dish Consumption Intentions," *Journal of Consumer Research* 34, no. 3 (2007): 301-14.

45. Anirban Mukhopadhyay, "Indulgence as Self-Reward for Prior Shopping Restraint: A Justification-Based Mechanism," *Journal of Consumer Psychology* 19, no. 3 (2009): 334-45. doi: 10.1016/j.jcps.2009.02.016.

46. Jonathon P. Schuldt and Norbert Schwarz, "The "Organic" Path to Obesity? Organic Claims Influence Calorie Judgments and Exercise Recommendations," *Judgment and Decision Making* 5, no. 3 (2010): 144-50.

47. Janet Polivy and C. Peter Herman, "Dieting and Binging: A Causal Analysis," *American Psychologist* 40, no. 2 (1985): 193-201. doi: 10.1037/0003-066X.40.2.193.

48. Melike M. Fourie, Henri G. L. Rauch, Barak E. Morgan, George F. R. Ellis, Esmè R. Jordaan, and Kevin G. F. Thomas, "Guilt and Pride Are Heartfelt, But Not Equally So," *Psychophysiology* 48, no. 7 (2011): 888-99. doi: 10.1111/j.1469-8986.2010.01157.x.

49. Michael J. A. Wohl, "I Forgive Myself, Now I Can Study: How Self-Forgiveness for Procrastinating Can Reduce Future Procrastination," *Personality and Individual Differences* 48, no. 7 (2010): 803-08. doi: 10.1016/j.paid.2010.01.029; Mark R. Leary, Eleanor B. Tate, Claire E. Adams, Ashley Batts Allen, and Jessica Hancock, "Self-Compassion and Reactions to Unpleasant Self-Relevant Events: The Implications of Treating Oneself Kindly," *Journal of Personality and Social Psychology* 92, no. 5 (2007): 887-904. doi: 10.1037/0022-3514.92.5.887;

Ashley Batts Allen and Mark R. Leary, "Self-Compassion, Stress, and Coping," *Social and Personality Psychology Compass* 4, no. 2 (2010): 107-18. doi: 10.1111/j.1751-9004.2009.00246.x.

50. Richard P. Bagozzi, Utpal M. Dholakia, and Suman Basuroy, "How Effortful Decisions Get Enacted: The Motivating Role of Decision Processes, Desires, and Anticipated Emotions," *Journal of Behavioral Decision Making* 16, no. 4 (2003): 273-95. doi: 10.1002/bdm.446; Melike M. Fourie, Henri G. L. Rauch, Barak E. Morgan, George F. R. Ellis, Esmè R. Jordaan, and Kevin G. F. Thomas, "Guilt and Pride Are Heartfelt, But Not Equally So," *Psychophysiology* 48, no. 7 (2011): 888-99. doi:10.1111/j.1469-8986.2010.01157.x.

51. HaeEun Chun; Vanessa M. Patrick, and Deborah J.MacInnis, "Making Prudent vs. Impulsive Choices: The Role of Anticipated Shame and Guilt on Consumer Self-Control," *Advances in Consumer Research* 34 (January 2007): 715.

52. Uzma Khan and Ravi Dhar, "Where There Is a Way, Is There a Will? The Effect of Future Choices on Self-Control," *Journal of Experimental Psychology* 136, no. 2 (2007): 277-88. doi: 10.1037/0096-3445.136.2.277.

53. Hal Ersner-Hershfield, G. Elliott Wimmer, and Brian Knutson, "Saving for the Future Self: Neural Measures of Future Self-Continuity Predict Temporal Discounting," *Social Cognitive and Affective Neuroscience* 4, no. 1 (2009): 85-92. doi: 10.1093/scan/nsn042.

54. Jan Peters and Christian Büchel, "Episodic Future Thinking Reduces Reward Delay Discounting through an Enhancement of Prefrontal-Mediotemporal Interactions," *Neuron* 66, no. 1 (2010): 138-48. doi: 10.1016/j.neuron.2010.03.026.

55. Elisa C. Murru and Kathleen A. Martin Ginis, "Imagining the Possibilities: The Effects of a Possible Selves Intervention on Self-Regulatory Efficacy and Exercise Behavior," *Journal of Sport and Exercise Physiology* 32, no. 4 (2010): 537-54.

56. Philippe Goldin, Wiveka Ramel, and James Gross, "Mindfulness Meditation Training and Self-Referential Processing in Social Anxiety Disorder: Behavioral and Neural Effects," *Journal of Cognitive Psychotherapy* 23, no. 3 (2009): 242; Philippe R. Goldin and James J. Gross, "Effects of Mindfulness-Based Stress Reduction (MBSR) on Emotion Regulation in Social Anxiety Disorder," *Emotion* 10, no. 1 (2010): 83-91. doi: 10.1037/a0018441.

57. Lee J. Markowitz and Jennifer L. S. Borton, "Suppression of Negative Self-Referent and Neutral Thoughts: A Preliminary Investigation," *Behavioural and Cognitive Psychotherapy* 30, no. 3 (2002): 271-77. doi:10.1017/S135246580200303X; Stefan G. Hofmann, Sanna Heering, Alice T. Sawyer, and Anu Asnaani, "How to Handle Anxiety: The Effects of Reappraisal, Acceptance, and Suppression Strategies on Anxious Arousal," *Behaviour Research and Therapy* 47, no. 5 (2009): 389-94. doi: 10.1016/j.brat.2009.02.010; Daniel M. Wegner and Sophia Zanakos, "Chronic Thought Suppression," *Journal of Personality* 62, no. 4 (1994): 615-40. doi: 10.1111/j.1467-6494.1994.tb00311.x; Peter Muris, Harald Merckelbach, and Robert Horselenberg, "Individual Differences in Thought Suppression. The White Bear Suppression Inventory: Factor Structure, Reliability, Validity and Correlates," *Behaviour Research and Therapy* 34, no. 5-6 (1996): 501-13. doi: 10.1016/0005-7967(96)00005-8; Daniel M.Wegner, Ralph Erber, and Sophia Zanakos, Ironic Processes in the Mental Control of Mood and Mood-Related Thought," *Journal of Personality and Social Psychology* 65, no. 6 (1993): 1093-104. doi: 10.1037/0022-3514.65.6.1093; James A.K. Erskine and George J. Georgiou, "Effects of Thought Suppression on Eating Behaviour in Restrained and Non-Restrained Eaters," *Appetite* 54, no. 3 (2010): 499-503. doi: 10.1016/j.appet.2010.02.001.

58. Rachel D. Barnes and Stacey Tantleff-Dunn, "Food for Thought: Examining the Relationship between Food Thought Suppression and Weight-Related Outcomes," *Eating Behaviors* 11, no. 3 (2010): 175-79. doi: 10.1016/j.eatbeh.2010.03.001.

59. Sarah Bowen and Alan Marlatt, "Surfing the Urge: Brief Mindfulness-Based Intervention for College Student Smokers," *Psychology of Addictive Behaviors* 23, no. 4 (2009): 666-71. doi: 10.1037/a0017127.

60. Veronika Job, Carol S. Dweck, and Gregory M. Walton, "Ego Depletion—Is It All in Your Head? Implicit Theories about Willpower Affect Self-Regulation," *Psychological Science* 21, no. 11 (2010): 1686-93. doi: 10.1177/0956797610384745.

61. Roy F. Baumeister, Todd F. Heatherton, and Dianne M. Tice, *Losing Control: How and Why People Fail at Self-Regulation* (San Diego: Academic Press, 1994).

62. *Ibid.*

63. Kathleen D. Vohs, Roy F. Baumeister, Brandon J. Schmeichel, Jean M. Twenge, Noelle M. Nelson, and Dianne M. Tice, "Making Choices Impairs Subsequent Self-Control: A Limited-Resource Account of Decision Making, Self-Regulation, and Active Initiative," *Journal of Personality and Social Psychology* 94, no. 5 (2008): 883-98. doi:

10.1037/0022-3514.94.5.883; Michael Inzlicht and Jennifer N. Gutsell, "Running on Empty: Neural Signals for Self-Control Failure," *Psychological Science* 18, no. 11: 933-37 (2007). doi: 10.1111/j.1467-9280.2007.02004.x.

64. Mark Muraven, Roy F. Baumeister, and Dianne M. Tice, "Longitudinal Improvement of Self-Regulation Through Practice: Building Self-Control Strength Through Repeated Exercise," *Journal of Social Psychology* 139, no. 4 (1999): 446-57. doi: :10.1080/00224549909598404; Mark Muraven, "Building Self-Control Strength: Practicing Self-Control Leads to Improved Self-Control Performance," *Journal of Experimental Social Psychology* 46, no. 2 (2010): 465-68. doi: 10.1016/j.jesp.2009.12.011; Megan Oaten and Ken Cheng, "Improvements in Self-Control from Financial Monitoring," *Journal of Economic Psychology* 28, no. 4 (2007): 487–501. doi: 10.1016/j.joep.2006.11.003; Roy F. Baumeister, Matthew Gailliot, C. Nathan DeWall, and Megan Oaten, "Self-Regulation and Personality: How Interventions Increase Regulatory Success, and How Depletion Moderates the Effects of Traits on Behavior," *Journal of Personality* 74, no. 6 (2006): 1773-1802. doi: 10.1111/j.1467-6494.2006.00428.x.

65. Suzanne C. Segerstrom, Jaime K. Hardy, Daniel R. Evans, and Natalie F. Winters, "Pause and Plan: Self-Regulation and the Heart," in *How Motivation Affects Cardiovascular Response: Mechanisms and Applications*, eds. Rex A. Wright and Guido H. E. Gendolla (Washington, DC: American Psychological Association, 2012), 181-98. doi.org/10.1037/13090-009.

66. Molly J. Crockett, Barbara R. Braams, Luke Clark, Philippe N. Tobler, Trevor W. Robbins, and Tobias Kalenscher, "Restricting Temptations: Neural Mechanisms of Precommitment," *Neuron* 79, no. 2 (2013): 391-401. doi: 10.1016/j.neuron.2013.05.028.

67. Ayelet Fishbach and Ravi Dhar, "Goals as Excuses or Guides: The Liberating Effect of Perceived Goal Progress on Choice," *Journal of Consumer Research* 32, no. 3 (2005): 370-77.

68. Ayelet Fishbach, Ravi Dhar, and Ying Zhang, "Subgoals as Substitutes or Complements: The Role of Goal Accessibility," *Journal of Personality and Social Psychology* 91, no. 2 (2006): 232-42. doi: 10.1037/0022-3514.91.2.232.

CHAPTER 12
GOING BEYOND "CLEAN EATING" THE DEFINITIVE GUIDE TO EFFECTIVE NUTRITION

1. Kevin D. Tipton and Robert R. Wolf, "Protein and Amino Acids for Athletes," *Journal of Sports Sciences* 22, no. 1 (2004): 65-79. doi: 10.1080/0264041031000140554.

2. Institute of Medicine, *Dietary Reference Intakes for Energy, Carbohydrate, Fiber, Fat, Fatty Acids, Cholesterol, Protein, and Amino Acids* (Washington, D.C.: National Academies Press, 2005).

3. Stuart M. Phillips and Luc J. C. Van Loon, "Dietary Protein for Athletes: From Requirements to Optimum Adaptation," *Journal of Sports Sciences* 29, no. S1 (2011): S29-S38. doi: 10.1080/02640414.2011.619204.

4. Peter W. Lemon, "Beyond the Zone: Protein Needs of Active Individuals," *Journal of the American College of Nutrition* 19, no. S5 (2000): 513S-21S.

5. Eric R. Helms, Caryn Zinn, David S. Rowlands, and Scott R. Brown, "A Systematic Review of Dietary Protein during Caloric Restriction in Resistance Trained Lean Athletes: A Case for Higher Intakes," *International Journal of Sport Nutrition and Exercise Metabolism* 24, no. 2 (2014): 127-38. doi: 10.1123/ijsnem.2013-0054.

6. Robert L. Rizek and Elizabeth M. Jackson, "Current Food Consumption Practices and Nutrient Sources in the American Diet," in *Animal Products in Human Nutrition*, ed. Donald Beitz (New York: Academic Press, 1982), 121-62. doi: 10.1016/B978-0-12-086380-8.50003-X.

7. Bilsborough, Shane, and Neil Mann. "A review of issues of dietary protein intake in humans." *International journal of sport nutrition and exercise metabolism* 16, no. 2 (2006): 129; Norton, Layne E., Gabriel J. Wilson, Donald K. Layman, Christopher J. Moulton, and Peter J. Garlick. "Leucine content of dietary proteins is a determinant of postprandial skeletal muscle protein synthesis in adult rats." *Nutr Metab* 9, no. 1 (2012): 67.

8. M. M. Suárez López, A. Kizlansky, and L. B. López, "Assessment of Protein Quality in Foods by Calculating the Amino Acids Score Corrected by Digestibility," [In Spanish], *Nutricion Hospitalaria* 21, no. 1 (2006): 47-51.

9. Anne Raben, Bente Kiens, Erik A. Richter, Lone B. Rasmussen, Birgit Svenstrup, Snezana Micic, and Paul Bennett, "Serum Sex Hormones and Endurance Performance after a Lacto-Ovo Vegetarian and a Mixed Diet," *Medicine and Science in Sports and Exercise* 24, no. 11 (1992): 1290-97; Mylène Aubertin-Leheudre and Herman

Adlercreutz, "Relationship between Animal Protein Intake and Muscle Mass Index in Healthy Women," *British Journal of Nutrition* 102, no. 12 (2009): 1803-10. doi: 10.1017/S0007114509991310.

10. Wayne W. Campbell, Marvin L. Barton Jr., Deanna Cyr-Campbell, Stephanie L. Davey, John L. Beard, Gianni Parise, and William J. Evans, "Effects of an Omnivorous Diet Compared with a Lactoovovegetarian Diet on Resistance-Training-Induced Changes in Body Composition and Skeletal Muscle in Older Men," *American Journal of Clinical Nutrition* 70, no. 6 (1999): 1032-39.

11. Vernon R. Young and Peter L. Pellett, "Plant Proteins in Relation to Human Protein and Amino Acid Nutrition," *American Journal of Clinical Nutrition* 59, supplement 5 (1994): 1203S-12S.

12. Layne E. Norton, Gabriel J. Wilson, Donald K. Layman, Christopher J. Moulton, and Peter J. Garlick, "Leucine Content of Dietary Proteins Is a Determinant of Postprandial Skeletal Muscle Protein Synthesis in Adult Rats," *Nutrition and Metabolism* 9, no. 1 (2012): 67. doi:10.1186/1743-7075-9-67; Satoshi Fujita, Hans C. Dreyer, Micah J. Drummond, Erin L. Glynn, Jerson G. Cadenas, Fumiaki Yoshizawa, Elena Volpi, and Blake B. Rasmussen, "Nutrient Signalling in the Regulation of Human Muscle Protein Synthesis," *Journal of Physiology* 582, pt. 2 (2007): 813-23. doi: 10.1113/jphysiol.2007.134593.

13. Jason E. Tang, Daniel R. Moore, Gregory W. Kujbida, Mark A. Tarnopolsky, and Stuart M. Phillips, "Ingestion of Whey Hydrolysate, Casein, or Soy Protein Isolate: Effects on Mixed Muscle Protein Synthesis at Rest and Following Resistance Exercise in Young Men," *Journal of Applied Physiology* 107, no. 3 (2009): 987-92. doi: 10.1152/japplphysiol.00076.2009; Yves Boirie, Martial Dangin, Pierre Gachon, Marie-Paule Vasson, Jean-Louis Maubois, and Bernard Beaufrère, "Slow and Fast Dietary Proteins Differently Modulate Postprandial Protein Accretion," *Proceedings of the National Academy of Sciences* 94, no. 26 (1997): 14930-35.

14. Martial Dangin, Yves Boirie, Clara Garcia-Rodenas, Pierre Gachon, Jacques Fauquant, Philippe Callier, Olivier Ballèvre, and Bernard Beaufrère, "The Digestion Rate of Protein Is an Independent Regulating Factor of Postprandial Protein Retention," *Endocrinology and Metabolism* 280, no. 2 (2001): E340-E348.

15. Ross G. Crittenden and Louise E. Bennett, "Cow's Milk Allergy: A Complex Disorder," *Journal of the American College of Nutrition* 24, no. S6 (2005): 582S-91S.

16. Boirie et al., "Slow and Fast Dietary Proteins Differently Modulate Postprandial Protein Accretion," 14930-35.

17. Kevin D. Tipton, Tabatha A. Elliott, Melanie G. Cree, Steven E. Wolf, Arthur P. Sanford, and Robert R. Wolfe, "Ingestion of Casein and Whey Proteins Result in Muscle Anabolism after Resistance Exercise," *Medicine and Science in Sports and Exercise* 36, no. 12 (2004): 2073-81. doi: 10.1249/01.MSS.0000147582.99810.C5; Daniel W. D. West, Nicholas A. Burd, Vernon G. Coffey, Steven K. Baker, Louise M. Burke, John A. Hawley, Daniel R. Moore, Trent Stellingwerff, and Stuart M. Phillips, "Rapid Aminoacidemia Enhances Myofibrillar Protein Synthesis and Anabolic Intramuscular Signaling Responses after Resistance Exercise," *American Journal of Clinical Nutrition* 94, no. 3: 795-803. doi: 10.3945/ajcn.111.013722; Boirie et al., "Slow and Fast Dietary Proteins Differently Modulate Postprandial Protein Accretion," 14930-35.

18. Peter T. Res, Bart Groen, Bart Pennings, Milou Beelen, Gareth A. Wallis, Annemie P. Gijsen, Joan M. Senden, and Luc J. van Loon, "Protein Ingestion before Sleep Improves Postexercise Overnight Recovery," *Medicine and Science of Sports and Exercise* 44, no. 8 (2012): 1560-9. doi: 10.1249/MSS.0b013e31824cc363.

19. Layne E. Norton, Gabriel J. Wilson, Donald K. Layman, Christopher J. Moulton, and Peter J. Garlick, "Leucine Content of Dietary Proteins Is a Determinant of Postprandial Skeletal Muscle Protein Synthesis in Adult Rats," *Nutrition and Metabolism* 9, no. 1 (2012): 67. doi:10.1186/1743-7075-9-67.

20. Shane Bilsborough and Neil Mann, "A Review of Issues of Dietary Protein Intake in Humans," *International Journal of Sport Nutrition and Exercise Metabolism* 16, no. 2 (2006): 129-52.

21. Jason E. Tang, Daniel R. Moore, Gregory W. Kujbida, Mark A. Tarnopolsky, and Stuart M. Phillips, "Ingestion of Whey Hydrolysate, Casein, or Soy Protein Isolate: Effects on Mixed Muscle Protein Synthesis at Rest and Following Resistance Exercise in Young Men," *Journal of Applied Physiology* 107 no. 3 (2009): 987-92. doi: 10.1152/japplphysiol.00076.2009.

22. Jorge E. Chavarro, Thomas L. Toth, Sonita M. Sadio, and Russ Hauser, "Soy Food and Isoflavone Intake in Relation to Semen Quality Parameters among Men from an Infertility Clinic," *Human Reproduction* 23, no. 11: 2584-90. doi: 10.1093/humrep/den243.

23. Laura K. Beaton, Brianne L. McVeigh, Barbara L. Dillingham, Johanna W. Lampe, and Alison M. Duncan, "Soy Protein Isolates of Varying Isoflavone Content Do Not Adversely Affect Semen Quality in Healthy Young Men," *Fertility and Sterility* 94, no. 5 (2010): 1717-22. doi: 10.1016/j.fertnstert.2009.08.055.

24. 133. Mark Messina, "Soybean Isoflavone Exposure Does Not Have Feminizing Effects on Men: A Critical Examination of the Clinical Evidence," *Fertility and Sterility* 93, no. 7 (2010): 2095-104. doi: 10.1016/j.fertnstert.2010.03.002; Jill M. Hamilton-Reeves, Gabriela Vazquez, Sue J. Duval, William R. Phipps, Mindy S. Kurzer, and Mark J. Messina, "Clinical Studies Show No Effects of Soy Protein or Isoflavones on Reproductive Hormones in Men: Results of a Meta-Analysis," *Fertility and Sterility* 94, no. 3 (2010): 997-1007. doi: 10.1016/j.fertnstert.2009.04.038.

25. Cara L. Frankenfeld, Charlotte Atkinson, Wendy K. Thomas, Alex Gonzalez, Tuija Jokela, Kristiina Wähälä, Stephen M. Schwartz, Shuying S. Lia, and Johanna W. Lampe, "High Concordance of Daidzein-Metabolizing Phenotypes in Individuals Measured 1 to 3 Years Apart," *British Journal of Nutrition* 94, no. 6 (2005): 873-76. doi: 10.1079/BJN20051565.

26. Bachua Liu, Liquiang Qin, Aiping Liu, Yuhui Shi, and Peiyu Wang, "Equol-Producing Phenotype and in Relation to Serum Sex Hormones among Healthy Adults in Beijing," [In Chinese], *Wei Sheng Yan Jiu* 40, no. 6 (2011): 727-31.

27. Chang Sun Hwang, Ho Seok Kwak, Hwa Jae Lim, Su Hee Lee, Young Soon Kang, Tae Boo Choe, Hor Gil Hur, and Ki Ok Han, "Isoflavone Metabolites and Their In Vitro Dual Functions: They Can Act as an Estrogenic Agonist or Antagonist Depending on the Estrogen Concentration," *Journal of Steroid Biochemistry and Molecular Biology* 101, nos. 4-5 (2006): 246-53. doi: 10.1016/j.jsbmb.2006.06.020.

28. David L. Brandon and Mendel Friedman, "Immunoassays of Soy Proteins," *Journal of Agricultural and Food Chemistry* 50, no. 22 (2002): 6635-42. doi: 10.1021/jf020186g; Sanae Hisayasu, Hideo Orimo, Setsuko Migita, Yuki Ikeda, Kumiko Satoh, Setsuko Shingo (Kanda), Yukihiko Hirai, and Yoshio Yoshino, "Soybean Protein Isolate and Soybean Lectin Inhibit Iron Absorption in Rats," *Journal of Nutrition* 122, no. 5 (1992): 1190-96; Brandon and Friedman, "Immunoassays of Soy Proteins," 6635-42.

29. James W. Anderson, Bryan M. Johnstone, and Margaret E. Cook-Newell, "Meta-Analysis of the Effects of Soy Protein Intake on Serum Lipids," *New England Journal of Medicine* 333, no. 5 (1995): 276-82. doi: 10.1056/NEJM199508033330502; Bruce J. Trock, Leena Hilakivi-Clarke, and Robert Clarke, "Meta-Analysis of Soy Intake and Breast Cancer Risk," *Journal of the National Cancer Institute* 98, no. 7 (2006): 459-71. doi: 10.1093/jnci/djj102; "Protein: Moving Closer to Center Stage," Harvard School of Public Health, accessed October 17, 2014, http://www.hsph.harvard.edu/nutritionsource/protein-full-story/.

30. Mário de Lemos, "Effects of Soy Phytoestrogens Genistein and Daidzein on Breast Cancer Growth," *Annals of Pharmacotherapy* 35, no. 9 (2001): 1118-21.

31. "Adoption of Genetically Engineered Crops in the U.S.," United States Department of Agriculture, last updated August 26, 2014, http://www.ers.usda.gov/data-products/adoption-of-genetically-engineered-crops-in-the-us.aspx#.VEkhkPldWWQ.

32. François Mariotti, Maria E. Pueyo, Daniel Tomé, Serge Bérot, Robert Benamouzig, and Sylvain Mahé, "The Influence of the Albumin Fraction on the Bioavailability and Postprandial Utilization of Pea Protein Given Selectively to Humans," *Journal of Nutrition* 131, no. 6 (2001): 1706-13.

33. James D. House, Jason Neufeld, and Gero Leson, "Evaluating the Quality of Protein from Hemp Seed (Cannabis sativa L.) Products Through the Use of the Protein Digestibility-Corrected Amino Acid Score Method," *Journal of Agricultural and Food Chemistry* 58, no. 22 (2010): 11801-07. doi: 10.1021/jf102636b.

34. Shane Bilsborough and Neil Mann, "A Review of Issues of Dietary Protein Intake in Humans," *International Journal of Sport Nutrition and Exercise Metabolism* 16, no. 2 (2006): 129-52.

35. Martin Storr, Daniel Sattler, Andreas Hahn, Volker Schusdziarra, and Hans-Dieter Allescher, "Endogenous CCK Depresses Contractile Activity within the Ascending Myenteric Reflex Pathway of Rat Ileum," *Neuropharmacology* 44, no. 4 (2003): 524-32. doi: 10.1016/S0028-3908(03)00028-5.

36. Institute of Medicine, *Dietary Reference Intakes for Energy, Carbohydrate, Fiber, Fat, Fatty Acids, Cholesterol, Protein, and Amino Acids* (Washington, D.C.: National Academies Press, 2005).

37. Daniel R. Moore, Meghann J. Robinson, Jessica L. Fry, Jason E. Tang, Elisa I. Glover, Sarah B. Wilkinson, Todd Prior, Mark A. Tarnopolsky, and Stuart M. Phillips, "Ingested Protein Dose Response of Muscle and Albumin Protein Synthesis after Resistance Exercise in Young Men," *American Journal of Clinical Nutrition* 89, no. 1 (2009): 161-68. doi: 10.3945/ajcn.2008.26401.

38. Marie-Agnès Arnal, Laurent Mosoni, Yves Boirie, Marie-Louise Houlier, Liliane Morin, Elisabeth Verdier, Patrick Ritz, Jean-Michel Antoine, Jacques Prugnaud, Bernard Beaufrère, and Philippe Patureau Mirand,

"Protein Feeding Pattern Does Not Affect Protein Retention in Young Women," *Journal of Nutrition* 130, no. 7 (2000): 1700-04.

39.   Maarten R. Soeters, Nicolette M. Lammers, Peter F. Dubbelhuis, Mariëtte Ackermans, Cora F. Jonkers-Schuitema, Eric Fliers, Hans P. Sauerwein, Johannes M. Aerts, and Mireille J. Serlie, "Intermittent Fasting Does Not Affect Whole-Body Glucose, Lipid, or Protein Metabolism," *American Journal of Clinical Nutrition* 90, no. 5 (2009): 1244-51. doi: 10.3945/ajcn.2008.27327.

40.   Arnal et al., "Protein Feeding Pattern Does Not Affect Protein Retention in Young Women," 1700-04.

41.   Madonna M. Mamerow, Joni A. Mettler, Kirk L. English, Shanon L. Casperson, Emily Arentson-Lantz, Melinda Sheffield-Moore, Donald K. Layman, and Douglas Paddon-Jones, "Dietary Protein Distribution Positively Influences 24-h Muscle Protein Synthesis in Healthy Adults," *Journal of Nutrition* 144, no. 6 (2014): 876-80. doi: 10.3945/jn.113.185280.

42.   T. Brock Symons, Melinda Sheffield-Moore, Robert R. Wolfe, and Douglas Paddon-Jones, "A Moderate Serving of High-Quality Protein Maximally Stimulates Skeletal Muscle Protein Synthesis in Young and Elderly Subjects," *Journal of the Academy of Nutrition and Dietetics* 109, no. 9 (2009): 1582-86. doi: 10.1016/j.jada.2009.06.369.

43.   Tracy J. Horton, Holy Drougas, Amy Brachey, George W. Reed, John C. Peters, and James O. Hill, "Fat and Carbohydrate Overfeeding in Humans: Different Effects on Energy Storage," *American Journal of Clinical Nutrition* 62, no. 1 (1995): 19-29.

44.   Robert A. Robergs, David R. Pearson, David L. Costill, William J. Fink, David D. Pascoe, Michael A. Benedict, Charles P. Lambert, and Jeffrey J. Zachweija, "Muscle Glycogenolysis during Differing Intensities of Weight-Resistance Exercise," *Journal of Applied Physiology* 70, no. 4 (1991): 1700-06.

45.   Sharon L. Miller and Robert R. Wolfe, "Physical Exercise as a Modulator of Adaptation to Low and High Carbohydrate and Low and High Fat Intakes," *European Journal of Clinical Nutrition* 53, no. S1 (1999): S112-19; Krista R. Howarth, Stuart M. Phillips, Maureen J. MacDonald, Douglas Richards, Natalie A. Moreau, and Martin J. Gibala, "Effect of Glycogen Availability on Human Skeletal Muscle Protein Turnover during Exercise and Recovery," *Journal of Applied Physiology* 109, no. 2 (2010): 431-38. doi: 10.1152/japplphysiol.00108.2009.

46.   George T. Macfarlane, Helen Steed, and Sandra Macfarlane, "Bacterial Metabolism and Health-Related Effects of Galacto-Oligosaccharides and Other Prebiotics," *Journal of Applied Microbiology* 104, no. 2 (2008): 305-44. doi: 10.1111/j.1365-2672.2007.03520.x.

47.   *Ibid.*

48.   "High Fructose Corn Syrup: Questions and Answers," U.S. Food and Drug Administration, last updated July 22, 2014, http://www.fda.gov/food/ingredientspackaginglabeling/foodadditivesingredients/ucm324856.htm.

49.   Carrie H. Ruxton, Fabienne J. Garceau, and Richard C. Cottrell, "Guidelines for Sugar Consumption in Europe: Is a Quantitative Approach Justified?" *European Journal of Clinical Nutrition* 53, no. 7 (1999): 503-13.

50.   Suzanne P. Murphy and Rachel K. Johnson, "The Scientific Basis of Recent US Guidance on Sugars Intake," *American Journal of Clinical Nutrition* 78, no. 4 (2003): 8275-335.

51.   Joanne F. Guthrie and Joan F. Morton, "Food Sources of Added Sweeteners in the Diets of Americans," *Journal of the Academy of Nutrition and Dietetics* 100, no. 1 (2000): 43-51. doi: 10.1016/S0002-8223(00)00018-3.

52.   Doreen P. DiMeglio and Richard D. Mattes, "Liquid Versus Solid Carbohydrate: Effects on Food Intake and Body Weight," *International Journal of Obesity* 24, no. 6 (2000): 794-800.

53.   John S. White, "Straight Talk about High-Fructose Corn Syrup: What It Is and What It Ain't," *American Journal of Clinical Nutrition* 88, no. 6 (2008): 17165-215. doi: 10.3945/ajcn.2008.25825B.

54.   Richard A. Forshee, Maureen L. Storey, David B. Allison, Walter H. Glinsmann, Gayle L. Hein, David R. Lineback, Sanford A. Miller, Theresa A. Nicklas, Gary A. Weaver, and John S. White, "A Critical Examination of the Evidence Relating High Fructose Corn Syrup and Weight Gain," *Critical Reviews and Food Science and Nutrition* 47, no. 6 (2007): 561-82. doi: 10.1080/10408390600846457.

55.   Victor Fulgoni III, "High-Fructose Corn Syrup: Everything You Wanted to Know, But Were Afraid to Ask," *American Journal of Clinical Nutrition* 88, no. 6 (2008): 17155. doi: 10.3945/ajcn.2008.25825A.

56.   Walter Willett, JoAnn Manson, and Simin Liu, "Glycemic Index, Glycemic Load, and Risk of Type 2 Diabetes," *American Journal of Clinical Nutrition* 76, no. 1 (2002): 2745-805.

57. Jergen Jeppesen, Patrica Schaaf, Clare Jones, M-Y Zhou, Y-D Ida Chen, and Gerald M. Reaven, "Effects of Low-Fat, High-Carbohydrate Diets on Risk Factors for Ischemic Heart Disease in Postmenopausal Women," *American Journal of Clinical Nutrition* 65, no. 4 (1997): 1027-33.

58. Gary Frost, Anthony Leeds, Geoffrey Trew, Raul Margara, and Anne Dornhorst, "Insulin Sensitivity in Women at Risk of Coronary Heart Disease and the Effect of a Low Glycemic Diet," *Metabolism—Clinical and Experimental* 47, no. 10 (1998): 1245-51. doi: 10.1016/S0026-0495(98)90331-6; Bente Kiens and Erik A. Richter, "Types of Carbohydrate in an Ordinary Diet Affect Insulin Action and Muscle Substrates in Humans," *American Journal of Clinical Nutrition* 63, no. 1 (1996): 47-53.

59. Thomas M. S. Wolever and Claudia Bolognesi, "Prediction of Glucose and Insulin Responses of Normal Subjects after Consuming Mixed Meals Varying in Energy, Protein, Fat, Carbohydrate and Glycemic Index," *American Journal of Clinical Nutrition* 126, no. 11 (1996): 2807-12.

60. Francis R. J. Bornet, Dominique Costagliola, Salwa W. Rizkalla, Anne Blayo, Anne-Marie Fontvielle, Marie-Joëlle Haardt, Martine Letanoux, Georges Tchobroutsky, and Gérard Slama, "Insulinemic and Glycemic Indexes of Six Starch-Rich Foods Taken Alone and in a Mixed Meal by Type 2 Diabetics," *American Journal of Clinical Nutrition* 45, no. 3 (1987): 588-95.

61. Sigrid A. Gibson, "Dietary Sugars Intake and Micronutrient Adequacy: A Systematic Review of the Evidence," *Nutrition Research Reviews* 20, no. 2 (2007): 121-31. doi: 10.1017/S0954422407797846.

62. *Ibid.*

63. Sander Kersten, "Mechanisms of Nutritional and Hormonal Regulation of Lipogenesis," *EMBO Reports* 2, no. 4 (2001): 282-86.

64. Bernardo Léo Wajchenberg, "Subcutaneous and Visceral Adipose Tissue: Their Relation to the Metabolic Syndrome," *Endocrine Reviews* 21, no. 6 (2000).

65. Alain Golay, Anne F. Allaz, Juan Ybarra, Paola Bianchi, Sergio Saraiva, Nouri Mensi, Ramon Gomis, and Nicholas de Tonnac, "Similar Weight Loss with Low-Energy Food Combining or Balanced Diets," *International Journal of Obesity* 24, no. 4 (2000): 492-96.

66. William S. Yancy Jr., Maren K. Olsen, John R. Guyton, Ronna P. Bakst, and Eric C. Westman, "Low-Carbohydrate, Ketogenic Diet versus a Low-Fat Diet to Treat Obesity and Hyperlipidemia: A Randomized, Controlled Trial," *Annals of Internal Medicine* 140, no. 10 (2004): 769-77.

67. Jeff S. Volek, Matthew J. Sharman, Ana L. Gómez, Daniel A. Judelson, Martyn R. Rubin, Greig Watson, Bulent Sokmen, Ricardo Silvestre, Duncan French, and William J. Kraemer, "Comparison of Energy-Restricted Very Low-Carbohydrate and Low-Fat Diets on Weight Loss and Body Composition in Overweight Men and Women," *Nutrition and Metabolism* 1 (2004): 13.

68. Frederick F. Samaha, Nayyar Iqbal, Prakash Seshadri, Kathryn L. Chicano, Denise A. Daily, Joyce McGrory, Terrence Williams, Monica Williams, Edward J. Gracely, and Linda Stern, "A Low-Carbohydrate as Compared with a Low-Fat Diet in Severe Obesity," *New England Journal of Medicine* 348 (May 22, 2003): 2074-81. doi: 10.1056/NEJMoa022637.

69. Stijn Soenen, Eveline A. P. Martens, Ananda Hochstenbach-Waelen, Sofie G. T. Lemmens, and Margriet S. Westerterp-Plantenga, "Normal Protein Intake Is Required for Body Weight Loss and Weight Maintenance, and Elevated Protein Intake for Additional Preservation of Resting Energy Expenditure and Fat Free Mass," *Journal of Nutrition* 143 no. 5 (2013): 591-96. doi: 10.3945/jn.112.167593; Helms et al., "A Systematic Review of Dietary Protein during Caloric Restriction in Resistance Trained Lean Athletes: A Case for Higher Intakes," 127-38.

70. Samuel Mettler, Nigel Mitchell, and Kevin D. Tipton, "Increased Protein Intake Reduces Lean Body Mass Loss during Weight Loss in Athletes," *Medicine and Science of Sports and Exercise* 42, no. (2010): 326-37. doi: 10.1249/MSS.0b013e3181b2ef8e.

71. Petra Stiegler and Adam Cunliffe, "The Role of Diet and Exercise for the Maintenance of Fat-Free Mass and Resting Metabolic Rate during Weight Loss," *Sports Medicine* 36, no. 3 (2006): 239-62.

72. Jo Smith and Lars McNaughton, "The Effects of Intensity of Exercise on Excess Postexercise Oxygen Consumption and Energy Expenditure in Moderately Trained Men and Women," *European Journal of Applied Physiology and Occupational Physiology* 67, no. 5 (1993): 420-25.

73. Tyler A. Churchward-Venne, Caoileann H. Murphy, Thomas M. Longland, and Stuart M. Phillips, "Role of Protein and Amino Acids in Promoting Lean Mass Accretion with Resistance Exercise and Attenuating Lean

Mass Loss during Energy Deficit in Humans," *Amino Acids* 45, no. 2 (2013): 231-40. doi: 10.1007/s00726-013-1506-0.

74. Donald K. Layman, Richard A. Boileau, Donna J. Erickson, James E. Painter, Harn Shiue, Carl Sather, and Demtra D. Christou, "A Reduced Ratio of Dietary Carbohydrate to Protein Improves Body Composition and Blood Lipid Profiles during Weight Loss in Adult Women," *Journal of Nutrition* 133, no. 2 (2003): 411-17; Mettler, Mitchell, and Tipton, "Increased Protein Intake Reduces Lean Body Mass Loss during Weight Loss in Athletes," 326-37.

75. Carol S. Johnston, Sherrie L. Tjonn, Pamela D. Swan, Andrea White, Heather Hutchins, and Barry Sears, "Ketogenic Low-Carbohydrate Diets Have No Metabolic Advantage Over Nonketogenic Low-Carbohydrate Diets," *American Journal of Clinical Nutrition* 83, no. 5 (2006): 1055-61; Shane A. Phillips, Jason W. Jurva, Amjad Q. Syed, Amina Q. Syed, Jacquelyn P. Kulinski, Joan Pleuss, Raymond G. Hoffmann, and David D. Gutterman, "Benefit of Low-Fat Over Low-Carbohydrate Diet on Endothelial Health in Obesity," *Hypertension* 51, no. 2 (2008): 376-82; Frank M. Sacks, George A. Bray, Vincent J. Carey, Steven R. Smith, Donna H. Ryan, Stephen D. Anton, Katherine McManus, Catherine M. Champagne, Louise M. Bishop, Nancy Laranjo, Meryl S. Leboff, Jennifer C. Rood, Lilian de Jonge, Frank L. Greenway, Catherine M. Loria, Eva Obarzanek, and Donald A. Williamson, "Comparison of Weight-Loss Diets with Different Compositions of Fat, Protein, and Carbohydrates," *New England Journal of Medicine* 360 (February 26, 2009): 859-73. doi: 10.1056/NEJMoa0804748; Cynthia A. Thomson, Alison T. Stopeck, Jennifer W. Bea, Ellen Cussler, Emily Nardi, Georgette Frey, and Patricia A. Thompson, "Changes in Body Weight and Metabolic Indexes in Overweight Breast Cancer Survivors Enrolled in a Randomized Trial of Low-Fat vs. Reduced Carbohydrate Diets," *Nutrition and Cancer* 62, no. 8 (2010): 1142-52. doi:10.1080/01635581.2010.513803.

76. Carol S. Johnston, Sherrie L. Tjonn, Pamela D. Swan, Andrea White, Heather Hutchins, and Barry Sears, "Ketogenic Low-Carbohydrate Diets Have No Metabolic Advantage over Nonketogenic Low-Carbohydrate Diets," *American Journal of Clinical Nutrition* 83, no. 5 (2006): 1055-61.

77. Frank M. Sacks, George A. Bray, Vincent J. Carey, Steven R. Smith, Donna H. Ryan, Stephen D. Anton, Katherine McManus, Catherine M. Champagne, Louise M. Bishop, Nancy Laranjo, Meryl S. Leboff, Jennifer C. Rood, Lilian de Jonge, Frank L. Greenway, Catherine M. Loria, Eva Obarzanek, and Donald A. Williamson, "Comparison of Weight-Loss Diets with Different Compositions of Fat, Protein, and Carbohydrates," *New England Journal of Medicine* no. 360 (February 26 2009): 859-73. doi: 10.1056/NEJMoa0804748.

78. Cynthia A. Thomson, Alison T. Stopeck, Jennifer W. Bea, Ellen Cussler, Emily Nardi, Georgette Frey, and Patricia A. Thompson, "Changes in Body Weight and Metabolic Indexes in Overweight Breast Cancer Survivors Enrolled in a Randomized Trial of Low-Fat vs. Reduced Carbohydrate Diets," *Nutrition and Cancer*, 62, no. 8 (2010): 1142-52. doi:10.1080/01635581.2010.513803.

79. Shane A. Phillips, Jason W. Jurva, Amjad Q. Syed, Amina Q. Syed, Jacquelyn P. Kulinski, Joan Pleuss, Raymond G. Hoffmann, David D. Gutterman, "Benefit of Low-Fat Over Low-Carbohydrate Diet on Endothelial Health in Obesity," *Hypertension* 51, no. 2 (2008): 376-82. doi: 10.1161/HYPERTENSIONAHA.107.101824.

80. David A. Fryburg, Linda A. Jahn, Stephen A. Hill, Diana M. Oliveras, and Eugene J. Barrett, "Insulin and Insulin-Like Growth Factor-I Enhance Human Skeletal Muscle Protein Anabolism during Hyperaminoacidemia by Different Mechanisms," *Journal of Clinical Investigation* 96, no. 4 (1995): 1722-29. doi:10.1172/JCI118217; Robert A. Gelfand and Eugene J. Barrett, "Effect of Physiologic Hyperinsulinemia on Skeletal Muscle Protein Synthesis and Breakdown in Man," *Journal of Clinical Investigation* 80, no. 1 (1987): 1-6. doi:10.1172/JCI113033.

81. Scott C. Denne, Edward A. Liechty, Ya Mei Liu, Ginger Brechtel, and Alain D. Baron, "Proteolysis in Skeletal Muscle and Whole Body in Response to Euglycemic Hyperinsulinemia in Normal Adults," *Endocrinology and Metabolism* 261, no. 6 (1991): E809-E814.

82. Andrew Creer, Philip Gallagher, Dustin Slivka, Bozena Jemiolo, William Fink, and Scott Trappe, "Influence of Muscle Glycogen Availability on ERK1/2 and Akt Signaling after Resistance Exercise in Human Skeletal Muscle," *Journal of Applied Physiology* 99, no. 3 (2005): 950-56. doi: 10.1152/japplphysiol.00110.2005.

83. Amy R. Lane, Joseph W. Duke, and Anthony C. Hackney, "Influence of Dietary Carbohydrate Intake on the Free Testosterone: Cortisol Ratio Responses to Short-Term Intensive Exercise Training," *European Journal of Applied Physiology* 108, no. 6 (2010): 1125-31.

84. Lyonel Benjamin, Peter Blanpied, and Linda Lamont, "Dietary Carbohydrate and Protein Manipulation and Exercise Recovery in Novice Weight-Lifters," *Journal of Exercise Physiology* 12, no. 6 (2009).

85. Krista R. Howarth, Stuart M. Phillips, Maureen J. MacDonald, Douglas Richards, Natalie A. Moreau, and Martin J. Gibala, "Effect of Glycogen Availability on Human Skeletal Muscle Protein Turnover during Exercise and Recovery," *Journal of Applied Physiology* 109, no. 2 (2010): 431-38. doi: 10.1152/japplphysiol.00108.2009.

86. Rajiv Chowdhury, Samantha Warnakula, Setor Kunutsor, Francesca Crowe, Heather A. Ward, Laura Johnson, Oscar H. Franco, Adam S. Butterworth, Nita G. Forouhi, Simon G. Thompson, Kay-Tee Khaw, Dariush Mozaffarian, John Danesh, and Emanuele Di Angelantonio, "Association of Dietary, Circulating, and Supplement Fatty Acids With Coronary Risk: A Systematic Review and Meta-Analysis," *Annals of Internal Medicine* 160, no. 6 (2014): 398-406. doi: 10.7326/M13-1788.

87. "Dietary Guidelines—2010," U.S. Department of Agriculture, accessed October 17, 2014, http://www.cnpp.usda.gov/dgas2010-dgacreport.htm.

88. Nathalie T. Bendsen, Ryan Christensen, Else M. Bartels, and Arne Astrup, "Consumption of Industrial and Ruminant Trans Fatty Acids and Risk of Coronary Heart Disease: A Systematic Review and Meta-Analysis of Cohort Studies," *European Journal of Clinical Nutrition* 65, no. 7 (2011): 773-83. doi:10.1038/ejcn.2011.34; Michael Lefevre, Jennifer C. Lovejoy, Steven R. Smith, James P. DeLany, Catherine Champagne, Marlene M. Most, Yvonne Denkins, Lilian de Jonge, Jennifer Rood, and George A. Bray, "Comparison of the Acute Response to Meals Enriched with Cis- or Trans-Fatty Acids on Glucose and Lipids in Overweight Individuals with Differing FABP2 Genotypes," *Metabolism—Clinical and Experimental* 54, no. 12 (2005): 1652-58. doi: 10.1016/j.metabol.2005.06.015; Dariush Mozaffarian, Tobias Pischon, Susan E. Hankinson, Nader Rifai, Kaumudi Joshipura, Walter C. Willett, and Eric B. Rimm, "Dietary Intake of Trans Fatty Acids and Systemic Inflammation in Women," *American Journal of Clinical Nutrition* 79, no. 4 (2004): 606-12; Jana Vrbíková, Bela Bendlová, Martin Hill, Markéta Vanková, Karel Vondra, and Luboslav Stárka, "Insulin Sensitivity and β-Cell Function in Women With Polycystic Ovary Syndrome," *Diabetes Care* 25, no. 7 (2002): 1217-22. doi:10.2337/diacare.25.7.1217; Jorge Salmerón, Frank B. Hu, JoAnn E. Manson, Meir J. Stampfer, Graham A. Colditz, Eric B. Rimm, and Walter C. Willett, "Dietary Fat Intake and Risk of Type 2 Diabetes in Women," *American Journal of Clinical Nutrition* 73, no. 6 (2001): 1019-26.

89. Institute of Medicine, *Dietary Reference Intakes for Energy, Carbohydrate, Fiber, Fat, Fatty Acids, Cholesterol, Protein, and Amino Acids* (Washington, D.C.: National Academies Press, 2005).

90. Institute of Medicine, *Dietary Reference Intakes: Water, Potassium, Sodium, Chloride, and Sulfate* (Washington, D.C.: National Academies Press, 2005).

91. Natural Resources Defense Council, "What's On Tap? Grading Drinking Water in U.S. Cities," last revised June 11, 2003, http://www.nrdc.org/water/drinking/uscities/contents.asp.

92. Martin Wagner, Michael P. Schlüsener, Thomas A. Ternes, and Jörg Oehlmann, "Identification of Putative Steroid Receptor Antagonists in Bottled Water: Combining Bioassays and High-Resolution Mass Spectrometry," *PLOS One* 8, no. 8 (2013): e72472. doi: 10.1371/journal.pone.0072472.

93. *Ibid.*

94. Roddy Scheer and Doug Moss, "Dirt Poor: Have Fruits and Vegetables Become Less Nutritious?" *Scientific American*, April 27, 2011, accessed October 17, 2014, http://www.scientificamerican.com/article.cfm?id=soil-depletion-and-nutrition-loss.

95. "Getting Your Vitamins and Minerals Through Diet," *Harvard Women's Health Watch*, July 2009, accessed October 17, 2014, http://www.health.harvard.edu/newsletters/Harvard_Womens_Health_Watch/2009/July/Getting-your-vitamins-and-minerals-through-diet.

96. Centers for Disease Control, *Sodium: The Facts*, accessed October 17, 2014, http://www.cdc.gov/salt/pdfs/Sodium_Fact_Sheet.pdf.

97. Institute of Medicine, *Dietary Reference Intakes: Water, Potassium, Sodium, Chloride, and Sulfate* (Washington, D.C.: National Academies Press, 2005).

98. *Ibid.*

99. Joanne L. Slavin, "Dietary Fiber: Classification, Chemical Analyses, and Food Sources," *Journal of the American Dietetic Association* 87, no. 9 (1987): 1164-71.

100. Alison M. Stephen and John H. Cummings, "Mechanism of Action of Dietary Fibre in the Human Colon," *Nature* 284, no. 5753 (1980): 283-4; Alfredo A. Rabassa and Arvey Rogers, "The Role of Short-Chain Fatty Acid Metabolism in Colonic Disorders," *American Journal of Gastroenterology* 87, no. 4 (1992): 419-23.

101. Slavin, "Dietary Fiber: Classification, Chemical Analyses, and Food Sources," 1164-71.

102. Medical College of Georgia, "Scientists Learn More about How Roughage Keeps You 'Regular,'" *Science Daily*, accessed October 17, 2014, http://www.sciencedaily.com/releases/2006/08/060823093156.htm.

103. Fabio Levi, Cristina Pasche, Franca Lucchini, Liliane Chatenoud, David R. Jacobs Jr., and Carlo La Vecchia, "Refined and Whole Grain Cereals and the Risk of Oral, Oesophageal and Laryngeal Cancer," *European Journal of Clinical Nutrition* 54, no. 6 (2000): 487-89.

104. 213. Dagfinn Aune, Doris S. M. Chan, Darren C. Greenwood, Ana Rita Vieira, Deborah A. Navarro Rosenblatt, Rui Vieira, and Teresa Norat, "Dietary Fiber and Breast Cancer Risk: A Systematic Review and Meta-Analysis of Prospective Studies," *Annals of Oncology* 23, no. 6 (2012): 1394-1402. doi: 10.1093/annonc/r589.

105. "Leading Causes of Death," Centers for Disease Control and Prevention, last updated July 14, 2014, http://www.cdc.gov/nchs/fastats/leading-causes-of-death.htm.

106. Mark A. Pereira, Eilis O'Reilly, Katarina Augustsson, Gary E. Fraser, Uri Goldbourt, Berit L. Heitmann, Goran Hallmans, Paul Knekt, Simin Liu, Pirjo Pietinen, Donna Spiegelman, June Stevens, Jarmo Virtamo, Walter C. Willett, and Alberto Ascherio, "Dietary Fiber and Risk of Coronary Heart Disease," *Archives of Internal Medicine: A Pooled Analysis of Cohort Studies* 164, no. 4 (2004): 370-76. doi:10.1001/archinte.164.4.370.

107. Eric B. Rimm, Alberto Ascherio, Edward Giovannucci, Donna Spiegelman, Meir J. Stampfer, and Walter C. Willett, "Vegetable, Fruit, and Cereal Fiber Intake and Risk of Coronary Heart Disease Among Men," *JAMA* 275, no. 6 (1996): 447-51. doi:10.1001/jama.1996.03530300031036.

108. Lisa Brown, Bernard Rosner, Walter W. Willett, and Frank M. Sacks, "Cholesterol-Lowering Effects of Dietary Fiber: A Meta-Analysis," *American Journal of Clinical Nutrition* 69, no. 1 (1999): 30-42.

109. "Metabolic Syndrome," MedlinePlus, accessed October 17, 2014, http://www.nlm.nih.gov/medlineplus/metabolicsyndrome.html.

110. Nicola M. McKeown, James B. Meigs, Simin Liu, Edward Saltzman, Peter W. F. Wilson, and Paul F. Jacques, "Carbohydrate Nutrition, Insulin Resistance, and the Prevalence of the Metabolic Syndrome in the Framingham Offspring Cohort," *Diabetes Care* 27 no. 2 (2004): 538-46. doi: 10.2337/diacare.27.2.538.

111. Manisha Chandalia, Abhimanyu Garg, Dieter Lutjohann, Klaus von Bergmann, Scott M. Grundy, and Linda J. Brinkley, "Beneficial Effects of High Dietary Fiber Intake in Patients with Type 2 Diabetes Mellitus," *New England Journal of Medicine* 342 (May 11, 2000): 1392-98. doi: 10.1056/NEJM200005113421903; Lawrence J. Appel, Thomas J. Moore, Eva Obarzanek, William M. Vollmer, Laura P. Svetkey, Frank M. Sacks, George A. Bray, Thomas M. Vogt, Jeffrey A. Cutler, Marlene M. Windhauser, Pao-Hwa Lin, Njeri Karanja, Denise Simons-Morton, Marjorie McCullough, Janis Swain, Priscilla Steele, Marguerite A. Evans, Edgar R. Miller, and David W. Harsha, "A Clinical Trial of the Effects of Dietary Patterns on Blood Pressure," *New England Journal of Medicine* 336 (April 17, 1997): 1117-24. doi: 10.1056/NEJM199704173361601; Cynthia M. Ripsin, Joseph M. Keenan, David R. Jacobs Jr., Patricia J. Elmer, Robert R. Welch, Linda Van Horn, Kiang Liu, Wilfred H. Turnbull, Forrest W. Thye, Mark Kestin, Maren Hegsted, Dennis M. Davidson, Michael H. Davidson, Lynn D. Dugan, Wendy Demark-Wahnefried, and Stephanie Beling, "Oat Products and Lipid Lowering: A Meta-analysis," *JAMA* 267, no. 24 (1992): 3317-25. doi: 10.1001/jama.1992.03480240079039; June Stevens, "Does Dietary Fiber Affect Food Intake and Body Weight?" *Journal of American Dietetic Assocation* 88, no. 8 (1988): 939-42, 945.

112. Supriya Krishnan, Lynn Rosenberg, Martha Singer, Frank B. Hu, Luc Djoussé, L. Adrienne Cupples, and Julie R. Palmer, "Glycemic Index, Glycemic Load, and Cereal Fiber Intake and Risk of Type 2 Diabetes in US Black Women," *Archives of Internal Medicine* 167, no. 21 (2007): 2304-09. doi:10.1001/archinte.167.21.2304; Teresa T. Fung, Frank B. Hu, Mark A. Pereira, Simin Liu, Meir J. Stampfer, Graham A. Colditz, and Walter C. Willett, "Whole-Grain Intake and the Risk of Type 2 Diabetes: A Prospective Study in Men," *American Journal of Clinical Nutrition* 76, no. 3 (2002): 535-40.

113. Matthias B. Schulze, Simin Liu, Eric B. Rimm, JoAnn E. Manson, Walter C. Willett, and Frank B. Hu, "Glycemic Index, Glycemic Load, and Dietary Fiber Intake and Incidence of Type 2 Diabetes in Younger and Middle-Aged Women," *American Journal of Clinical Nutrition* 80, no. 2 (2004): 348-56; Simin Liu, Walter C. Willett, Meir J. Stampfer, Frank B. Hu, Mary Franz, Laura Sampson, Charles H. Hennekens, and JoAnn E. Manson, "A Prospective Study of Dietary Glycemic Load, Carbohydrate Intake, and Risk of Coronary Heart Disease in US Women," *American Journal of Clinical Nutrition* 71, no. 6 (2000): 1455-61.

114. Walid H. Aldoori, Edward L. Giovannucci, Helaine R. H. Rockett, Laura Sampson, Eric B. Rimm, and Walter C. Willett, "A Prospective Study of Dietary Fiber Types and Symptomatic Diverticular Disease in Men," *Journal of Nutrition* 128, no. 4 (1998): 714-19.

115. Yikyung Park, Amy F. Subar, Albert Hollenbeck, and Arthur Schatzkin, "Dietary Fiber Intake and Mortality in the NIH-AARP Diet and Health Study," *Archives of Internal Medicine* 171, no. 12 (2011): 1061-68. doi:10.1001/archinternmed.2011.18.

116. Institute of Medicine, *Dietary Reference Intakes for Energy, Carbohydrate, Fiber, Fat, Fatty Acids, Cholesterol, Protein, and Amino Acids* (Washington, D.C.: National Academies Press, 2005).

117. 21 C.F.R. § 101.9, also available at http://www.accessdata.fda.gov/scripts/cdrh/cfdocs/cfcfr/cfrsearch.cfm?fr=101.9.

CHAPTER 13

HOW TO MAXIMIZE YOUR GAINS WITH PRE- AND POST-WORKOUT NUTRITION

1. Jay R. Hoffman, Nicholas A. Ratamess, Christopher P. Tranchina, Stefanie L. Rashti, Jie Kang, and Avery D. Faigenbaum, "Effect of Protein-Supplement Timing on Strength, Power, and Body-Composition Changes in Resistance-Trained Men," *International Journal of Sport Nutrition and Exercise Metabolism* 19, no. 2 (2009): 172-85; Lex B. Verdijk, Richard A. M. Jonkers, Benjamin G. Gleeson, Milou Beelen, Kenneth Meijer, Hans H. C. M. Savelberg, Will K. W. H. Wodzig, Paul Dendale, and Luc J. C. van Loon, "Protein Supplementation before and after Exercise Does Not Further Augment Skeletal Muscle Hypertrophy after Resistance Training in Elderly Men," *American Journal of Clinical Nutrition* 89, no. 2 (2009): 608-16. doi: 10.3945/ajcn.2008.26626.

2. Louise M. Burke, John A. Hawley, Megan L. Ross, Daniel R. Moore, Stuart M. Phillips, Gary R. Slater, Trent Stellingwerff, Kevin D. Tipton, Andrew P. Garnham, and Vernon G. Coffey, "Preexercise Aminoacidemia and Muscle Protein Synthesis after Resistance Exercise," *Medicine and Science of Sports and Exercise* 44, no. 10 (2012): 1968-77. doi: 10.1249/MSS.0b013e31825d28fa; Kevin D. Tipton, Blake B. Rasmussen, Sharon L. Miller, Steven E. Wolf, Sharla K. Owens-Stovall, Bart E. Petrini, and Robert R. Wolfe, "Timing of Amino Acid-Carbohydrate Ingestion Alters Anabolic Response of Muscle to Resistance Exercise," *American Journal of Physiology—Endocrinology and Metabolism*, 281, no. 2 (2001): E197-E206.

3. Denise M. Surina, Wolfgang Langhans, Ruth Pauli, and Caspar Wenk, "Meal Composition Affects Postprandial Fatty Acid Oxidation," *American Journal of Physiology—Regulatory, Integrative and Comparative Physiology* 264, no. 6 (1993): R1065-70.

4. Kevin D. Tipton, Tabatha A. Elliott, Melanie G. Cree, Asle A. Aarsland, Arthur P. Sanford, and Robert R. Wolfe, "Stimulation of Net Muscle Protein Synthesis by Whey Protein Ingestion before and after Exercise," *American Journal of Physiology—Endocrinology and Metabolism* 292, no. 1 (2007): E71-E76. doi: 10.1152/ajpendo.00166.2006.

5. Martial Dangin, Yves Boirie, Clara Garcia-Rodenas, Pierre Gachon, Jacques Fauquant, Philippe Callier, Olivier Ballèvre, and Bernard Beaufrère, "The Digestion Rate of Protein Is an Independent Regulating Factor of Postprandial Protein Retention," *Endocrinology and Metabolism* 280, no. 2 (2001): E340-E348.

6. Yves Boirie, Martial Dangin, Pierre Gachon, Marie-Paule Vasson, Jean-Louis Maubois, and Bernard Beaufrère, "Slow and Fast Dietary Proteins Differently Modulate Postprandial Protein Accretion," *Proceedings of the National Academy of Sciences* 94, no. 26 (1997): 14930-35.

7. Sharon L. Miller and Robert R. Wolfe, "Physical Exercise as a Modulator of Adaptation to Low and High Carbohydrate and Low and High Fat Intakes," *European Journal of Clinical Nutrition* 53, no. S1 (1999): S112-19.

8. Kostas Tsintzas, Clyde Williams, Dumitru Constantin-Teodosiu, Eric Hultman, Leslie Boobis, and Paul Greenhaff, "Carbohydrate Ingestion prior to Exercise Augments the Exercise-Induced Activation of the Pyruvate Dehydrogenase Complex in Human Skeletal Muscle," *Experimental Physiology* 85, no. 5 (2000): 581-86; Satoshi Fujita, Hans C. Dreyer, Micah J. Drummond, Erin L. Glynn, Elena Volpi, and Blake B. Rasmussen, "Essential Amino Acid and Carbohydrate Ingestion before Resistance Exercise Does Not Enhance Postexercise Muscle Protein Synthesis," *Journal of Applied Physiology* 106, no. 5 (2009): 1730-39. doi: 10.1152/japplphysiol.90395.2008.

9. Luca Mondazzi and Enrico Arcelli, "Glycemic Index in Sport Nutrition," *Journal of the American College of Nutrition* 28, supplement 4 (2009): 455S-63S.

10. Raymond D. Starling, Todd A. Trappe, Allen C. Parcell, Chad G. Kerr, William J. Fink, and David L. Costill, "Effects of Diet on Muscle Triglyceride and Endurance Performance," *Journal of Applied Physiology* 82, no. 4 (1997): 1185-89.

11. Louise M. Burke, Damien J. Angus, Gregory R. Cox, Nicola K. Cummings, Mark A. Febbraio, Kathryn Gawthorn, John A. Hawley, Michelle Minehan, David T. Martin, and Mark Hargreaves, "Effect of Fat Adaptation and Carbohydrate Restoration on Metabolism and Performance during Prolonged Cycling," *Journal of Applied Physiology* 89, no. 6 (2000): 2413-21.

12. Mark Hargreaves, John A. Hawley, and Asker Jeukendrup, "Pre-Exercise Carbohydrate and Fat Ingestion: Effects on Metabolism and Performance," *Journal of Sports Sciences* 22, no. 1 (2004): 31-38. doi:10.1080/02640410310 00140536.

13. Vinod Kumar, Philip Atherton, Kenneth Smith, and Michael J. Rennie, "Human Muscle Protein Synthesis and Breakdown during and after Exercise," *Journal of Applied Physiology* 106, no. 6 (2009): 2026-39. doi: 10.1152/japplphysiol.91481.2008.

14. Hannu T. Pitkanen, Tarja Nykanen, Juha Knuutinen, Kaisa Lahti, Olavi Keinanen, Marrku Alen, Paavo V. Komi, and Antti A. Mero, "Free Amino Acid Pool and Muscle Protein Balance after Resistance Exercise," *Medicine and Science of Sports and Exercise* 35, no. 5 (2003): 784-92.

15. Kevin D. Tipton, Arny A. Ferrando, Stuart M. Phillips, David Doyle Jr., and Robert R. Wolfe, "Postexercise Net Protein Synthesis in Human Muscle from Orally Administered Amino Acids," *American Journal of Physiology—Endocrinology and Metabolism* 276, no. 4 (1999): E628-34.

16. G. Biolo, Kevin D. Tipton, S. Klein, and Robert R. Wolfe, "An Abundant Supply of Amino Acids Enhances the Metabolic Effect of Exercise on Muscle Protein," *American Journal of Physiology—Endocrinology and Metabolism* 273, no. 1 (1997): E122-29.

17. Birgitte Esmarck, Jesper L. Andersen, Steen Olsen, Erik A. Richter, Masashi Mizuno, and Michael Kjær, "Timing of Postexercise Protein Intake Is Important for Muscle Hypertrophy with Resistance Training in Elderly Humans," *The Journal of Physiology* 535, pt. 1 (2001): 301-11. doi: 10.1111/j.1469-7793.2001.00301.x.

18. Paul J. Cribb and Alan Hayes, "Effects of Supplement Timing and Resistance Exercise on Skeletal Muscle Hypertrophy," *Medicine and Science of Sports and Exercise* 38, no. 11 (2006): 1918-25. doi: 10.1249/01.mss.0000233790.08788.3e.

19. Daniel R. Moore, Meghann J. Robinson, Jessica L. Fry, Jason E. Tang, Elisa I. Glover, Sarah B. Wilkinson, Todd Prior, Mark A. Tarnopolsky, and Stuart M. Phillips, "Ingested Protein Dose Response of Muscle and Albumin Protein Synthesis after Resistance Exercise in Young Men," *American Journal of Clinical Nutrition* 89, no. 1 (2009): 161-68. doi: 10.3945/ajcn.2008.26401.

20. Peter W. Lemon, "Beyond the Zone: Protein Needs of Active Individuals," *Journal of the American College of Nutrition* 19, no. S5 (2000): 513S-21S.

21. Wayne W. Campbell, Todd A. Trappe, Robert R. Wolfe, and William J. Evans, "The Recommended Dietary Allowance for Protein May Not Be Adequate for Older People to Maintain Skeletal Muscle," *Journal of Gerontology: Biological Sciences and Medical Sciences*, 56 no. 6 (2001): M373-80.

22. David L. Russell-Jones and A. Margot Umpleby, "The Hormonal Control of Protein Metabolism," *Baillière's Clinical Endocrinology and Metabolism* 10, no. 4 (1996): 551-70.

23. Jens Juel Christiansen, Christian B. Djurhuus, Claus H. Gravholt, Per Iversen, Jens Sandahl Christiansen, Ole Schmitz, Jørgen Weeke, Jens Otto Lunde Jørgensen, and Niels Møller, "Effects of Cortisol on Carbohydrate, Lipid, and Protein Metabolism: Studies of Acute Cortisol Withdrawal in Adrenocortical Failure," *Journal of Clinical Endocrinology and Metabolism* 92, no. 9 (2007): 3553-59. doi: 10.1210/jc.2007-0445.

24. René Koopman, Anton J. M. Wagenmakers, Ralph J. F. Manders, Antoine H. G. Zorenc, Joan M. G. Senden, Marchel Gorselink, Hans A. Keizer, and Luc J. C. van Loon, "Combined Ingestion of Protein and Free Leucine with Carbohydrate Increases Postexercise Muscle Protein Synthesis in Vivo in Male Subjects," *American Journal of Physiology—Endocrinology and Metabolism* 288, no. 4 (2005): E645-53. doi: 10.1152/ajpendo.00413.2004.

25. Robert A. Gelfand and Eugene J. Barrett, "Effect of Physiologic Hyperinsulinemia on Skeletal Muscle Protein Synthesis and Breakdown in Man," *Journal of Clinical Investigation* 80, no. 1 (1987): 1-6. doi:10.1172/JCI113033.

26. Scott C. Denne, Edward A. Liechty, Ya Mei Liu, Ginger Brechtel, and Alain D. Baron, "Proteolysis in Skeletal Muscle and Whole Body in Response to Euglycemic Hyperinsulinemia in Normal Adults," *Endocrinology and Metabolism* 261, no. 6 (1991): E809-E814.

27. Krista R. Howarth, Stuart M. Phillips, Maureen J. MacDonald, Douglas Richards, Natalie A. Moreau, and Martin J. Gibala, "Effect of Glycogen Availability on Human Skeletal Muscle Protein Turnover during Exercise and Recovery," *Journal of Applied Physiology* 109, no. 2 (2010): 431-38. doi: 10.1152/japplphysiol.00108.2009.

28. Paul L. Greenhaff, Leonidas G. Karagounis, Nick Peirce, Elizabeth J. Simpson, Matthew Hazell, Robert Layfield, Henning Wackerhage, Kenneth Smith, Pamela Atherton, Anna Selby, and Michael J. Rennie, "Disassociation between the Effects of Amino Acids and Insulin on Signaling, Ubiquitin Ligases, and Protein Turnover in Human Muscle," *American Journal of Physiology—Endocrinology and Metabolism* 295, no. 3 (2008): E595-E604. doi: 10.1152/ajpendo.90411.2008.

29. Orla Power, Aine Hallihan, and Philip Jakeman, "Human Insulinotropic Response to Oral Ingestion of Native and Hydrolysed Whey Protein," *Amino Acids* 37, no. 2 (2009): 333-39. doi: 10.1007/s00726-008-0156-0.

30. Brunella Capaldo, Amalia Gastaldelli, Salvatore Antoniello, Maria Auletta, Francesco Pardo, Demetrio Ciociaro, Raffaele Guida, Ele Ferrannini, and Luigi Saccà, "Splanchnic and Leg Substrate Exchange after Ingestion of a Natural Mixed Meal in Humans," *Diabetes* 48, no. 5 (1999): 958-66. doi: 10.2337/diabetes.48.5.958.

31. Sharon L. Miller and Robert R. Wolfe, "Physical Exercise as a Modulator of Adaptation to Low and High Carbohydrate and Low and High Fat Intakes," *European Journal of Clinical Nutrition* 53, no. S1 (1999): S112-19; Howarth, et al. "Effect of Glycogen Availability on Human Skeletal Muscle Protein Turnover during Exercise and Recovery," 431-38.

32. Robert A. Robergs, David R. Pearson, David L. Costill, William J. Fink, David D. Pascoe, Michael A. Benedict, Charles P. Lambert, and Jeffrey J. Zachweija, "Muscle Glycogenolysis during Differing Intensities of Weight-Resistance Exercise," *Journal of Applied Physiology* 70, no. 4 (1991): 1700-06; J. L. Ivy, "Glycogen Resynthesis after Exercise: Effect of Carbohydrate Intake," *International Journal of Sports Medicine* 19, no. S2 (1998): S142-45. doi: 10.1055/s-2007-971981.

33. *Ibid.*

34. *Ibid.*

CHAPTER 14
BUILD THE BODY YOU WANT EATING THE FOODS YOU LOVE THE BIGGER LEANER STRONGER "DIET"

1. Sophie B. P. Chargé and Michael A. Rudnicki, "Cellular and Molecular Regulation of Muscle Regeneration," *Physiological Reviews* 84, no. 1 (2004). doi: 10.1152/physrev.00019.2003.

2. Ivan Bautmans, Katrien Van Puyvelde, and Tony Mets, "Sarcopenia and Functional Decline: Pathophysiology, Prevention and Therapy," *Acta Clinica Belgica* 64, no. 4 (2009): 303-16.

3. Blake B. Rasmussen and Stuart M. Phillips, "Contractile and Nutritional Regulation of Human Muscle Growth," *Exercise Sport Sciences Reviews* 31, no. 3 (2003): 127-31.

4. Roberto Cangemi, Alberto J. Friedmann, John O. Holloszy, and Luigi Fontana, "Long-Term Effects of Calorie Restriction on Serum Sex-Hormone Concentrations in Men," *Aging Cell* 9, no. 2 (2010): 236-42. doi: 10.1111/j.1474-9726.2010.00553.x; Stefan M. Pasiakos, Lisa M. Vislocky, John W. Carbone, Nicholas Altieri, Karen Konopelski, Hedley C. Freake, Jeffrey M. Anderson, Arny A. Ferrando, Robert R. Wolfe, and Nancy R. Rodriguez, "Acute Energy Deprivation Affects Skeletal Muscle Protein Synthesis and Associated Intracellular Signaling Proteins in Physically Active Adults," *Journal of Nutrition* 140, no. 4 (2010): 745-51. doi: 10.3945/jn.109.118372.

5. Eric R. Helms, Caryn Zinn, David S. Rowlands, and Scott R. Brown, "A Systematic Review of Dietary Protein during Caloric Restriction in Resistance Trained Lean Athletes: A Case for Higher Intakes," *International Journal of Sport Nutrition and Exercise Metabolism* 24, no. 2 (2014): 127-38. doi: 10.1123/ijsnem.2013-0054; Jo C. Bruusgaard, Ingun B. Johansen, Ingrid M. Egner, Zaheer A. Rana, and Kristian Gundersen, "Myonuclei Acquired by Overload Exercise Precede Hypertrophy and Are Not Lost on Detraining," *Proceedings of the National Academy of Sciences* 107, no. 34 (2009): 15111–16. doi: 10.1073/pnas.0913935107.

6. David J. Dyck, George J. F. Heigenhauser, and Clinton R. Bruce, "The Role of Adipokines as Regulators of Skeletal Muscle Fatty Acid Metabolism and Insulin Sensitivity," *Acta Physiologica* 186, no. 1 (2006): 5-16.

7. Jin Zhang, Christopher J. Hupfeld, Susan S. Taylor, Jerrold M. Olefsky, and Roger Y. Tsien, "Insulin Disrupts Bold Beta-Adrenergic Signalling to Protein Kinase A in Adipocytes," *Nature* 437, no. 7058 (2005): 569-73. doi:10.1038/nature04140.

8. Xiaonan Wang, Zhaoyong Hu, Junping Hu, Jie Du, and William E. Mitch, "Insulin Resistance Accelerates Muscle Protein Degradation: Activation of the Ubiquitin-Proteasome Pathway by Defects in Muscle Cell Signaling," *Endocrinology* 147, no. 9 (2006): 4160-68. doi: 10.1210/en.2006-0251.

9. Sabine Rohrmann, Meredith S. Shiels, David S. Lopez, Nader Rifai, William G. Nelson, Norma Kanarek, Eliseo Guallar, Andy Menke, Corinne E. Joshu, Manning Feinleib, Siobhan Sutcliffe, and Elizabeth A. Platz, "Body Fatness and Sex Steroid Hormone Concentrations in US Men: Results from NHANES III," *Cancer Causes and Control* 22, no. 8 (2011): 1141-51. doi: 10.1007/s10552-011-9790-z.

10. Sylvia Santosa and Michael D. Jensen, "Adipocyte Fatty Acid Storage Factors Enhance Subcutaneous Fat Storage in Postmenopausal Women," *Diabetes* 62, no. 3 (2013): 775-82. doi: 10.2337/db12-0912.

11. Raphaëlle L. Santarellia, Fabrice Pierrea, and Denis E. Corpeta, "Processed Meat and Colorectal Cancer: A Review of Epidemiologic and Experimental Evidence," *Nutrition and Cancer* 60, no. 2 (2008): 131-44. doi:10.1080/01635580701684872.

12. Darren M. Opland, Gina M. Leinninger, and Martin G. Myers Jr., "Modulation of the Mesolimbic Dopamine System by Leptin," *Brain Research* 1350 (September 2, 2010): 65-70. doi:10.1016/j.brainres.2010.04.028.

13. Harvey L. Katzeff, Maureen O'Connell, Edward S. Horton, Elliot Danforth Jr., James B. Young, and Lewis Landsberg, "Metabolic Studies in Human Obesity during Overnutrition and Undernutrition: Thermogenic and Hormonal Responses to Norepinephrine," *Metabolism* 35, no. 2 (1986): 166-75.

14. Jon F. Davis, Derrick L. Choi, and Stephen C. Benoit, "Insulin, Leptin and Reward," *Trends in Endocrinology and Metabolism* 21, no. 2 (2010): 68-74. doi: 10.1016/j.tem.2009.08.004; Jon F. Davis, "Adipostatic Regulation of Motivation and Emotion," *Discovery Medicine* 9, no. 48 (2010): 462-67; Gary J. Hausman and C. Richard Barb, "Adipose Tissue and the Reproductive Axis: Biological Aspects," *Endocrine Development* 19 (2010): 31-44. doi:10.1159/000316895.

15. Eric Jéquier, "Leptin Signaling, Adiposity, and Energy Balance," *Annals of the New York Academy of Sciences* 967, no. 1 (2002): 379-88. doi: 10.1111/j.1749-6632.2002.tb04293.x.

16. Rolando B. Ceddia, "Direct Metabolic Regulation in Skeletal Muscle and Fat Tissue by Leptin: Implications for Glucose and Fatty Acids Homeostasis," *International Journal of Obesity* 29, 1175-83 (2005). doi:10.1038/sj.ijo.0803025.

17. Mirjam Dirlewanger, Véronique di Vetta, Eliane Guenat, P. Battilana, Gérald Seematter, Philippe Schneiter, Eric Jéquier, and Luc Tappy, "Effects of Short-Term Carbohydrate or Fat Overfeeding on Energy Expenditure and Plasma Leptin Concentrations in Healthy Female Subjects," *International Journal of Obesity* 24, no. 11 (2000): 1413-18; George A. Bray, Steven R. Smith, Lilian de Jonge, Hui Xie, Jennifer Rood, Corby K. Martin, Marlene Most, Courtney Brock, Susan Mancuso, and Leanne M. Redman, "Effect of Dietary Protein Content on Weight Gain, Energy Expenditure, and Body Composition during Overeating: A Randomized Controlled Trial," *JAMA* 307 no. 1 (2012): 47-55. doi: 10.1001/jama.2011.1918; Peter J. Havel, Raymond Townsend, Leslie Chaump, and Karen Teff, "High-Fat Meals Reduce 24-h Circulating Leptin Concentrations in Women," *Diabetes* 48, no. 2 (1999): 334-41. doi: 10.2337/diabetes.48.2.334; Sven Röjdmark, Jan Calissendorff, and Kerstin Brismar, "Alcohol Ingestion Decreases Both Diurnal and Nocturnal Secretion of Leptin in Healthy Individuals," *Clinical Endocrinology* 55.5 (2001): 639-47.

18. John J. Shelmet, George A. Reichard, Charles L. Skutches, Robert D. Hoeldtke, Oliver E. Owen, and Guenther Boden, "Ethanol Causes Acute Inhibition of Carbohydrate, Fat, and Protein Oxidation and Insulin Resistance," *Journal of Clinical Investigation* 81, no. 4 (1988): 1137-45. doi:10.1172/JCI113428.

CHAPTER 15
HOW TO EAT HEALTHY FOODS ON A BUDGET

1. Anna Yukhananov, "Eating Healthy Food Costs More Money in U.S.," *Reuters*, August 4, 2011, accessed October 17, 2014, http://www.reuters.com/article/2011/08/04/us-food-costs-idUSTRE7734L620110804.

2. Sabine Rohrmann, Kim Overvad, H. Bas Bueno-de-Mesquita, Marianne U. Jakobsen, Rikke Egeberg, Anne Tjønneland, Laura Nailler, Marie-Christine Boutron-Ruault, Françoise Clavel-Chapelon, Vittorio Krogh, Domenico Palli, Salvatore Panico, Rosario Tumino, Fulvio Ricceri, Manuela M. Bergmann, Heiner Boeing, Kuanrong Li, Rudolf Kaaks, Kay-Tee Khaw, Nicholas J. Wareham, Francesca L. Crowe, Timothy J. Key, Androniki Naska, Antonia Trichopoulou, Dimitirios Trichopoulos, Max Leenders, Petra H. M. Peeters, Dagrun Engeset, Christine L. Parr, Guri Skeie, Paula Jakszyn, María-José Sánchez, José M. Huerta, M. Luisa Redondo, Aurelio

Barricarte, Pilar Amiano, Isabel Drake, Emily Sonestedt, Göran Hallmans, Ingegerd Johansson, Veronika Fedirko, Isabelle Romieux, Pietro Ferrari, Teresa Norat, Anne C. Vergnaud, Elio Riboli, and Jakob Linseisen, "Meat Consumption and Mortality—Results from the European Prospective Investigation into Cancer and Nutrition," *BMC Medicine* 11 (2013): 63. doi:10.1186/1741-7015-11-63.

3.   Hyun-Jeong Cho, Hye-Seon Ham, Dong-Seok Lee, and Hwa-Jin Park, "Effects of Proteins from Hen Egg Yolk on Human Platelet Aggregation and Blood Coagulation," *Biological and Pharmaceutical Bulletin* 26 No. 10 (2003): 1388-92. doi:10.1248/bpb.26.138; Elizabeth F. Goodrow, Thomas A. Wilson, Susan Crocker Houde, Rohini Vishwanathan, Patrick A. Scollin, Garry Handelman, and Robert J. Nicolosi, "Consumption of One Egg Per Day Increases Serum Lutein and Zeaxanthin Concentrations in Older Adults without Altering Serum Lipid and Lipoprotein Cholesterol Concentrations," *Journal of Nutrition* 136, no. 10 (2006): 2519-24.

4.   Frank B. Hu, Meir J. Stampfer, Eric B. Rimm, JoAnn E. Manson, Alberto Ascherio, Graham A. Colditz, Bernard A. Rosner, Donna Spiegelman, Frank E. Speizer, Frank M. Sacks, Charles H. Hennekens, and Walter C. Willett, "A Prospective Study of Egg Consumption and Risk of Cardiovascular Disease in Men and Women," *JAMA* 281, no. 15 (1999): 1387-94. doi:10.1001/jama.281.15.1387; Gisella Mutungi, Joseph Ratliff, Michael Puglisi, Moises Torres-Gonzalez, Ushma Vaishnav, Jose O. Leite, Erin Quann, Jeff S. Volek, and Maria Luz Fernandez," Dietary Cholesterol from Eggs Increases Plasma HDL Cholesterol in Overweight Men Consuming a Carbohydrate-Restricted Diet, *Journal of Nutrition* 138, no. 2 (2008): 272-76.

5.   Alison Kamil and C.-Y. Oliver Chen, "Health Benefits of Almonds beyond Cholesterol Reduction," *Journal of Agricultural and Food Chemistry* 60, no. 27 (2012): 6694-02. doi: 10.1021/jf2044795; Richard D. Mattes, Penny M. Kris-Etherton, and Gary D. Foster, "Impact of Peanuts and Tree Nuts on Body Weight and Healthy Weight Loss in Adults," *Journal of Nutrition* 138, no. 9 (2008): 1741S-1745S.

6.   Vikkie A. Mustad, Terry D. Etherton, Allen D. Cooper, Andrea M. Mastro, Thomas A. Pearson, Satya S. Jonnalagadda, and Penny M. Kris-Etherton, "Reducing Saturated Fat Intake Is Associated with Increased Levels of LDL Receptors on Mononuclear Cells in Healthy Men and Women," *Journal of Lipid Research* 38, no. 3 (1997): 459-68.

7.   William C. Stanley, Erinne R. Dabkowski, Rogerio F. Ribeiro Jr., and Kelly A. O'Connell, "Dietary Fat and Heart Failure: Moving From Lipotoxicity to Lipoprotection," *Circulation Research* 110, no. 5: 764-76 (2010). doi: 10.1161/CIRCRESAHA.111.253104; Tina Sartorius, Caroline Ketterer, Stephanie Kullmann, Michelle Balzer, Carola Rotermund, Sonja Binder, Manfred Hallschmid, Jürgen Machann, Fritz Schick, Veronika Somoza, Hubert Preissl, Andreas Fritsche, Hans-Ulrich Häring, and Anita M. Hennige, "Monounsaturated Fatty Acids Prevent the Aversive Effects of Obesity on Locomotion, Brain Activity, and Sleep Behavior," *Diabetes* 61, no. 7 (2012): 1669-79. doi: 10.2337/db11-1521.

8.   Rajkumar Paul, Paresh Kulkarni, and N. Vijaya Ganesh, "Avocado Fruit (*Persea americana Mill*) Exhibits Chemo-Protective Potentiality against Cyclophosphamide Induced Genotoxicity in Human Lymphocyte Culture," *Journal of Experimental Therapeutics and Oncology* 9, no. 3 (2011): 221-30.

9.   David S. Ludwig, Joseph A. Majzoub, Ahmad Al-Zahrani, Gerard E. Dallal, Isaac Blanco, and Susan B. Roberts, "High Glycemic Index Foods, Overeating, and Obesity," *Pediatrics* 103, no. 3 (1999): e26. doi: 10.1542/peds.103.3.e26.

10.   Alan W. Barclay, Peter Petocz, Joanna McMillan-Price, Victoria M. Flood, Tania Prvan, Paul Mitchell, and Jennie C. Brand-Miller, "Glycemic Index, Glycemic Load, and Chronic Disease Risk—A Meta-Analysis of Observational Studies," *American Journal of Clinical Nutrition* 87, no. 3 (2008): 627-37.

11.   Thomas M. S. Wolever, Susan M. Tosh, Alison L. Gibbs, Jennie Brand-Miller, Alison M. Duncan, Valerie Hart, Benoît Lamarche, Barbara A. Thomson, Ruedi Duss, and Peter J. Wood, "Physicochemical Properties of Oat β-glucan Influence Its Ability to Reduce Serum LDL Cholesterol in Humans: A Randomized Clinical Trial," *American Journal of Clinical Nutrition* 92, no. 4 (2010): 723-32. doi: 10.3945/ajcn.2010.29174.

12.   Laura Gabriela Sánchez-Lozada, MyPhuong Le, Mark Segal, and Richard J. Johnson, "How Safe Is Fructose for Persons with or without Diabetes?" *American Journal of Clinical Nutrition* 88, no. 55 (2008): 1189-90. doi: 10.3945/ajcn.2008.26812.

CHAPTER 16
THE BIGGER LEANER STRONGER TRAINING PHILOSOPHY

1.   Shane Schwanbeck, Philip D. Chilibeck, and Gordon Binsted, "A Comparison of Free Weight Squat to Smith Machine Squat Using Electromyography," *Journal of Strength and Conditioning Research* 23, no. 9 (2009): 2588-

91. doi: 10.1519/JSC.0b013e3181b1b181; Evan E. Schick, Jared W. Coburn, Lee E. Brown, Daniel A. Judelson, Andy V. Khamoui, Thanh Tam Tran, and Brandon P. Uribe, "A Comparison of Muscle Activation between a Smith Machine and Free Weight Bench Press," *Journal of Strength and Conditioning Research*, 24, no. 3 (2010): 779-84. doi: 10.1519/JSC.0b013e3181cc2237.

2.   Mathias Wernbom, Jesper Augustsson, and Roland Thomeé, "The Influence of Frequency, Intensity, Volume and Mode of Strength Training on Whole Muscle Cross-Sectional Area in Humans," *Sports Medicine* 37, no. 3 (2007): 225-64.

3.   William J. Kraemer, Kent Adams, Enzo Cafarelli, Gary A. Dudley, Cathryn Dooly, Matthew S. Feigenbaum, Steven J. Fleck, Barry Franklin, Andrew C. Fry, Jay R. Hoffman, Robert U. Newton, Jeffrey Potteiger, Michael H. Stone, Nicholas A. Ratamess, and Travis Triplett-McBride, "American College of Sports Medicine Position Stand: Progression Models in Resistance Training for Healthy Adults," *Medicine and Science in Sports and Exercise*, 41, no. 3 (2009): 687-708. doi: 10.1249/MSS.0b013e3181915670.

4.   Matthew R. Rhea, Brent A. Alvar, Lee N. Burkett, and Stephen D. Ball, "A Meta-Analysis to Determine the Dose Response for Strength Development," *Medicine and Science in Sports and Exercise* 35, no. 3 (2003): 456-64.

5.   Gerson E. Campos, Thomas J. Luecke, Heather K. Wendeln, Kumika Toma, Fredrick C. Hagerman, Thomas F. Murray, Kerry E. Ragg, Nicholas A. Ratamess, William J. Kraemer, and Robert S. Staron, "Muscular Adaptations in Response to Three Different Resistance-Training Regimens: Specificity of Repetition Maximum Training Zones," *European Journal of Applied Physiology* 88, no. 1-2 (2002): 50-60.

6.   Tácito P. Souza-Junior, Jeffrey M. Willardson, Richard Bloomer, Richard D. Leite, Steven J. Fleck, Paulo R. Oliveira, and Roberto Simão, "Strength and Hypertrophy Responses to Constant and Decreasing Rest Intervals in Trained Men Using Creatine Supplementation," *Journal of the International Society of Sports Nutrition* 8, no. 1 (2011): 17. doi: 10.1186/1550-2783-8-17.

7.   Robert Buresh, Kris Berg, and Jeffrey French, "The Effect of Resistive Exercise Rest Interval on Hormonal Response, Strength, and Hypertrophy with Training," *Journal of Strength and Conditioning Research* 23, no. 1 (2009): 62-71. doi: 10.1519/JSC.0b013e318185f14a.

8.   Belmiro Freitas de Salles, Roberto Simão, Fabrício Miranda, Jefferson da Silva Novaes, Adriana Lemos, and Jeffrey M. Willardson, "Rest Interval between Sets in Strength Training," *Sports Medicine* 39, no. 9 (2009): 765-77. doi: 10.2165/11315230-000000000-00000.

9.   Jeffrey M. Willardson and Lee N. Burkett, "The Effect of Different Rest Intervals between Sets on Volume Components and Strength Gains," *Journal of Strength and Conditioning Research* 22, no. 1 (2008): 146-52. doi: 10.1519/JSC.0b013e31815f912d.

10. Jeffrey M. Willardson and Lee N. Burkett, "The Effect of Rest Interval Length on Bench Press Performance with Heavy vs. Light Loads," *Journal of Strength and Conditioning Research* 20, no. 2 (2006): 396-99.

11. Jeffrey B. Kreher and Jennifer B. Schwartz, "Overtraining Syndrome," *Sports Health* 4, no. 2 (2012): 128-38. doi: 10.1177/1941738111434406.

12. Alan St. Clair Gibson, Michael I. Lambert, and Timothy D. Noakes, "Neural Control of Force Output during Maximal and Submaximal Exercise," *Sports Medicine* 31, no. 9 (2001): 637-50. doi: 10.2165/00007256-200131090-00001.

13. Gary A. Sforzo, Beth G. McManis, Dennis Black, D. Luniewski, and Kent Scriber, "Resilience to Exercise Detraining in Healthy Older Adults," *Journal of the American Geriatrics Society* 43, no. 3 (1995): 209-15.

14. Samuel A. Headley, Kelley Henry, Bradley C. Nindl, Brian A. Thompson, William J. Kraemer, and Margaret T. Jones, "Effects of Lifting Tempo on One Repetition Maximum and Hormonal Responses to a Bench Press Protocol," *Journal of Strength Conditioning Research*, 25, no. 2 (2011): 406-13. doi: 10.1519/JSC.0b013e3181bf053b.

15. Disa L. Hatfield, William J. Kraemer, Barry A. Spiering, Keijo Häkkinen, Jeff S. Volek, Tomoko Shimano, Luuk P. Spreuwenberg, Ricardo Silvestre, Jakob L. Vingren, Maren S. Fragala, Ana L. Gómez, Steven J. Fleck, Robert U. Newton, and Carl M. Maresh, "The Impact of Velocity of Movement on Performance Factors in Resistance Exercise," *Journal of Strength and Conditioning Research* 20, no. 4 (2006): 760-66; Alfred L. Goldberg, Joseph D. Etlinger, David F. Goldspink, and Charles Jablecki, "Mechanism of Work-Induced Hypertrophy of Skeletal Muscle," *Medicine and Science in Sports* 7, no. 3 (1975): 185-98.

16. Joanne Munn, Robert D. Herbert, Mark J. Hancock, and Simon C. Gandevia, "Resistance Training for Strength: Effect of Number of Sets and Contraction Speed," *Medicine and Science of Sports and Exercise* 37, no. 9 (2005): 1622-26.

17. Hatfield, et al. "The Impact of Velocity of Movement on Performance Factors in Resistance Exercise," 760-66.

18. Christopher M. Neils, Brian E. Udermann, Glenn A. Brice, Jason B. Winchester, and Michael R. McGuigan, "Influence of Contraction Velocity in Untrained Individuals over the Initial Early Phase of Resistance Training," *Journal of Strength and Conditioning Research* 19, no. 4 (2005): 883-87.

19. Eonho Kim, Alexis Dear, Steven L. Ferguson, Dongil Seo, and Michael G. Bemben, "Effects of 4 Weeks of Traditional Resistance Training vs. Superslow Strength Training on Early Phase Adaptations in Strength, Flexibility, and Aerobic Capacity in College-Aged Women," *Journal of Strength and Conditioning Research* 25, no. 11 (2011): 3006-13. doi: 10.1519/JSC.0b013e318212e3a2.

20. Riana R. Pryor, Gary A. Sforzo, and Daniel L. King, "Optimizing Power Output by Varying Repetition Tempo," *Journal of Strength and Conditioning Research*, 25, no. 11 (2005): 3029-34. doi: 10.1519/JSC.0b013e31820f50cb.

21. Said Ahmaidi, Phillipe Granier, Z. Taoutaou, Jacques Mercier, Hervé Dubouchaud, and Christian Préfaut, "Effects of Active Recovery on Plasma Lactate and Anaerobic Power Following Repeated Intensive Exercise," *Medicine and Science of Sports and Exercise* 28, no. 4 (1996): 450-56.

22. Christian Frøsig and Erik A. Richter, "Improved Insulin Sensitivity after Exercise: Focus on Insulin Signaling," *Obesity* 17, no. S3: S15-S20. doi: 10.1038/oby.2009.383; John J. Dubé, Katelyn Fleishman, Valentin Rousson, Bret H. Goodpaster, and Francesca Amati, "Exercise Dose and Insulin Sensitivity: Relevance for Diabetes Prevention," *Medicine and Science of Sports and Exercise* 44, no. 5 (2012): 793-9. doi: 10.1249/MSS.0b013e31823f679f.

23. David J. Brillon, Baohui Zheng, Robert G. Campbell, and Dwight E. Matthews, "Effect of Cortisol on Energy Expenditure and Amino Acid Metabolism in Humans," *American Journal of Physiology—Endocrinology and Metabolism* 268, no. 3 (1995): E501-13.

24. Edward L. Melanson, Paul S. MacLean, and James O. Hill, "Exercise Improves Fat Metabolism in Muscle But Does Not Increase 24-h Fat Oxidation," *Exercise and Sport Sciences Reviews* 37, no. 2 (2009): 93-101. doi: 10.1097/JES.0b013e31819c2f0b.

25. Jeffrey C. Gergley, "Comparison of Two Lower-Body Modes of Endurance Training on Lower-Body Strength Development While Concurrently Training," *Journal of Strength Conditioning Research* 23, no. 3 (2009): 979-87. doi: 10.1519/JSC.0b013e3181a0629d.

26. John P. McCarthy, Myron A. Pozniak, and James C. Agre, "Neuromuscular Adaptations to Concurrent Strength and Endurance Training," *Medicine and Science of Sports and Exercise* 34, no. 3 (2002): 511-19.

27. Rebecca E. Macpherson, Tom J. Hazell, T. Dylan Olver, Don H. Paterson, and Peter W. Lemon, "Run Sprint Interval Training Improves Aerobic Performance But Not Maximal Cardiac Output," *Medicine and Science of Sports and Exercise*, 43, no. 1 (2011): 115-22. doi: 10.1249/MSS.0b013e3181e5eacd.

28. Angelo Tremblay, Jean-Aimé Simoneau, and Claude Bouchard, "Impact of Exercise Intensity on Body Fatness and Skeletal Muscle Metabolism," *Metabolism* 43, no. 7 (1994): 814-18. doi: 10.1016/0026-0495(94)90259-3; Jeffrey W. King, "A Comparison of the Effects of Interval Training vs. Continuous Training on Weight Loss and Body Composition in Obese Pre-Menopausal Women" (Thesis, East Tennessee State University, 2001), http://static.ow.ly/docs/Interval Training v Continuous Training_5gS.pdf; Margarita S. Treuth, Gary R. Hunter, and Michael Williams, "Effects of Exercise Intensity on 24-h Energy Expenditure and Substrate Oxidation," *Medicine and Science of Sports and Exercise* 28, no. 9 (1996): 1138-43; E. Gail Trapp, Donald J. Chisholm, Judith Freund, and Stephen H. Boutcher, "The Effects of High-Intensity Intermittent Exercise Training on Fat Loss and Fasting Insulin Levels of Young Women," *International Journal of Obesity* 32, no. 4 (2008): 684-691. doi:10.1038/sj.ijo.0803781.

29. Stephen H. Boutcher, "High-Intensity Intermittent Exercise and Fat Loss," *Journal of Obesity* 2011 (2011). doi: 10.1155/2011/868305.

30. Jeffrey C. Gergley, "Comparison of Two Lower-Body Modes of Endurance Training on Lower-Body Strength Development While Concurrently Training," *Journal of Strength Conditioning Research* 23, no. 3 (2009): 979-87. doi: 10.1519/JSC.0b013e3181a0629d.

31. John A. Hawley, "Molecular Responses to Strength and Endurance Training: Are They Incompatible?" *Applied Physiology, Nutrition, and Metabolism*, 34, no. 3 (2009): 355-61. doi: 10.1139/H09-023.

32. Gustavo A. Nader, "Concurrent Strength and Endurance Training: From Molecules to Man," *Medicine and Science of Sports and Exercise* 38, no. 11 (2006): 1965-70; Michael Leveritt, Peter J. Abernethy, Benjamin K. Barry, and Peter A. Logan, "Concurrent Strength and Endurance Training. A Review," *Sports Medicine* 28, no. 6 (1999): 413-27; Keijo Häkkinen, Markku Alen, William J. Kraemer, Esteban Gorostiaga, Mikel Izquierdo, Heikki

Rusko, Jussi Mikkola, Arja Häkkinen, Heli Valkeinen, E. Kaarakainen, Saara Romu, V. Erola, Juha Ahtiainen, and Leena Paavolainen, "Neuromuscular Adaptations during Concurrent Strength and Endurance Training versus Strength Training," *European Journal of Applied Physiology* 89, no. 1 (2003): 42-52. doi: 10.1007/s00421-002-0751-9.

CHAPTER 17
THE BIGGER LEANER STRONGER TRAINING PROGRAM

1. Paul Comfort, Anne-Marie F. Haigh, and Martyn J. Matthews, "Are Changes in Maximal Squat Strength During Preseason Training Reflected in Changes in Sprint Performance in Rugby League Players?" *Journal of Strength Conditioning Research* 26, no. 3 (2012): 772-76. doi: 10.1519/JSC.0b013e31822a5cbf; Hagen Hartmann, Klaus Wirth, Markus Klusemann, Josip Dalic, Christiane Matuschek, and Dietmar Schmidtbleicher, "Influence of Squatting Depth on Jumping Performance," *Journal of Strength Conditioning Research* 26, no. 12 (2012): 3243-61. doi: 10.1519/JSC.0b013e31824ede62.

2. James Shinkle, Thomas W. Nesser, Timothy J. Demchak, and David M. McMannus, "Effect of Core Strength on the Measure of Power in the Extremities," *Journal of Strength Conditioning Research* 26, no. 2 (2012): 373-80. doi: 10.1519/JSC.0b013e31822600e5.

3. Rafael F. Escamilla, "Knee Biomechanics of the Dynamic Squat Exercise," *Medicine and Science of Sports and Exercise* 33, no. 1 (2001): 127-41.

4. Takeo Nagura, Chris O. Dyrby, Eugene J. Alexander, and Thomas P. Andriacchi, "Mechanical Loads at the Knee Joint during Deep Flexion," *Journal of Orthopedic Research* 20, no. 4 (2002): 881-86. doi: 10.1016/S0736-0266(01)00178-4.

5. Danielle E. Toutoungi, Tung-Wu Lu, Alberto Leardini, Fabio Catani, and John J. O'Connor, "Cruciate Ligament Forces in the Human Knee during Rehabilitation Exercises," *Clinical Biomechanics* 15, no. 3 (2000): 176-87. doi: 10.1016/S0268-0033(99)00063-7.

6. Rafael F. Escamilla, Glenn S. Fleisig, Naiquan Zheng, Jeffrey E. Lander, Steven W. Barrentine, James R. Andrews, Brian W. Bergemann, and Claude T. Moorman, "Effects of Technique Variations on Knee Biomechanics during the Squat and Leg Press," *Medicine and Science of Sports and Exercise* 33, no. 9 (2001): 1552-66.

7. Frank R. Noyes, David L. Butler, Edward S. Grood, Ronald F. Zernicke, and Mohamed S. Hefzy "Biomechanical Analysis of Human Ligament Grafts Used in Knee-Ligament Repairs and Reconstructions," *Journal of Bone and Joint Surgery* 66, no. 3 (1984): 344-52.

8. Amos Race and Andrew A. Amis, "The Mechanical Properties of the Two Bundles of the Human Posterior Cruciate Ligament," *Journal of Biomechanics* 27, no. 1 (1994): 13-24. doi: 10.1016/0021-9290(94)90028-0; Jim P. Vakos, Arthur J. Nitz, A. Joseph Threlkeld, Robert Shapiro, and Terry S. Horn, "Electromyographic Activity of Selected Trunk and Hip Muscles during a Squat Lift: Effect of Varying the Lumbar Posture," *Spine* 19, no. 6 (1976): 687-95; Valdeci Carlos Dionisio, Gil Lúcio Almeida, Marcos Duarte, and Rogério Pessoto Hirata, "Kinematic, Kinetic and EMG Patterns during Downward Squatting," *Journal of Electromyography and Kinesiology* 18, no. 1 (2008): 134-43. doi: 10.1016/j.jelekin.2006.07.010.

9. Rafael F. Escamilla, "Knee Biomechanics of the Dynamic Squat Exercise," *Medicine and Science of Sports and Exercise* 33, no. 1 (2001): 127-41.

10. NSCA Position Paper, "The Squat Exercise in Athletic Conditioning: A Position Statement and Review of the Literature," *National Strength and Conditioning Association Journal* 13, no. 5 (1991): 51-58.

11. James Watkins, *Structure and Function of the Musculoskeletal System* (Champaign, IL: Human Kinetics, 2010).

12. Jim P. Vakos, Arthur J. Nitz, A. Joseph Threlkeld, Robert Shapiro, and Terry S. Horn, "Electromyographic Activity of Selected Trunk and Hip Muscles during a Squat Lift: Effect of Varying the Lumbar Posture," *Spine* 19, no. 6 (1976): 687-95.

13. Shane Schwanbeck, Philip D. Chilibeck, and Gordon Binsted, "A Comparison of Free Weight Squat to Smith Machine Squat Using Electromyography," *Journal of Strength and Conditioning Research* 23, no. 9 (2009): 2588-91. doi: 10.1519/JSC.0b013e3181b1b181.

14. Antonio La Torre, Carlo Castagna, Elisa Gervasoni, Emiliano Cè, Susanna Rampichini, Maurizio Ferrarin, and Giampiero Merati, "Acute Effects of Static Stretching on Squat Jump Performance at Different Knee Starting Angles," *Journal of Strength and Conditioning Research* 24, no. 3 (2010): 687-94. doi: 10.1519/

JSC.0b013e3181c7b443; Stephen B. Thacker, Julie Gilchrist, Donna F. Stroup, and C. Dexter Kimsey, "The Impact of Stretching on Sports Injury Risk: A Systematic Review of the Literature," *Medicine and Science in Sports and Exercise* 36, no. 3 (2004): 371-78.

15. Jonathan C. Gullett, Mark D. Tillman, Gregory M. Gutierrez, and John W. Chow, "A Biomechanical Comparison of Back and Front Squats in Healthy Trained Individuals," *Journal of Strength and Conditioning Research* 23, no. 1 (2009): 284-92. doi: 10.1519/JSC.0b013e31818546bb.

16. Carly M. Green and Paul Comfort, "The Affect of Grip Width on Bench Press Performance and Risk of Injury," *Strength and Conditioning Journal* 29, no. 5 (2007): 10-14. doi: 10.1519/00126548-200710000-00001.

17. Chris Barnett, Vaughan Kippers, and Peter Turner, "Effects of Variations of the Bench Press Exercise on the EMG Activity of Five Shoulder Muscles," *Journal of Strength and Conditioning Research* 9, no. 4 (1995): 222-27. doi: 10.1519/1533-4287(1995)0092.3.CO;2.

18. Juan C. Colado, Carlos Pablos, Ivan Chulvi-Medrano, Xavier Garcia-Masso, Jorgez Flandez, and David G. Behm, "The Progression of Paraspinal Muscle Recruitment Intensity in Localized and Global Strength Training Exercises Is Not Based on Instability Alone," *Archives of Physical Medicine and Rehabilitation* 92, no. 11 (2011): 1875-83. doi: 10.1016/j.apmr.2011.05.015.

19. Jacek Cholewicki and Stuart M. McGill, "Lumbar Posterior Ligament Involvement during Extremely Heavy Lifts Estimated from Fluoroscopic Measurements," *Journal of Biomechanics* 25, no. 1 (1992): 17-28. doi: 10.1016/0021-9290(92)90242-S.

20. Rafael F. Escamilla, Tracy M. Lowry, Daryl C. Osbahr, and Kevin P. Speer, "Biomechanical Analysis of the Deadlift during the 1999 Special Olympics World Games," *Medicine and Science of Sports and Exercise* 33, no. 8 (2001): 1345-53. doi: 10.1097/00005768-200108000-00016.

21. Juan C. Colado, Carlos Pablos, Ivan Chulvi-Medrano, Xavier Garcia-Masso, Jorgez Flandez, and David G. Behm, "The Progression of Paraspinal Muscle Recruitment Intensity in Localized and Global Strength Training Exercises Is Not Based on Instability Alone," *Archives of Physical Medicine and Rehabilitation* 92, no. 11 (2011): 1875-83. doi: 10.1016/j.apmr.2011.05.015.

22. Paul A. Swinton, Arthur Stewart, Ioannis Agouris, Justin W. L. Keogh, and Ray Lloyd, "A Biomechanical Analysis of Straight and Hexagonal Barbell Deadlifts Using Submaximal Loads," *Journal of Strength and Conditioning Research* 25, no. 7 (2011): 2000-09. doi: 10.1519/JSC.0b013e3181e73f87.

23. *Ibid.*

24. Valdinar de Araújo Rocha Júnior, Paulo Gentil, Elke Oliveira, and Jake do Carmo, "Comparison among the EMG Activity of the Pectoralis Major, Anterior Deltoidis and Triceps Brachii during the Bench Press and Peck Deck Exercises," [In Spanish], *Revista Brasileira de Medicina do Esporte* 13, no. 1 (2007): 51-54. doi: 10.1590/S1517-86922007000100012.

25. Jose Antonio, "Nonuniform Response of Skeletal Muscle to Heavy Resistance Training: Can Bodybuilders Induce Regional Muscle Hypertrophy," *Journal of Strength and Conditioning Research* 14, no. 1 (2000): 102–13.

26. *Ibid.*

27. Philip D. Gollnick, Bertil Sjödin, Jan Karlsson, Eva Jansson, and Bengt Saltin, "Human Soleus Muscle: A Comparison of Fiber Composition and Enzyme Activities with Other Leg Muscles," *European Journal of Physiology* 348, no. 3 (1974): 247-55.

28. Per Olof Åstrand, Kaare Rodahl, Hans Dahl, and Sigmund B. Strømme, *Textbook of Work Physiology: Physiological Bases of Exercise* (Champaign, IL: Human Kinetics, 2003).

29. Nicolle Hamlyn, David G. Behm, and Warren B. Young, "Trunk Muscle Activation during Dynamic Weight-Training Exercises and Isometric Instability Activities," *Journal of Strength and Conditioning Research* 21, no. 4 (2007): 1108-12.

30. Jason M. Martuscello, James L. Nuzzo, Candi Ashley, Bill I. Campbell, John J. Orriola, and John Mayer, "Systematic Review of Core Muscle Activity during Physical Fitness Exercises," *Journal of Strength and Conditioning Research* 27, no. 6 (2013): 1684-98. doi: 10.1519/JSC.0b013e318291b8da.

31. James L. Nuzzo, Grant O. McCaulley, Prue Cormie, Michael J. Cavill, and Jeffrey M. McBride, "Trunk Muscle Activity during Stability Ball and Free Weight Exercises," *Journal of Strength and Conditioning Research* 22, no. 1 (2008): 95-102. doi: 10.1519/JSC.0b013e31815ef8cd.

CHAPTER 21
HOW TO PREVENT WORKOUT INJURIES

1. Fitzgerald, B., and G. R. McLatchie. "Degenerative joint disease in weight-lifters. Fact or fiction?." *British journal of sports medicine* 14, no. 2-3 (1980): 97-101.

2. Zachary Y. Kerr, Christy L. Collins, and R. Dawn Comstock, "Epidemiology of Weight Training-Related Injuries Presenting to United States Emergency Departments, 1990 to 2007," *American Journal of Sports Medicine* 38, no. 4 (2010): 765-71. doi: 10.1177/0363546509351560.

3. Michael H. Stone, "Muscle Conditioning and Muscle Injuries," *Medicine and Science of Sports and Exercise* 22, no. 4 (1990): 457-62.

4. Kerr, Collins, and Comstock, "Epidemiology of Weight Training-Related Injuries Presenting to United States Emergency Departments, 1990 to 2007," 765-71.

5. *Ibid.*

6. Ronei S. Pinto, Naiara Gomes, Regis Radaelli, Cíntia E. Botton, Lee E. Brown, and Martim Bottaro, "Effect of Range of Motion on Muscle Strength and Thickness," *Journal of Strength and Conditioning Research* 26, no. 8 (2012): 2140-45. doi: 10.1519/JSC.0b013e31823a3b15.

7. Sam K. Morton, James R. Whitehead, Ronald H. Brinkert, and Dennis J. Caine, "Resistance Training vs. Static Stretching: Effects on Flexibility and Strength," *Journal of Strength and Conditioning Research* 25, no. 12 (2011): 3391-98. doi: 10.1519/JSC.0b013e31821624aa.

8. Jason B. Winchester, Arnold G. Nelson, Dennis Landin, Michael A. Young, and Irving C. Schexnayder, "Static Stretching Impairs Sprint Performance in Collegiate Track and Field Athletes," *Journal of Strength and Conditioning Research* 22, no. 1 (2008): 13-19. doi: 10.1519/JSC.0b013e31815ef202; Antonio La Torre, Carlo Castagna, Elisa Gervasoni, Emiliano Cè, Susanna Rampichini, Maurizio Ferrarin, and Giampiero Merati, "Acute Effects of Static Stretching on Squat Jump Performance at Different Knee Starting Angles," *Journal of Strength and Conditioning Research* 24, no. 3 (2010): 687-94. doi: 10.1519/JSC.0b013e3181c7b443.

9. Lawrence Hart, "Effect of Stretching on Sport Injury Risk: A Review," *Clinical Journal of Sport Medicine* 15, no. 2 (2005): 113; Peter C. D. Macpherson, M. Anthony Schork, and James A. Faulkner, "Contraction-Induced Injury to Single Fiber Segments from Fast and Slow Muscles of Rats by Single Stretches," *American Journal of Physiology—Cell Physiology* 271, no. 5 (1996): C1438-46; Marjorie A. Moore and Robert S. Hutton, "Electromyographic Investigation of Muscle Stretching Techniques," *Medicine and Science of Sports and Exercise* 12, no. 5 (1980): 322-29. doi: 10.1249/00005768-198012050-00004.

10. Danny J. McMillian, Josef H. Moore, Brian S. Hatler, and Dean C. Taylor, "Dynamic vs. Static-Stretching Warm Up: The Effect on Power and Agility Performance," *Journal of Strength and Conditioning Research* 20, no. 3 (2006): 492-99.

11. Katherine Herman, Christian Barton, Peter Malliaras, and Dylan Morrissey, "The Effectiveness of Neuromuscular Warm-Up Strategies, that Require No Additional Equipment, for Preventing Lower Limb Injuries during Sports Participation: A Systematic Review," *BMC Medicine*, 10 (July 19, 2012): 75. doi: 10.1186/1741-7015-10-75.

12. Michel P. J. van den Bekerom, Peter A. A. Struijs, Leendert Blankevoort, Lieke Welling, C. Niek van Dijk, and Gino M. M. J. Kerkhoffs, "What Is the Evidence for Rest, Ice, Compression, and Elevation Therapy in the Treatment of Ankle Sprains in Adults?" *Journal of Athletic Training* 47, no. 4 (2012): 435-43.

13. *Ibid.*

14. *Ibid.*

CHAPTER 22
THE NO-BS GUIDE TO SUPPLEMENTS WHAT WORKS, WHAT DOESN'T, AND WHAT TO WATCH OUT FOR

1. Dawson-Hughes, Bess, A. Mithal, J-P. Bonjour, Steven Boonen, Peter Burckhardt, GE-H. Fuleihan, R. G. Josse, P. T. A. M. Lips, J. Morales-Torres, and Noriko Yoshimura. "IOF position statement: vitamin D recommendations for older adults." *Osteoporosis International* 21, no. 7 (2010): 1151-1154; Wang, Thomas J., Michael J. Pencina, Sarah L. Booth, Paul F. Jacques, Erik Ingelsson, Katherine Lanier, Emelia J. Benjamin, Ralph B. D'Agostino, Myles Wolf, and Ramachandran S. Vasan. "Vitamin D deficiency and risk of cardiovascular disease." *Circulation* 117, no. 4 (2008): 503-511; Pilz, Stefan, Harald Dobnig, Joachim E. Fischer, Britta Wellnitz, Ursula Seelhorst, Bernhard O. Boehm, and Winfried März. "Low vitamin D levels predict stroke in patients referred to coronary angiography." *Stroke* 39, no. 9 (2008): 2611-2613; Giovannucci, Edward. "Epidemiological evidence for vitamin D and colorectal cancer." *Journal of Bone and Mineral Research* 22, no. S2 (2007): V81-V85; Hyppönen, Elina, Esa Läärä, Antti Reunanen, Marjo-Riitta Järvelin, and Suvi M. Virtanen. "Intake of vitamin D and risk of type 1 diabetes: a birth-cohort study." *The Lancet* 358, no. 9292 (2001): 1500-1503; Munger, Kassandra L., Lynn I. Levin, Bruce W. Hollis, Noel S. Howard, and Alberto Ascherio. "Serum 25-hydroxyvitamin D levels and risk of multiple sclerosis." *Jama* 296, no. 23 (2006): 2832-2838; Nnoaham, Kelechi E., and Aileen Clarke. "Low serum vitamin D levels and tuberculosis: a systematic review and meta-analysis." *International journal of epidemiology* 37, no. 1 (2008): 113-119; Cannell, J. J., R. Vieth, J. C. Umhau, M. F. Holick, W. B. Grant, S. Madronich, C. F. Garland, and E. Giovannucci. "Epidemic influenza and vitamin D." *Epidemiology and infection* 134, no. 06 (2006): 1129-1140.

2. Michael Holick, "Vitamin D Is Essential to the Modern Indoor Lifestyle," *Science News* 178, no. 9 (2010): 32; Michael Holick, "Vitamin D Is Essential to the Modern Indoor Lifestyle," *Science News* 178, no. 9 (2010): 32; Michael F. Holick, "Vitamin D: Evolutionary, Physiological and Health Perspectives," *Current Drug Targets* 12, no. 1 (2011): 4-18. doi: 10.2174/138945011793591635.

3. *Ibid.*

4. Matthias Wacker and Michael F. Holick, "Vitamin D—Effects on Skeletal and Extraskeletal Health and the Need for Supplementation," *Nutrients* 5, no. 1 (2013): 111-48. doi: 10.3390/nu5010111.

5. Michael F. Holick, "Vitamin D: Importance in the Prevention of Cancers, Type 1 Diabetes, Heart Disease, and Osteoporosis," *American Journal of Clinical Nutrition* 79, no. 3 (2004): 362-71; Anne C. Looker, Clifford L. Johnson, David A. Lacher, Christine M. Pfeiffer, Rosemary L. Schleicher, and Christopher T. Sempos, "Vitamin D Status: United States, 2001–2006," *NCHS Data Brief* 59 (March 2011), http://www.cdc.gov/nchs/data/databriefs/db59.pdf.

6. Kimberly Y. Z. Forrest and Wendy L. Stuhldreher, "Prevalence and Correlates of Vitamin D Deficiency in US Adults," *Nutrition Research* 31, no. 1 (2011): 48-54. doi: 10.1016/j.nutres.2010.12.001.

7. Vitaly Terushkin, Anna Bender, Estee L. Psaty, Ola Engelsen, Steven Q. Wang, and Allan C. Halpern, "Estimated Equivalency of Vitamin D Production from Natural Sun Exposure versus Oral Vitamin D Supplementation across Seasons at Two US Latitudes," *Journal of the American Academy of Dermatology* 62, no. 6 (2010): 929. e1-e9. doi: 10.1016/j.jaad.2009.07.028.

8. A. Catharine Ross, JoAnn E. Manson, Steven A. Abrams, John F. Aloia, Patsy M. Brannon, Steven K. Clinton, Ramon A. Durazo-Arvizu, J. Christopher Gallagher, Richard L. Gallo, Glenville Jones, Christopher S. Kovacs, Susan T. Mayne, Clifford J. Rosen, and Sue A. Shapses, "The 2011 Report on Dietary Reference Intakes for Calcium and Vitamin D from the Institute of Medicine: What Clinicians Need to Know," *Journal of Clinical Endocrinology and Metabolism* 96, no. 1 (2011): 53-58. doi: 10.1210/jc.2010-2704.

9. Robert P. Heaney and Michael F. Holick, "Why the IOM Recommendations for Vitamin D Are Deficient," *Journal of Bone and Mineral Research* 26, no. 3 (2011): 455-57. doi: 10.1002/jbmr.328.

10. Michael F. Holick, Neil C. Binkley, Heike A. Bischoff-Ferrari, Catherine M. Gordon, David A. Hanley, Robert P. Heaney, M. Hassan Murad, and Connie M. Weaver, "Evaluation, Treatment, and Prevention of Vitamin D Deficiency: An Endocrine Society Clinical Practice Guideline," *Journal of Clinical Endocrinology and Metabolism* 96, no. 7 (2011): 1911-30. doi: 10.ef1210/jc.2011-0385.

11. Bich Tran, Bruce K. Armstrong, John B. Carlin, Peter R. Ebeling, Dallas R. English, Michael G. Kimlin, Bayzidur Rahman, Jolieke C. van der Pols, Alison Venn, Val Gebski, David C. Whiteman, Penelope M. Webb, and Rachel E. Neale, "Recruitment and Results of a Pilot Trial of Vitamin D Supplementation in the General Population of Australia," *Journal of Clinical Endocrinology and Metabolism* 97, no. 12 (2012): 4473-80. doi: 10.1210/jc.2012-2682; Michael F. Holick, *The Vitamin D Solution: A 3-Step Strategy to Cure Our Most Common Health Problems* (New York: Penguin, 2010).

12. Holick, et al., "Evaluation, Treatment, and Prevention of Vitamin D Deficiency: An Endocrine Society Clinical Practice Guideline," 1911-30.

13. Farrell Jr, H. M., et al. "Nomenclature of the proteins of cows' milk—sixth revision." Journal of Dairy Science 87.6 (2004): 1641-1674.

14. Potier, Mylne, and Daniel Tom. "Comparison of digestibility and quality of intact proteins with their respective hydrolysates." Journal of AOAC International 91.4 (2008): 1002-1005.

15. Potier, Mylne, and Daniel Tom. "Comparison of digestibility and quality of intact proteins with their respective hydrolysates." Journal of AOAC International 91.4 (2008): 1002-1005.

16. *Ibid.*

17. http://www.fda.gove/downloads/NewsEvents/MeetingsConferencesWorkshops/UCM1 63645.ppt

18. Scot R. Kimball and Leonard S. Jefferson, "Signaling Pathways and Molecular Mechanisms through which Branched Chain Amino Acids Mediate Translational Control of Protein Synthesis," *Journal of Nutrition* 136, no. 1 (2006): 2275-315.

19. Masako Doi, Ippei Yamaoka, Tetsuya Fukunaga, and Mitsuo Nakayama, "Isoleucine, a Potent Plasma Glucose-Lowering Amino Acid, Stimulates Glucose Uptake in C2C12 Myotubes," *Biochemical and Biophysical Research Communications* 312, no. 4 (2003): 1111-17. doi: 10.1016/j.bbrc.2003.11.039.

20. Myrlene A. Staten, Denis M. Bier, and Dwight E. Mathews, "Regulation of Valine Metabolism in Man: A Stable Isotope Study," *American Journal of Clinical Nutrition* 40, no. 6 (1984): 1224-34.

21. Phillip C. Calder, "Branched-Chain Amino Acids and Immunity," *Journal of Nutrition* 136, no. 1 (2006): 2885-935.

22. Romain Meeusen and Phil Watson, "Amino Acids and the Brain: Do They Play a Role in 'Central Fatigue'?" *International Journal of Sport Nutrition and Exercise Metabolism* 17, supplement (2007): S37-46.

23. Glyn Howatson, Michael Hoad, Stuart Goodall, Jamie Tallent, Phillip G. Bell, and Duncan N. French, "Exercise-Induced Muscle Damage Is Reduced in Resistance-Trained Males by Branched Chain Amino Acids: A Randomized, Double-Blind, Placebo Controlled Study," *Journal of the International Society of Sports Nutrition* 9, no. 20 (2012): doi:10.1186/1550-2783-9-20.

24. Eva Blomstrand, Jörgen Eliasson, Håkan K. R. Karlsson, and Rickard Köhnke, "Branched-Chain Amino Acids Activate Key Enzymes in Protein Synthesis after Physical Exercise," *Journal of Nutrition* 136, no. 1 (2006): 269S-73S.

25. Agnès Mourier, André Xavier Bigard, Eric de Kerviler, Bernard Roger, Helene Legrand, and Charles Y. Guezennec, "Combined Effects of Caloric Restriction and Branched-Chain Amino Acid Supplementation on Body Composition and Exercise Performance in Elite Wrestlers," *International Journal of Sports Medicine* 18, no. 1 (1997): 47-55. doi: 10.1055/s-2007-972594.

26. Yoshiharu Shimomura, Yuko Yamamoto, Gustavo Bajotto, Juichi Sato, Taro Murakami, Noriko Shimomura, Hisamine Kobayashi, and Kazunori Mawatari, "Nutraceutical Effects of Branched-Chain Amino Acids on Skeletal Muscle," *Journal of Nutrition* 136, no. 2 (2006): 529S-32S.

27. Carwyn P. M. Sharp and David R. Pearson, "Amino Acid Supplements and Recovery from High-Intensity Resistance Training," *Journal of Strength and Conditioning Research* 24, no. 4 (2010): 1125-30. doi: 10.1519/JSC.0b013e3181c7c655.

28. Antti Mero, "Leucine Supplementation and Intensive Training," *Sports Medicine* 27, no. 6 (1999): 347-58. doi: 10.2165/00007256-199927060-00001.

29. Juha J. Hulmi, Christopher M. Lockwood, and Jeffrey R. Stout, "Effect of Protein/Essential Amino Acids and Resistance Training on Skeletal Muscle Hypertrophy: A Case for Whey Protein," *Nutrition and Metabolism* 7 (June 2010): 51. doi:10.1186/1743-7075-7-51.

30. Yu Li Lydia Law, Wee Sian Ong, Tsien Lin Gillian Yap, Su Ching Joselin Lim, and Ee Von Chia, "Effects of Two and Five Days of Creatine Loading on Muscular Strength and Anaerobic Power in Trained Athletes," *Journal of Strength and Conditioning Research* 23, no. 3 (2009): 906-14.

31. Jim Stoppani, Timothy Scheett, James Pena, Chuck Rudolph, and Derek Charlebois, "Consuming a Supplement Containing Branched-Chain Amino Acids during a Resistance-Training Program Increases Lean Mass, Muscle Strength and Fat Loss," *Journal of the International Society of Sports Nutrition* 6, no. S1 (2009): P1. doi:10.1186/1550-2783-6-S1-P1.

32. Scivation, January 26, 2009 (7:27 a.m.), "Groundbreaking Xtend Study Results Are In!" Bodybuilding (forum), http://forum.bodybuilding.com/showthread.php?t=113689801&p=279437771#post279437771.

33. Alan Aragon, "Alan's Vault," accessed October 17, 2014, http://alanaragon.com/researchreview.

34. Wim Derave, Ann Mertens, Erik Muls, Karel Pardaens, and Peter Hespel, "Effects of Post-Absorptive and Postprandial Exercise on Glucoregulation in Metabolic Syndrome," *Obesity* 15, no. 3 (2007): 704-11. doi: 10.1038/oby.2007.548; William J. Kraemer, Steven J. Fleck, Carl M. Maresh, Nicholas A. Ratamess, Scott E. Gordon, Kenneth L. Goetz, Everett A. Harman, Peter N. Frykman, Jeff S. Volek, Scott A. Mazzetti, Andrew C. Fry, Louis J. Marchitelli, and John F. Patton, "Acute Hormonal Responses to a Single Bout of Heavy Resistance Exercise in Trained Power Lifters and Untrained Men," *Canadian Journal of Applied Physiology* 24, no. 6 (1999): 524-37.

35. Hannu T. Pitkanen, Tarja Nykanen, Juha Knuutinen, Kaisa Lahti, Olavi Keinanen, Marrku Alen, Paavo V. Komi, and Antti A. Mero, "Free Amino Acid Pool and Muscle Protein Balance after Resistance Exercise," *Medicine and Science of Sports and Exercise* 35, no. 5 (2003): 784-92.

36. Glyn Howatson, Michael Hoad, Stuart Goodall, Jamie Tallent, Phillip G. Bell, and Duncan N. French, "Exercise-Induced Muscle Damage Is Reduced in Resistance-Trained Males by Branched Chain Amino Acids: A Randomized, Double-Blind, Placebo Controlled Study," *Journal of the International Society of Sports Nutrition* 9, no. 20 (2012): doi:10.1186/1550-2783-9-20; Yi Zhang, Hisamine Kobayashi, Kazunori Mawatari, Juichi Sato, Gustavo Bajotto, Yasuyuki Kitaura, and Yoshiharu Shimomura, "Effects of Branched-Chain Amino Acid Supplementation on Plasma Concentrations of Free Amino Acids, Insulin, and Energy Substrates in Young Men," *Journal of Nutritional Science and Vitaminology* 57, no. 1 (2011): 114-17. doi: 10.3177/jnsv.57.114.

37. Eric S. Rawson and Jeff S. Volek, "Effects of Creatine Supplementation and Resistance Training on Muscle Strength and Weightlifting Performance," *Journal of Strength and Conditioning Research* 17, no. 4 (2003): 822-31.

38. Joan M. Eckerson, Jeffrey R. Stout, Geri A. Moore, Nancy J. Stone, Kate A. Iwan, and Amy N. Gebauer, "Effect of Creatine Phosphate Supplementation on Anaerobic Working Capacity and Body Weight after Two and Six Days of Loading in Men and Women," *Journal of Strength and Conditioning Research* 19, no. 4 (2005): 756. doi: 10.1519/R-16924.1; Settar Kocak and Unal Karli, "Effects of High Dose Oral Creatine Supplementation on Anaerobic Capacity of Elite Wrestlers," *Journal of Sports Medicine and Physical Fitness* 43, no. 4 (2003): 488-92; Reinaldo Abunasser Bassit, Carlos Hermano da Justa Pinheiro, Kaio Fernando Vitzel, Antônio José Sproesser, Leonardo R. Silveira, and Rui Curi, "Effect of Short-Term Creatine Supplementation on Markers of Skeletal Muscle Damage after Strenuous Contractile Activity," *European Journal of Applied Physiology* 108, no. 5 (2010): 945-55; Ronaldo V. T. Santos, Reinaldo A. Bassit, Erico C. Caperuto, and Luis F. B. P. Costa Rosa, "The Effect of Creatine Supplementation upon Inflammatory and Muscle Soreness Markers after a 30km Race," *Life Sciences* 75, no. 16 (2004): 1917-24. doi: 10.1016/j.lfs.2003.11.036; Jacques R. Poortmans and Marc Francaux, "Adverse Effects of Creatine Supplementation: Fact or Fiction?" *Sports Medicine* 30, no. 3 (2000): 155-70; Ronald L. Terjung, Priscilla Clarkson, E. Randy Eichner, Paul L. Greenhaff, Peter J. Hespel, Richard G. Israel, William J. Kraemer, Ronald A. Meyer, Lawrence L. Spriet, Mark A. Tarnopolsky, Anton J. M. Wagenmakers, and Melvin H. Williams," American College of Sports Medicine Roundtable: The Physiological and Health Effects of Oral Creatine Supplementation," *Medicine and Science of Sports Exercise* 32, no. 3 (2000): 706-17; Wyndie M. Yoshizumi and Candy Tsourounis, "Effects of Creatine Supplementation on Renal Function," *Journal of Herbal Pharmacology* 4, no. 1 (2004): 1-7.

39. Emiliana Bizzarini and Luisa De Angelis, "Is the Use of Oral Creatine Supplementation Safe? *Journal of Sports Medicine and Physical Fitness* 44, no. 4 (2004): 411-6; Geert J. Groeneveld, Cornelis Beijer, Jan H. Veldink, Sandra Kalmijn, John H. Wokke, and Leonard H. van den Berg, "Few Adverse Effects of Long-Term Creatine Supplementation in a Placebo-Controlled Trial," *International Journal of Sports Medicine* 26, no. 4 (2005): 307-13. doi: 10.1055/s-2004-817917.

40. Marc Francaux and Jacques R. Poortmans, "Side Effects of Creatine Supplementation in Athletes," *International Journal of Sports Physiology Performance* 1, no. 4 (2006): 311-23; Ralf Jäger, Roger C. Harris, Martin Purpura, and Marc Francaux, "Comparison of New Forms of Creatine in Raising Plasma Creatine Levels," *Journal of the International Society of Sports Nutrition* 4 (2007): 17. doi: 10.1186/1550-2783-4-17.

41. Ambrish Pandit, Pinal Mistry, P. Dib, A. Nikolaidis, and Alekha K. Dash, "Equilibrium Solubility Studies of Creatine Nitrate, Creatine Monohydrate and Buffered Creatine," Poster presented at the FIP Pharmaceutical Sciences World Congress 2010 in Association with the AAPS Annual Meeting and Exposition, New Orleans, LA, November 2010.

42. Heike A. Bischoff-Ferrari, Andrew Shao, Bess Dawson-Hughes, John Hathcock, Edward Giovannucci, and Walter C. Willett, "Benefit-Risk Assessment of Vitamin D Supplementation," *Osteoporos International* 21, no.

7 (2010): 1121-32. doi: 10.1007/s00198-009-1119-3; Glaura S. A. Fernandes, Carla D. B. Fernandez, Kleber E. Campos, Débora C. Damasceno, Janete A. Anselmo-Franci, and Wilma DG Kempinas, "Vitamin C Partially Attenuates Male Reproductive Deficits in Hyperglycemic Rats," *Reproductive Biology and Endocrinology* 9 (July 27, 2011): 100. doi: 10.1186/1477-7827-9-100.

43. Michael G. Bemben and Hugh S. Lamont, "Creatine Supplementation and Exercise Performance: Recent Findings," *Sports Medicine* 35, no. 2 (2005): 107-25.

44. Alexander L. Green, Eric Hultman, Ian A. Macdonald, Dean A. Sewell, and Paul L. Greenhaff, "Carbohydrate Ingestion Augments Skeletal Muscle Creatine Accumulation during Creatine Supplementation in Humans," *American Journal of Physiology—Endocrinology and Metabolism* 271, no. 5 (1996): E821-26.

45. Gery R. Steenge, J. Lambourne, Anna Casey, Ian A. Macdonald, and Paul L. Greenhaff, "Stimulatory Effect of Insulin on Creatine Accumulation in Human Skeletal Muscle," *American Journal of Physiology—Endocrinology and Metabolism* 275, no. 6 (1998): E974-79.

46. Gery R. Steenge, Elizabeth J. Simpson, and Paul L. Greenhaff, "Protein- and Carbohydrate-Induced Augmentation of Whole Body Creatine Retention in Humans," *Journal of Applied Physiology* 89, no. 3 (2000): 1165-71.

47. Jose Antonio and Victoria Ciccone, "The Effects of Pre versus Post Workout Supplementation of Creatine Monohydrate on Body Composition and Strength," *Journal of the International Society of Sports Nutrition* 10, no. 36 (2013): doi:10.1186/1550-2783-10-36.

48. Kamiel Vandenberghe, Nanna Gillis, Marc Van Leemputte, Paul Van Hecke, Florent Vanstapel, and Peter Hespel, "Caffeine Counteracts the Ergogenic Action of Muscle Creatine Loading," *Journal of Applied Physiology* 80, no. 2 (1996): 452-57.

49. Mike Doherty, Paul M. Smith, R. C. Richard Davison, Michael G. Hughes, "Caffeine Is Ergogenic after Supplementation of Oral Creatine Monohydrate," *Medicine and Science of Sports and Exercise* 34, no. 11 (2002): 1785-92.

50. Chia-Lun Lee, Jung-Charng Lin, and Ching-Feng Cheng, "Effect of Caffeine Ingestion after Creatine Supplementation on Intermittent High-Intensity Sprint Performance," *European Journal of Applied Physiology* 111, no. 8 (2011): 1669-77. doi: 10.1007/s00421-010-1792-0.

51. John A. Rockwell, Janet Walberg-Rankin, and Ben Toderico, "Creatine Supplementation Affects Muscle Creatine during Energy Restriction," *Medicine and Science of Sports and Exercise* 33, no. 1 (2001): 61-68.

52. Pilz, S., S. Frisch, H. Koertke, J. Kuhn, J. Dreier, B. Obermayer-Pietsch, E. Wehr, and A. Zittermann. "Effect of vitamin D supplementation on testosterone levels in men." Hormone and Metabolic Research 43, no. 03 (2011): 223-225; Fernandes GS, Fernandez CD, Campos KE, Damasceno DC, Anselmo-Franci JA, Kempinas WD. Vitamin C partially attenuates male reproductive deficits in hyperglycemic rats. Reprod Biol Endocrinol. 2011 Jul 27;9:100. doi: 10.1186/1477-7827-9-100; Ananda S. Prasad, Christos S. Mantzoros, Frances W. Beck, Joseph W. Hess, and George J. Brewer, "Zinc Status and Serum Testosterone Levels of Healthy Adults," Nutrition 12, no. 5 (1996): 344-48; Vedat Cinar, Abdulkerim K. Baltaci, Rasim Mogulkoc, and Mehmet Kilic, "Testosterone Levels in Athletes at Rest and Exhaustion: Effects of Calcium Supplementation," Biological Trace Element Research 129, no. 1-3 (2009): 65-69. doi: 10.1007/s12011-008-8294-5; Vedat Cinar, Yahya Polat, Abdulkerim K. Baltaci, and Rasim Mogulkoc, "Effects of Magnesium Supplementation on Testosterone Levels of Athletes and Sedentary Subjects at Rest and after Exhaustion," Biological Trace Element Research 140, no. 1 (2011): 18-23. doi: 10.1007/s12011-010-8676-3.

53. Vladimir K. Neychev and Vanyo I. Mitev, "The Aphrodisiac Herb *Tribulus terrestris* Does Not Influence the Androgen Production in Young Men," *Journal of Ethnopharmacology*, 101, no. 1-3 (2005): 319-23. doi: 10.1016/j.jep.2005.05.017; Jose Antonio, John Uelmen, Rodrigo Rodriguez, and Conrad P. Earnest, "The Effects of *Tribulus terrestris* on Body Composition and Exercise Performance in Resistance-Trained Males," *International Journal of Sport Nutrition and Exercise Metabolism* 10, no. 2 (2000): 208-15; Shane Rogerson, Christopher J. Riches, Carl Jennings, Robert P. Weatherby, Rudi A. Meir, and Sonya M. Marshall-Gradisnik, "The Effect of Five Weeks of *Tribulus terrestris* Supplementation on Muscle Strength and Body Composition during Preseason Training in Elite Rugby League Players," *Journal of Strength and Conditioning Research* 21, no. 2 (2007): 348-53; Karsten Koehler, Maria Kristina Parr, Hans Geyer, Joachim Mester, and Wilhelm Schänzer, "Serum Testosterone and Urinary Excretion of Steroid Hormone Metabolites after Administration of a High-Dose Zinc Supplement," *European Journal of Clinical Nutrition* 63, no. 1 (2009): 65-70; Leila Shafiei Neek, Abas Ali Gaeini, and Siroos Choobineh, "Effect of Zinc and Selenium Supplementation on Serum Testosterone and Plasma Lactate in Cyclist after an Exhaustive Exercise Bout," *Biological Trace Element Research* 144, no. 1-3 (2011): 454-62. doi: 10.1007/s12011-011-9138-2.

54. Koehler, K., M. K. Parr, H. Geyer, J. Mester, and W. Schänzer. "Serum testosterone and urinary excretion of steroid hormone metabolites after administration of a high-dose zinc supplement." *European journal of clinical nutrition* 63, no. 1 (2007): 65-70.

55. Enza Topo, Andrea Soricelli, Antimo D'Aniello, Salvatore Ronsini, and Gemma D'Aniello, "The Role and Molecular Mechanism of D-aspartic Acid in the Release and Synthesis of LH and Testosterone in Humans and Rats." *Reproductive Biology Endocrinology* 7 (October 27, 2009): 120. doi: 10.1186/1477-7827-7-120; Michael E. Powers, Joshua F. Yarrow, Sean C. McCoy, and Stephen E. Borst, "Growth Hormone Isoform Responses to GABA Ingestion at Rest and after Exercise," *Medicine and Science of Sports and Exercise* 40, no. 1 (2008): 104-10. doi: 10.1249/mss.0b013e318158b518.

56. Franco Cavagnini, Cecilia Invitti, Matteo Pinto, Caterina Maraschini, Anna Di Landro, Antonella Dubini, and Antonella Marelli, "Effect of Acute and Repeated Administration of Gamma Aminobutyric Acid (GABA) on Growth Hormone and Prolactin Secretion in Man," Acta Endocrinologica 93, no. 2 (1980): 149-54. doi: 10.1530/acta.0.0930149.

57. Paula J. Robson, Andrew K. Blannin, Neil P. Walsh, Linda M. Castell, and Michael Gleeson, "Effects of Exercise Intensity, Duration and Recovery on In Vitro Neutrophil Function in Male Athletes," International Journal of Sports Medicine 20, no. 2 (1999): 128-35; Philip Babij, Stella M. Matthews, and Michael J. Rennie, "Changes in Blood Ammonia, Lactate and Amino Acids in Relation to Workload during Bicycle Ergometer Exercise in Man," European Journal of Applied Physiology and Occupational Physiology 50, no. 3 (1983): 405-11. doi: 10.1007/BF00423246.

58. Linda M. Castell, "Can Glutamine Modify the Apparent Immunodepression Observed after Prolonged, Exhaustive Exercise?" Nutrition 18, no. 5 (2002): 371-75; Mark Parry-Billings, Richard Budgett, Yiannis Koutedakis, Eva Blomstrand, Stephen Brooks, Clyde Williams, Philip C. Calder, Stephen Pilling, Robert Baigrie, and Eric A. Newsholme, "Plasma Amino Acid Concentrations in the Overtraining Syndrome: Possible Effects on the Immune System," Medicine and Science in Sports and Exercise 24, no. 12 (1992): 1353; Philip C. Calder and Parveen Yaqoob, "Glutamine and the Immune System," Amino Acids 17, no. 3 (1999): 227-41; Jacqueline Carvalho-Peixoto, Robson Cardilo Alves, and Luiz-Claudio Cameron, "Glutamine and Carbohydrate Supplements Reduce Ammonemia Increase during Endurance Field Exercise," Applied Physiology, Nutrition, and Metabolism 32, no. 6 (2007): 1186-90; Alessandra Favano, Paulo Roberto Santos-Silva, Eduardo Yoshio Nakano, André Pedrinelli, Arnaldo José Hernandez, and Julia Maria D'Andrea Greve, "Peptide Glutamine Supplementation for Tolerance of Intermittent Exercise in Soccer Players," Clinics-Universidade de Sao Paulo 63, no. 1 (2008): 27-32; Kori J. Kingsbury, Louise Kay, and Magnus Hjelm, "Contrasting Plasma Free Amino Acid Patterns in Elite Athletes: Association with Fatigue and Infection," British Journal of Sports Medicine 32, no. 1 (1998): 25-32; Vinicius Fernandes Cruzat, Marcelo Macedo Rogero, and Julio Tirapegui, "Effects of Supplementation with Free Glutamine and the Dipeptide Alanyl-Glutamine on Parameters of Muscle Damage and Inflammation in Rats Submitted to Prolonged Exercise," Cell Biochemistry and Function 28, no. 1 (2010): 24-30; Adriana Bassini-Cameron, André Nascimento Monteiro, André Gomes, João Pedro S. Werneck-De-Castro, and Luiz-Claudio Cameron, "Glutamine Protects against Increases in Blood Ammonia in Football Players in an Exercise Intensity-Dependent Way," British Journal of Sports Medicine 42, no. 4 (2008): 260-66.

59. Margaret M. Jepson, Peter C. Bates, P. Broadbent, Jennifer M. Pell, and D. Joe Millward, "Relationship between Glutamine Concentration and Protein Synthesis in Rat Skeletal Muscle," American Journal of Physiology-Endocrinology and Metabolism 255, no. 2 (1988): E166-72; Peter A. MacLennan, Ken Smith, Brian V. Weryk, Peter W. Watt, and Michael J. Rennie, "Inhibition of Protein Breakdown by Glutamine in Perfused Rat Skeletal Muscle," FEBS Letters 237, no. 1 (1988): 133-36; Regis G. Hankard, Morey W. Haymond, and Dominique Darmaun, "Effect of Glutamine on Leucine Metabolism in Humans," American Journal of Physiology-Endocrinology and Metabolism 271, no. 4 (1996): E748-54;

60. Sarah B. Wilkinson, "Addition of Glutamine to Essential Amino Acids and Carbohydrate Does Not Enhance Anabolism in Young Human Males Following Exercise," *Applied Physiology, Nutrition, and Metabolism* 31 no. 5 (2006): 518-29;

61. Cameron et al., "Glutamine Protects against Increases in Blood Ammonia in football Players in an Exercise Intensity-Dependent Way," 260-66.

62. Thiago S. Álvares, Cláudia M. Meirelles, Yagesh N. Bhambhani, Vânia M. F. Paschoalin, and Paulo S. C. Gomes, "L-Arginine as a Potential Ergogenic Aid in Healthy Subjects," Sports Medicine 41, no. 3 (2011): 233-48. doi: 10.2165/11538590-000000000-00000; Antoni Sureda, Alfredo Córdova, Miguel D. Ferrer, Pedro Tauler, Gerardo Pérez, Josep A. Tur, and Antoni Pons, "Effects of L-Citrulline Oral Supplementation on Polymorphonuclear Neutrophils Oxidative Burst and Nitric Oxide Production after Exercise," *Free Radical Research* 43, no. 9 (2009): 828-35. doi: 10.1080/10715760903071664; Guilherme Giannini Artioli, Bruno Gualano, Abbie Smith,

Jeffrey Stout, and Antonio H. Lancha Jr., "Role of Beta-Alanine Supplementation on Muscle Carnosine and Exercise Performance," *Medicine and Science of Sports and Exercise*, 42, no. 6 (2010): 1162-73. doi: 10.1249/ MSS.0b013e3181c74e38; Nancy R. Rodriguez, Nancy M. Di Marco, and Susie Langley, "American College of Sports Medicine Position Stand: Nutrition and Athletic Performance," *Medicine and Science of Sports and Exercise* 41, no. 3 (2009): 709-31. doi: 10.1249/MSS.0b013e31890eb86.

63. Loren Cordain, S. Boyd Eaton, Anthony Sebastian, Neil Mann, Staffan Lindeberg, Bruce A. Watkins, James H. O'Keefe, and Janette Brand-Miller, "Origins and Evolution of the Western Diet: Health Implications for the 21st Century," *American Journal of Clinical Nutrition* 81, no. 2 (2005): 341-54.

64. Arja T. Erkkilä and Sarah L. Booth, "Vitamin K Intake and Atherosclerosis," *Current Opinion in Lipidology* 19, no. 1 (2008): 39-42. doi: 10.1097/MOL.0b013e3282f1c57f; Bess Dawson-Hughes, Ambrish Mithal, Jean-Phillipe Bonjour, Steven Boonen, Peter Burckhardt, Ghada El-Hajj Fuleihan, Robert G. Josse, Paul Lips, Jorge Morales-Torres, and Noriko Yoshimura, "IOF Position Statement: Vitamin D Recommendations for Older Adults," *Osteoporosis International* 21, no. 7 (2010): 1151-54. doi: 10.1007/s00198-010-1285-3.

65. Nico S. Rizzo, Karen Jaceldo-Siegl, Joan Sabate, and Gary E. Fraser, "Nutrient Profiles of Vegetarian and Nonvegetarian Dietary Patterns," *Journal of the Academy of Nutrition and Dietetics* 113, no. 12 (2013): 1610-19. doi: 10.1016/j.jand.2013.06.349; Peter Clarys, Tom Deliens, Inge Huybrechts, Peter Deriemaeker, Barbara Vanaelst, Willem De Keyzer, Marcel Hebbelinck, and Patrick Mullie, "Comparison of Nutritional Quality of the Vegan, Vegetarian, Semi-Vegetarian, Pesco-Vegetarian and Omnivorous Diet," *Nutrients* 6, no. 3 (2014): 1318-32. doi:10.3390/nu6031318; Steven A. Abrams, "Setting Dietary Reference Intakes with the Use of Bioavailability Data: Calcium," *American Journal of Clinical Nutrition* 91, no. 5 (2010): 1474S-77S. doi: 10.3945/ ajcn.2010.28674H.

66. Marie-Cécile Nollevaux, Yves Guiot, Yves Horsmans, Isabelle Leclercq, Jacques Rahier, André P. Geubel, and Christine Sempoux, "Hypervitaminosis A-Induced Liver Fibrosis: Stellate Cell Activation and Daily Dose Consumption," *Liver International* 26, no. 2 (2006): 182-86. doi: 10.1111/j.1478-3231.2005.01207.x.

67. Edgar R. Miller III, Roberto Pastor-Barriuso, Darshan Dalal, Rudolph A. Riemersma, Lawrence J. Appel, and Eliseo Guallar, "Meta-Analysis: High-Dosage Vitamin E Supplementation May Increase All-Cause Mortality," *Annals of Internal Medicine* 142, no. 1 (2005): 37-46. doi:10.7326/0003-4819-142-1-200501040-00110.

68. Maret G. Traber, Angelika Elsner, and Regina Brigelius-Flohé, "Synthetic as Compared with Natural Vitamin E Is Preferentially Excreted as α-CEHC in Human Urine: Studies Using Deuterated α-Tocopheryl Acetates," *FEBS Letters* 437, no. 1-2 (1998): 145-48. doi: 10.1016/S0014-5793(98)01210-1; Francesco Scaglione and Giscardo Panzavolta, "Folate, Folic Acid and 5-Methyltetrahydrofolate Are Not the Same Thing," *Xenobiotica* 44, no. 5 (2014): 480-88. doi:10.3109/00498254.2013.845705.

69. Marketdata Enterprises Inc., "The U.S. Weight Loss Market: 2014 Status Report and Forecast," February 1, 2014, http://www.marketresearch.com/Marketdata-Enterprises-Inc-v416/Weight-Loss-Status-Forecast-8016030/; Cynthia L. Ogden, Margaret D. Carroll, Brian K. Kit, and Katherine M. Flegal, "Prevalence of Childhood and Adult Obesity in the United States," *JAMA* 311, no. 8 (2014): 806-14. doi:10.1001/jama.2014.732.

70. Arne Astrup, Soren Toubro, Stephen Cannon, Pia Hem, Leif Breum, and Joop Madsen, "Caffeine: A Double-Blind, Placebo-Controlled Study of Its Thermogenic, Metabolic, and Cardiovascular Effects in Healthy Volunteers," *American Journal of Clinical Nutrition* 51, no. 5 (1990): 759-67; Todd A. Astorino, Riana L. Rohmann, and Kelli Firth, "Effect of Caffeine Ingestion on One-Repetition Maximum Muscular Strength," *European Journal of Applied Physiology* 102, no. 2 (2008): 127-32. doi: 10.1007/s00421-007-0557-x; Travis W. Beck, Terry J. Housh, Richard J. Schmidt, Glen O. Johnson, Dona J. Housh, Jared W Coburn, and Moh H. Malek, "The Acute Effects of a Caffeine-Containing Supplement on Strength, Muscular Endurance, and Anaerobic Capabilities," *Journal of Strength and Conditioning Research* 20, no. 3 (2006): 506-10. doi: 10.1519/18285.1; Ricardo Mora-Rodríguez, Jesús García Pallarés, Álvaro López-Samanes, Juan Fernando Ortega, and Valentín E. Fernández-Elías, "Caffeine Ingestion Reverses the Circadian Rhythm Effects on Neuromuscular Performance in Highly Resistance-Trained Men," *PLOS One* 7, no. 4 (2012): e33807. doi: 10.1371/journal.pone.0033807.

71. Kyoung Sik Park, "Raspberry Ketone Increases Both Lipolysis and Fatty Acid Oxidation in 3T3-L1 Adipocytes," *Planta Medica* 76, no. 15 (2010): 1654-58. doi: 10.1055/s-0030-1249860; Chie Morimoto, Yurie Satoh, Mariko Hara, Shintaro Inoue, Takahiro Tsujita, and Hiromichi Okuda, "Anti-Obese Action of Raspberry Ketone," *Life Sciences* 77, no. 2 (2005): 194-204. doi: 10.1016/j.lfs.2004.12.029.

72. Park, "Raspberry Ketone increases Both Lipolysis and Fatty Acid Oxidation in 3T3 L1 Adipocytes, 1654-58.

73. Morimoto et al., "Anti-Obese Action of Raspberry Ketone," 194-204.

74. Hector L. Lopez, Tim N. Ziegenfuss, Jennifer E. Hofheins, Scott M. Habowski, Shawn M. Arent, Joseph P. Weir, and Arny A. Ferrando, "Eight Weeks of Supplementation with a Multi-Ingredient Weight Loss Product Enhances Body Composition, Reduces Hip and Waist Girth, and Increases Energy Levels in Overweight Men and Women," *Journal of the International Society of Sports and Nutrition* 10, no. 1 (2013): 22. doi: 10.1186/1550-2783-10-22.

75. Steffany Haaz, Kevin R. Fontaine, Gary Cutter, Nita Limdi, Suzanne Perumean-Chaney, and David B. Allison, "*Citrus aurantium* and Synephrine Alkaloids in the Treatment of Overweight and Obesity: An Update," *Obesity Reviews* 7, no. 1 (2006): 79-88. doi: 10.1111/j.1467-789X.2006.00195.x; Christine M. Brown, John C. McGrath, John M. Midgley, A. G. Muir, J. W. O'Brien, C. Mohan Thonoor, Clyde M. Williams, and V. G. Wilson, "Activities of Octopamine and Synephrine Stereoisomers on Alpha-Adrenoceptors," *British Journal of Pharmacology* 93, no. 2 (1988): 417–29; Réjeanne Gougeon, Kathy Harrigan, Jean-François Tremblay, Philip Hedrei, Marie Lamarche, and José A. Morais, "Increase in the Thermic Effect of Food in Women by Adrenergic Amines Extracted from Citrus Aurantium," *Obesity Research* 13, no. 7 (2005): 1187-94.

76. John G. Seifert, Aaron Nelson, Julia Devonish, Edmund R. Burke, and Sidney J. Stohs, "Effect of Acute Administration of an Herbal Preparation on Blood Pressure and Heart Rate in Humans," *International Journal of Medical Sciences* 8 no. 3 (2011): 192-97. doi:10.7150/ijms.8.192.

77. R. Nageswara Rao and Kunnumpurath K. Sakariah, "Lipid-Lowering and Antiobesity Effect of (−)Hydroxycitric Acid," *Nutrition Research* 8, no. 2 (1988): 209-12. doi: 10.1016/S0271-5317(88)80024-1; John M. Lowenstein, "Effect of (-)-Hydroxycitrate on Fatty Acid Synthesis by Rat Liver in Vivo, *Journal of Biological Chemistry* 246, no. 3 (1971): 629-32.

78. Igho Onakpoya, Shao Kang Hung, Rachel Perry, Barbara Wider, and Edzard Ernst, "The Use of Garcinia Extract (Hydroxycitric Acid) as a Weight Loss Supplement: A Systematic Review and Meta-Analysis of Randomised Clinical Trials," *Journal of Obesity* 2011 (2011): 509038. doi: 10.1155/2011/509038.

79. Chung S. Yang, Joshua D. Lambert, and Shengmin Sang, "Antioxidative and Anti-Carcinogenic Activities of Tea Polyphenols, *Archives of Toxicology* 83, no. 1 (2009): 11-21. doi: 10.1007/s00204-008-0372-0.

80. Kevin C. Maki, Matthew S. Reeves, Mildred Farmer, Koichi Yasunaga, Noboru Matsuo, Yoshihisa Katsuragi, Masanori Komikado, Ichiro Tokimitsu, Donna Wilder, Franz Jones, Jeffrey B. Blumberg, and Yolanda Cartwright, "Green Tea Catechin Consumption Enhances Exercise-Induced Abdominal Fat Loss in Overweight and Obese Adults," *Journal of Nutrition* 139, no. 2 (2009): doi: 10.3945/jn.108.098293.

81. Rick Hursel, Wolfgang Viechtbauer, and Margriet S. Westerterp-Plantenga, "The Effects of Green Tea on Weight Loss and Weight Maintenance: A Meta-Analysis," *International Journal of Obesity* 33 (2009): 956-61. doi:10.1038/ijo.2009.135; Michelle C. Venables, Carl J. Hulston, Hannah R. Cox, and Asker E. Jeukendrup, "Green Tea Extract Ingestion, Fat Oxidation, and Glucose Tolerance in Healthy Humans," *American Journal of Clinical Nutrition* 87, no. 3 (2008): 778-84; Kevin C. Maki, Matthew S. Reeves, Mildred Farmer, Koichi Yasunaga, Noboru Matsuo, Yoshihisa Katsuragi, Masanori Komikado, Ichiro Tokimitsu, Donna Wilder, Franz Jones, Jeffrey B. Blumberg, and Yolanda Cartwright, "Green Tea Catechin Consumption Enhances Exercise-Induced Abdominal Fat Loss in Overweight and Obese Adults," *Journal of Nutrition* 139, no. 2 (2009): doi: 10.3945/jn.108.098293; Bao Ting Zhu, Jae-Yoon Shim, Mime Nagai, and Hyoung-Woo Bai, "Molecular Modelling Study of the Mechanism of High-Potency Inhibition of Human Catechol-O-Methyltransferase by (−)-Epigallocatechin-3-O-Gallate," *Xenobiotica* 38, no. 2 (2008): 130-46. doi:10.1080/00498250701744641.

82. Frank Thielecke, Gabriele Rahn, Jana Böhnke, Frauke Adams, Andreas L. Birkenfeld, Jens Jordan, and Michael Boschmann, "Epigallocatechin-3-Gallate and Postprandial Fat Oxidation in Overweight/Obese Male Volunteers: A Pilot Study," *European Journal of Clinical Nutrition* 64, no. 7 (2010): 704-13. doi:10.1038/ejcn.2010.47.

83. Olivia J. Phung, William L. Baker, Leslie J. Matthews, Michael Lanosa, Alicia Thorne, and Craig I. Coleman, "Effect of Green Tea Catechins with or without Caffeine on Anthropometric Measures: A Systematic Review and Meta-Analysis," *American Journal of Clinical Nutrition* 91, no. 1 (2010): 73-81. doi: 10.3945/ajcn.2009.28157.

84. H-H. Sherry Chow, Iman A. Hakim, Donna R. Vining, James A. Crowell, James Ranger-Moore, Wade M. Chew, Catherine A. Celaya, Steven R. Rodney, Yukihiko Hara, and David S. Alberts, "Effects of Dosing Condition on the Oral Bioavailability of Green Tea Catechins after Single-Dose Administration of Polyphenon E in Healthy Individuals," *Clinical Cancer Research* 11, no. 12 (2005): 4627-33. doi: 10.1158/1078-0432.CCR-04-2549.

85. National Center for Complementary and Alternative Medicine, "Acai," last modified November 23, 2012, http://nccam.nih.gov/health/acai/ataglance.htm.

86. Igho Onakpoya, Rohini Terry, and Edzard Ernst, "The Use of Green Coffee Extract as a Weight Loss Supplement: A Systematic Review and Meta-Analysis of Randomised Clinical Trials," *Gastroenterology Research and Practice* 2011 (2011): 382852. doi: 10.1155/2011/382852.

87. Jeff S. Volek, William J. Kraemer, Martyn R. Rubin, Ana L. Gómez, Nicholas A. Ratamess, and Paula Gaynor, "L-Carnitine L-Tartrate Supplementation Favorably Affects Markers of Recovery from Exercise Stress," *American Journal of Physiology—Endocrinology and Metabolism* 282, no. 2 (2002): E474-82. doi: 10.1152/ajpendo.00277.2001.

88. Francis B. Stephens, Dumitru Constantin-Teodosiu, and Paul L. Greenhaff, "New Insights Concerning the Role of Carnitine in the Regulation of Fuel Metabolism in Skeletal Muscle," *Journal of Physiology* 581, pt. 2 (2007): 431-44. doi: 10.1113/jphysiol.2006.125799.

89. Mariano Malaguarnera, Lisa Cammalleri, Maria Pia Gargante, Marco Vacante, Valentina Colonna, and Massimo Motta, "L-Carnitine Treatment Reduces Severity of Physical and Mental Fatigue and Increases Cognitive Functions in Centenarians: A Randomized and Controlled Clinical Trial," *American Journal of Clinical Nutrition* 86, no. 6 (2007): 1738-44; Rudolph G. Villani, Jenelle Gannon, Megan Self, and Peter A. Rich, "L-Carnitine Supplementation Combined with Aerobic Training Does Not Promote Weight Loss in Moderately Obese Women," *International Journal of Sport Nutrition and Exercise Metabolism* 10, no. 2 (2000): 199-207.

90. Corinna Brandsch and Klaus Eder, "Effect of L-Carnitine on Weight Loss and Body Composition of Rats Fed a Hypocaloric Diet," *Annals of Nutrition and Metabolism* 46, no. 5 (2002): 205-10. doi: 10.1159/000065408; Sheri Melton, Michael J. Keenan, C. E. Stanciu, Maren Hegsted, E. M. Zablah-Pimentel, Carol E. O'Neil, Paula Gaynor, Andrea O. Schaffhauser, Kevin Owen, Rhonda D. Prisby, L . L. LaMotte, and J. M. Fernandez, "L-Carnitine Supplementation Does Not Promote Weight Loss in Ovariectomized Rats Despite Endurance Exercise," *International Journal of Vitamin Nutrition Research* 75, no. 2 (2005): 156-60.

91. Fabrizio Ceci, Carlo Cangiano, M. Cairella, Antonia Cascino, Maria Del Ben, Maurizio Muscaritoli, Lucio Sibilia, and Filippo Rossi-Fanelli, "The Effects of Oral 5-Hydroxytryptophan Administration on Feeding Behavior in Obese Adult Female Subjects," *Journal of Neural Transmission* 76, no. 2 (1989): 109-17.

92. Richard J. Wurtman and Judith J. Wurtman, "Brain Serotonin, Carbohydrate-Craving, Obesity and Depression," *Obesity Research* 3, supplement 4 (1995): 477S-80S.

93. Donal A. Walsh and Scott M. Van Patten, "Multiple Pathway Signal Transduction by the cAMP-Dependent Protein Kinase," *FASEB Journal* 8, no. 15 (1994): 1227-36; Irene Litosch, Thomas H. Hudson, Ira Mills, Shih-Ying Li, and John N. Fain, "Forskolin as an Activator of Cyclic AMP Accumulation and Lipolysis in Rat Adipocytes," *Molecular Pharmacology* 22, no. 1 (1982): 109-15.

94. Litosch et al., "Forskolin as an Activator of Cyclic AMP Accumulation and Lipolysis in Rat Adipocytes," 109-15.

95. Walsh and Patten, "Multiple Pathway Signal Transduction by the cAMP-Dependent Protein Kinase," 1227-36.

96. Michael P. Godard, Brad A. Johnson, and Scott R. Richmond, "Body Composition and Hormonal Adaptations Associated with Forskolin Consumption in Overweight and Obese Men," *Obesity Research* 18, no. 8 (2005): 1335-43.

97. Mark J. Millan, Adrian Newman-Tancredi, Valérie Audinot, Didier Cussac, Françoise Lejeune, Jean Paul Nicolas, Francis Cogé, Jean Pierre Galizzi, Jean Albert Boutin, Jean-Michel Rivet, Anne Dekeyne, and Alain Gobert, "Agonist and Antagonist Actions of Yohimbine as Compared to Fluparoxan at Alpha(2)-Adrenergic Receptors (AR)s, Serotonin (5-HT)(1A), 5-HT(1B), 5-HT(1D) and Dopamine D(2) and D(3) Receptors. Significance for the Modulation of Frontocortical Monoaminergic Transmission and Depressive States," *Synapse* 35, no. 2 (2000): 79-95; Sergej M. Ostojic, "Yohimbine: The Effects on Body Composition and Exercise Performance in Soccer Players, *Research in Sports Medicine* 14, no. 4 (2006): 289-99.

98. Jean Galitzky, Mohammed Taouis, Michel Berlan, Daniel Rivière, Michel Garrigues, and Max Lafontan, "Alpha 2-Antagonist Compounds and Lipid Mobilization: Evidence for a Lipid Mobilizing Effect of Oral Yohimbine in Healthy Male Volunteers," *European Journal of Clinical Investigation* 18, no. 6 (1988): 587-94.

99. Nevio Cimolai and Tomas Cimolai, "Yohimbine Use for Physical Enhancement and Its Potential Toxicity," *Journal of Dietary Supplements* 8, no. 4 (2011): 346-54. doi: 10.3109/19390211.2011.615806.

100. Michael R. Goldberg, Alan S. Hollister, and David Robertson, "Influence of Yohimbine on Blood Pressure, Autonomic Reflexes, and Plasma Catecholamines in Humans," *Hypertension* 5, no. 5 (1983): 772-78.

101. Gordon I. Smith, Philip Atherton, Dominic N. Reeds, B. Selma Mohammed, Debbie Rankin, Michael J. Rennie, and Bettina Mittendorfer, "Omega-3 Polyunsaturated Fatty Acids Augment the Muscle Protein Anabolic

Response to Hyperinsulinaemia–Hyperaminoacidaemia in Healthy Young and Middle-Aged Men and Women," *Clinical Science* 121, no. 6 (2011): 267-78; Bakhtiar Tartibian, Behzad Hajizadeh Maleki, and Asghar Abbas, "The Effects of Ingestion of Omega-3 Fatty Acids on Perceived Pain and External Symptoms of Delayed Onset Muscle Soreness in Untrained Men," *Clinical Journal of Sport Medicine* 19, no. 2 (2009): 115-19. doi: 10.1097/JSM.0b013e31819b51b3; Richard J. Bloomer, Douglas E. Larson, Kelsey H. Fisher-Wellman, Andrew J. Galpin, and Brian K. Schilling, "Effect of Eicosapentaenoic and Docosahexaenoic Acid on Resting and Exercise-Induced Inflammatory and Oxidative Stress Biomarkers: A Randomized, Placebo Controlled, Cross-Over Study," *Lipids in Health and Disease* 8 (August 19, 2009):36. doi:10.1186/1476-511X-8-36; Janice K. Kiecolt-Glasera, Martha A. Beluryc, Rebecca Andridged, William B. Malarkey, and Ronald Glasera, "Omega-3 Supplementation Lowers Inflammation and Anxiety in Medical Students: A Randomized Controlled Trial," *Brain, Behavior, and Immunity* 25, no. 8 (2011): 1725-34; Alfons Ramel, J. Alfredo Martinez, Mairead Kiely, Narcisa M. Bandarra, and Inga Thorsdottir, "Moderate Consumption of Fatty Fish Reduces Diastolic Blood Pressure in Overweight and Obese European Young Adults during Energy Restriction," *Nutrition* 26, no. 2 (2010): 168-74. doi: 10.1016/j.nut.2009.04.002. M. Elizabeth Sublette, Steven P. Ellis, Amy L. Geant, and J. John Mann, "Meta-Analysis of the Effects of Eicosapentaenoic Acid (EPA) in Clinical Trials in Depression," *Journal of Clinical Psychiatry* 72, no. 12 (2011): 1577-84. doi: 10.4088/JCP.10m06634; Tomohito Hamazaki, Miho Itomura, Shigeki Sawazaki, and Yoko Nagao, "Anti-Stress Effects of DHA," *Biofactors* 13, no. 1-4 (2000): 41-45; Fulvio Lauretani, Marcello Maggio, Francesco Pizzarelli, Stefano Michelassi, Carmelinda Ruggiero, Gian Paulo Ceda, Stefania Bandinelli, and L. Ferrucci, "Omega-3 and Renal Function in Older Adults," *Current Pharmaceutical Design* 15, no. 36 (2009): 4149-56. doi: 10.2174/138161209789909719; Artemis P. Simopoulos, "The Importance of the Ratio of Omega-6/Omega-3 Essential Fatty Acids," *Biomedicine and Pharmacotherapy* 56, no. 8 (2002): 365-79; Ka He, Eric B. Rimm, Anwar Merchant, Bernard A. Rosner, Meir J. Stampfer, Walter C. Willett, and Alberto Ascherio, "Fish Consumption and Risk of Stroke in Men," *JAMA* 288, no. 24 (2002): 3130-36. doi: 10.1001/jama.288.24.3130; Tao Huang, Subhachai Bhulaidok, Zhenzhen Cai, Tongcheng Xu, Fang Xu, Mark L. Wahlqvist, and Duo Li, "Plasma Phospholipids n-3 Polyunsaturated Fatty Acid Is Associated with Metabolic Syndrome," *Molecular Nutrition and Food Research* 54, no. 11 (2010): 1628-35. doi: 10.1002/mnfr.201000025; Steen B. Haugaard, Allan Vaag, Huiling Mu, and Sten Madsbad, "Skeletal Muscle Structural Lipids Improve during Weight-Maintenance after a Very Low Calorie Dietary Intervention," *Lipids in Health and Disease* 8 (August 13, 2009): 34. doi:10.1186/1476-511X-8-34; Rajesh Narendran, William G. Frankle, Neale S. Mason, Matthew F. Muldoon, and Bita Moghaddam, "Improved Working Memory but No Effect on Striatal Vesicular Monoamine Transporter Type 2 after Omega-3 Polyunsaturated Fatty Acid Supplementation," *PLOS One* 7, no. 10 (2012): e46832. doi: 10.1371/journal.pone.0046832; Matthew F. Muldoon, Christopher M. Ryan, Lei Sheu, Jeffrey K. Yao, Sarah M. Conklin, and Stephen B. Manuck, "Serum Phospholipid Docosahexaenonic Acid Is Associated with Cognitive Functioning during Middle Adulthood," *Journal of Nutrition* 140, no. 4 (2010): 848-53. doi: 10.3945/jn.109.119578; Jonathan D. Buckley and Peter R. C. Howe, "Anti-Obesity Effects of Long-Chain Omega-3 Polyunsaturated Fatty Acids," *Obesity Reviews* 10, no. 6 (2009): 648-59. doi: 10.1111/j.1467-789X.2009.00584.x; Charles Couet, Jacques Delarue, Patrick Ritz, Jean Michel Antoine, and Fernand Lamisse, "Effect of Dietary Fish Oil on Body Fat Mass and Basal Fat Oxidation in Healthy Adults," *International Journal of Obesity and Related Metabolic Disorders* 21, no. 8 (1997): 637-43.

102. Simopoulos, "The Importance of the Ratio of Omega-6/Omega-3 Essential Fatty Acids," 365-79.

103. Bernhard Beckermann, Manfred Beneke, and Isabell Seitz, "Comparative Bioavailability of Eicosapentaenoic Acid and Docasahexaenoic Acid from Triglycerides, Free Fatty Acids and Ethyl Esters in Volunteers," [in German], *Arzneimittelforschung* 40, no. 6 (1990): 700-04.

104. Jørn Dyerberg, Poul Madsen, Jørn M. Møller, Inge Aardestrup, and Erik B. Schmidt, "Bioavailability of Marine n-3 Fatty Acid Formulations," *Prostaglandins, Leukotrienes and Essential Fatty Acids* 83, no. 3 (2010): 137-41. doi: 10.1016/j.plefa.2010.06.007.

105. Catherine A. Best and Michael Laposata, "Fatty Acid Ethyl Esters: Toxic Non-Oxidative Metabolites of Ethanol and Markers of Ethanol Intake," *Frontiers in Bioscience* 8 (January 1, 2003): e202-17.

106. Penny M. Kris-Etherton, William S. Harris, and Lawrence J. Appel, "Fish Consumption, Fish Oil, Omega-3 Fatty Acids, and Cardiovascular Disease AHA Scientific Statement," *Circulation* 106 (2002): 2747-57. doi: 10.1161/01.CIR.0000038493.65177.94.

107. Hsueh-Kuan Lu, Chin-Cheng Hsieh, Jen-Jung Hsu, Yuh-Kuan Yang, and Hong-Nong Chou, "Preventive Effects of Spirulina platensis on Skeletal Muscle Damage under Exercise-Induced Oxidative Stress," *European Journal of Applied Physiology* 98, no. 2 (1998): 220-26; Maria Kalafati, Athanasios Z. Jamurtas, Michalis G. Nikolaidis, Vassilis Paschalis, Anastasios A. Theodorou, Giorgos K. Sakellariou, Yiannis Koutedakis, and Dimitris Kouretas, "Ergogenic and Antioxidant Effects of Spirulina Supplementation in Humans," *Medicine and Science of Sports and Exercise* 42, no. 1 (2010): 142-51. doi: 10.1249/MSS.0b013e3181ac7a45; Jaspal Sandhu, Dheera Bhardwaj,

and Shweta Shenoy, "Efficacy of Spirulina Supplementation on Isometric Strength and Isometric Endurance of Quadriceps in Trained and Untrained Individuals—A Comparative Study," Ibnosina Journal of Medicine and Biomedical Sciences 2, no. 2 (2010): 79-86; Eun Hee Lee, Ji-Eun Park, Young-Ju Choi, Kap-Bum Huh, and Wha-Young Kim, "A Randomized Study to Establish the Effects of Spirulina in Type 2 Diabetes Mellitus Patients," Nutrition Research and Practice 2, no. 4 (2008): 295-300. doi: 10.4162/nrp.2008.2.4.295; Patricia V. Torres-Duran, Aldo Ferreira-Hermosillo, and Marco A. Juarez-Oropeza, "Antihyperlipemic and Antihypertensive Effects of Spirulina maxima in an Open Sample of Mexican Population: A Preliminary Report," Lipids in Health and Disease 6 (November 26, 2007): 33. doi:10.1186/1476-511X-6-33; Panam Parikh, Uliyar Mani, and Uma Iyer, "Role of Spirulina in the Control of Glycemia and Lipidemia in Type 2 Diabetes Mellitus," Journal of Medicinal Food 4, no. 4 (2001): 193-99. doi: 10.1089/10966200152744463; Hee Jung Park, Yun Jung Lee, Han Kyoung Ryu, Mi Hyun Kim, Hye Won Chung, and Wha Young Kim, "A Randomized Double-Blind, Placebo-Controlled Study to Establish the Effects of Spirulina in Elderly Koreans," Annals of Nutrition and Metabolism 52, no. 4 (2008): 322-28. doi:10.1159/000151486; Cemal Cingi, Meltem Conk-Dalay, Hamdi Cakli, and Cengiz Bal, "The Effects of Spirulina on Allergic Rhinitis," European Archives of Oto-Rhino-Laryngology 265, no. 10 (2008): 1219-23. doi: 10.1007/s00405-008-0642-8; Azabji-Kenfack Marcel, Loni G. Ekali, Sobngwi Eugene, Onana E. Arnold, Edie D. Sandrine, Denis Von der Weid, Emmanuel Gbaguidi, Jeanne Ngogang, and Jean C. Mbanya, "The Effect of Spirulina platensis versus Soybean on Insulin Resistance in HIV-Infected Patients: A Randomized Pilot Study," Nutrients 3, no. 7 (2011): 712-24. doi:10.3390/nu3070712.

CHAPTER 24
FREQUENTLY ASKED QUESTIONS

1. Chad M. Kerksick, Colin D. Wilborn, Bill I. Campbell, Michael D. Roberts, Christopher J. Rasmussen, Michael Greenwood, and Richard B. Kreider, "Early-Phase Adaptations to a Split-Body, Linear Periodization Resistance Training Program in College-Aged and Middle-Aged Men," Journal of Strength and Conditioning Research 23, no. 3 (2009): 962-71. doi: 10.1519/JSC.0b013e3181a00baf.

2. Gary R. Hunter, John P. McCarthy, and Marcas M. Bamman, "Effects of Resistance Training on Older Adults," Sports Medicine 34, no. 5 (2004): 329-48; Wojtek J. Chodzko-Zajko, David N. Proctor, Maria A. Fiatarone Singh, Christopher T. Minson, Claudio R. Nigg, George J. Salem, and James S. Skinner, "American College of Sports Medicine Position Stand: Exercise and Physical Activity for Older Adults," Medicine and Science in Sports and Exercise, 41, no. 7 (2009): 1510-30.

3. James Fell and Dafydd Williams, "The Effect of Aging on Skeletal-Muscle Recovery from Exercise: Possible Implications for Aging Athletes," Journal of Aging and Physical Activity 16, no. 1 (2008): 97-115.

4. Marie-Pierre St-Onge and Dympna Gallagher, "Body Composition Changes with Aging: The Cause or the Result of Alterations in Metabolic Rate and Macronutrient Oxidation?" Nutrition 26, no. 2 (2010): doi: 10.1016/j.nut.2009.07.004.

5. Alfonso J. Cruz-Jentoft, Jean Pierre Baeyens, Jürgen M. Bauer, Yves Boirie, Tommy Cederholm, Francesco Landi, Finbarr C. Martin, Jean-Pierre Michel, Yves Rolland, Stéphane M. Schneider, Eva Topinková, Maurits Vandewoude, and Mauro Zamboni, "Sarcopenia: European Consensus on Definition and Diagnosis: Report of the European Working Group on Sarcopenia in Older People," Age Ageing 39, no. 4 (2010): 412-23. doi: 10.1093/ageing/afq034.

6. Roger G. Eston, Jane Mickleborough, and Vasilios Baltzopoulos, "Eccentric Activation and Muscle Damage: Biomechanical and Physiological Considerations during Downhill Running," British Journal of Sports Medicine 29, no. 2 (1995): 89-94; Kyle L. Flann, Paul C. LaStayo, Donald A. McClain, Mark Hazel, and Stan L. Lindstedt, "Muscle Damage and Muscle Remodeling: No Pain, No Gain?" Journal of Experimental Biology 214, pt. 4 (2011): 674-79. doi: 10.1242/jeb.050112.

7. Kazunori Nosaka, Mike Newton, and Paul Sacco, "Delayed-Onset Muscle Soreness Does Not Reflect the Magnitude of Eccentric Exercise-Induced Muscle Damage," Scandinavian Journal of Medicine and Science in Sports 12, no. 6 (2002): 337-46. doi: 10.1034/j.1600-0838.2002.10178.x.

8. Regina M. Crameri, Per Aagaard, Klaus Qvortrup, Henning Langberg, J. Olesen, and Michael Kjær, "Myofibre Damage in Human Skeletal Muscle: Effects of Electrical Stimulation versus Voluntary Contraction," Journal of Physiology 583 (August 15, 2007): 365-80. doi: 10.1113/jphysiol.2007.128827.

9. Nicolette C. Bishop and Michael Gleeson, "Acute and Chronic Effects of Exercise on Markers of Mucosal Immunity," Frontiers in Bioscience 14 (January 1, 2009): 4444-56.

10. E. Angela Murphy, J. Mark Davis, Martin D. Carmichael, J. David Gangemi, Abdul Ghaffar, and Eugene P. Mayer, "Exercise Stress Increases Susceptibility to Influenza Infection," *Brain, Behavior, and Immunity* 22, no. 8 (2008): 1152-55. doi: 10.1016/j.bbi.2008.06.004.

11. Stephen A. Martin, Brandt D. Pence, and Jeffrey A. Woods, "Exercise and Respiratory Tract Viral Infections," *Exercise and Sport Sciences Review* 37, no. 4 (2009): 157-64. doi: 10.1097/JES.0b013e3181b7b57b.

12. John J. Shelmet, George A. Reichard, Charles L. Skutches, Robert D. Hoeldtke, Oliver E. Owen, and Guenther Boden, "Ethanol Causes Acute Inhibition of Carbohydrate, Fat, and Protein Oxidation and Insulin Resistance," *Journal of Clinical Investigation* 81, no. 4 (1988): 1137-45. doi:10.1172/JCI113428.

INDEX

17967519R00197

Printed in Great Britain
by Amazon